HAWORTH Social Work Practice
Carlton E. Munson, DSW, Senior Editor

GROUP WORK: SKILLS AND STRATEGIES FOR EFFECTIVE INTERVENTIONS, SECOND EDITION by Sondra Brandler and Camille P. Roman. (1999). "A clear, basic description of what group work requires, including what skills and techniques group workers need to be effective." *Hospital and Community Psychiatry* (from the first edition)

TEENAGE RUNAWAYS: BROKEN HEARTS AND "BAD ATTITUDES" by Laurie Schaffner. (1999).

CELEBRATING DIVERSITY: COEXISTING IN A MULTICULTURAL SOCIETY by Benyamin Chetkow-Yanoov. (1999). "Makes a valuable contribution to peace theory and practice." *Ian Harris, EdD, Executive Secretary, Peace Education Committee, International Peace Research Association*

SOCIAL WELFARE POLICY ANALYSIS AND CHOICES by Hobart A. Burch. (1999). "Will become the landmark text in its field for many decades to come." *Sheldon Rahn, DSW, Founding Dean and Emeritus Professor of Social Policy and Social Administration, Faculty of Social Work, Wilfrid Laurier University, Canada*

SOCIAL WORK PRACTICE: A SYSTEMS APPROACH, SECOND EDITION by Benyamin Chetkow-Yanoov. (1999)."Highly recommended as a primary text for any and all introductory social work courses." *Ram A. Cnaan, PhD, Associate Professor, School of Social Work, University of Pennsylvania*

CRITICAL SOCIAL WELFARE ISSUES: TOOLS FOR SOCIAL WORK AND HEALTH CARE PROFESSIONALS edited by Arthur J. Katz, Abraham Lurie, and Carlos M. Vidal. (1997). "Offers hopeful agendas for change, while navigating the societal challenges facing those in the human services today." *Book News Inc.*

SOCIAL WORK IN HEALTH SETTINGS: PRACTICE IN CONTEXT, SECOND EDITION edited by Toba Schwaber Kerson. (1997). "A first-class document. . . . It will be found among the steadier and lasting works on the social work aspects of American health care." *Hans S. Falck, PhD, Professor Emeritus and Former Chair, Health Specialization in Social Work, Virginia Commonwealth University*

PRINCIPLES OF SOCIAL WORK PRACTICE: A GENERIC PRACTICE APPROACH by Molly R. Hancock. (1997). "Hancock's discussions advocate reflection and self-awareness to create a climate for client change." *Journal of Social Work Education*

NOBODY'S CHILDREN: ORPHANS OF THE HIV EPIDEMIC by Steven F. Dansky. (1997). "Professionally sound, moving, and useful for both professionals and interested readers alike." *Ellen G. Friedman, ACSW, Associate Director of Support Services, Beth Israel Medical Center, Methadone Maintenance Treatment Program*

SOCIAL WORK APPROACHES TO CONFLICT RESOLUTION: MAKING FIGHTING OBSOLETE by Benyamin Chetkow-Yanoov. (1996). "Presents an examination of the nature and cause of conflict and suggests techniques for coping with conflict." *Journal of Criminal Justice*

FEMINIST THEORIES AND SOCIAL WORK: APPROACHES AND APPLICATIONS by Christine Flynn Saulnier. (1996). "An essential reference to be read repeatedly by all educators and practitioners who are eager to learn more about feminist theory and practice." *Nancy R. Hooyman, PhD, Dean and Professor, School of Social Work, University of Washington, Seattle*

THE RELATIONAL SYSTEMS MODEL FOR FAMILY THERAPY: LIVING IN THE FOUR REALITIES by Donald R. Bardill. (1996). "Engages the reader in quiet, thoughtful conversation on the timeless issue of helping families and individuals." *Christian Counseling Resource Review*

SOCIAL WORK INTERVENTION IN AN ECONOMIC CRISIS: THE RIVER COMMUNITIES PROJECT by Martha Baum and Pamela Twiss. (1996). "Sets a standard for universities in terms of the types of meaningful roles they can play in supporting and sustaining communities." *Kenneth J. Jaros, PhD, Director, Public Health Social Work Training Program, University of Pittsburgh*

FUNDAMENTALS OF COGNITIVE-BEHAVIOR THERAPY: FROM BOTH SIDES OF THE DESK by Bill Borcherdt. (1996). "Both beginning and experienced practitioners . . . will find a considerable number of valuable suggestions in Borcherdt's book." *Albert Ellis, PhD, President, Institute for Rational-Emotive Therapy, New York City*

BASIC SOCIAL POLICY AND PLANNING: STRATEGIES AND PRACTICE METHODS by Hobart A. Burch. (1996). "Burch's familiarity with his topic is evident and his book is an easy introduction to the field." *Readings*

THE CROSS-CULTURAL PRACTICE OF CLINICAL CASE MANAGEMENT IN MENTAL HEALTH edited by Peter Manoleas. (1996). "Makes a contribution by bringing together the cross-cultural and clinical case management perspectives in working with those who have serious mental illness." *Disability Studies Quarterly*

FAMILY BEYOND FAMILY: THE SURROGATE PARENT IN SCHOOLS AND OTHER COMMUNITY AGENCIES by Sanford Weinstein. (1995). "Highly recommended to anyone concerned about the welfare of our children and the breakdown of the American family." *Jerrold S. Greenberg, EdD, Director of Community Service, College of Health & Human Performance, University of Maryland*

PEOPLE WITH HIV AND THOSE WHO HELP THEM: CHALLENGES, INTEGRATION, INTERVENTION by R. Dennis Shelby. (1995). "A useful and compassionate contribution to the HIV psychotherapy literature." *Public Health*

THE BLACK ELDERLY: SATISFACTION AND QUALITY OF LATER LIFE by Marguerite Coke and James A. Twaite. (1995). "Presents a model for predicting life satisfaction in this population." *Abstracts in Social Gerontology*

BUILDING ON WOMEN'S STRENGTHS: A SOCIAL WORK AGENDA FOR THE TWENTY-FIRST CENTURY edited by Liane V. Davis. (1994). "The most lucid and accessible overview of the related epistemological debates in the social work literature." *Journal of the National Association of Social Workers*

NOW DARE EVERYTHING: TALES OF HIV-RELATED PSYCHOTHERAPY by Steven F. Dansky. (1994). "A highly recommended book for anyone working with persons who are HIV positive. . . . Every library should have a copy of this book." *AIDS Book Review Journal*

INTERVENTION RESEARCH: DESIGN AND DEVELOPMENT FOR HUMAN SERVICE edited by Jack Rothman and Edwin J. Thomas. (1994). "Provides a useful framework for the further examination of methodology for each separate step of such research." *Academic Library Book Review*

FORENSIC SOCIAL WORK: LEGAL ASPECTS OF PROFESSIONAL PRACTICE by Robert L. Barker and Douglas M. Branson. (1993). "The authors combine their expertise to create this informative guide to address legal practice issues facing social workers." *Newsletter of the National Organization of Forensic Social Work*

CLINICAL SOCIAL WORK SUPERVISION, SECOND EDITION by Carlton E. Munson. (1993). "A useful, thorough, and articulate reference for supervisors and for 'supervisees' who are wanting to understand their supervisor or are looking for effective supervision." *Transactional Analysis Journal*

ELEMENTS OF THE HELPING PROCESS: A GUIDE FOR CLINICIANS by Raymond Fox. (1993). "Filled with helpful hints, creative interventions, and practical guidelines." *Journal of Family Psychotherapy*

IF A PARTNER HAS AIDS: GUIDE TO CLINICAL INTERVENTION FOR RELATIONSHIPS IN CRISIS by R. Dennis Shelby. (1993). "A welcome addition to existing publications about couples coping with AIDS, it offers intervention ideas and strategies to clinicians." *Contemporary Psychology*

GERONTOLOGICAL SOCIAL WORK SUPERVISION by Ann Burack-Weiss and Frances Coyle Brennan. (1991). "The creative ideas in this book will aid supervisors working with students and experienced social workers." *Senior News*

SOCIAL WORK THEORY AND PRACTICE WITH THE TERMINALLY ILL by Joan K. Parry. (1989). "Should be read by all professionals engaged in the provision of health services in hospitals, emergency rooms, and hospices." *Hector B. Garcia, PhD, Professor, San Jose State University School of Social Work*

THE CREATIVE PRACTITIONER: THEORY AND METHODS FOR THE HELPING SERVICES by Bernard Gelfand. (1988). "[Should] be widely adopted by those in the helping services. It could lead to significant positive advances by countless individuals." *Sidney J. Parnes, Trustee Chairperson for Strategic Program Development, Creative Education Foundation, Buffalo, NY*

MANAGEMENT AND INFORMATION SYSTEMS IN HUMAN SERVICES: IMPLICATIONS FOR THE DISTRIBUTION OF AUTHORITY AND DECISION MAKING by Richard K. Caputo. (1987). "A contribution to social work scholarship in that it provides conceptual frameworks that can be used in the design of management information systems." *Social Work*

Hobart A. Burch, PhD

Social Welfare Policy Analysis and Choices

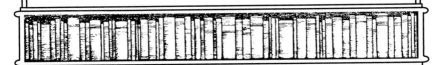

More pre-publication
REVIEWS, COMMENTARIES, EVALUATIONS . . .

"**A**n original and stimulating guide to the world of social welfare policy that influences professional efforts to improve social well-being. It is valuable for the beginning student of policy, as a refresher for the expert, and as a window for the interested public. It is unique in the clear way it helps the reader understand the processes of making choices through the maze of diverse values, histories, cultures, attitudes, and powers of interest groups as our open society seeks to improve well-being for all.

The framework presents the dilemmas of preference and effective intervention: what is true—facts and beliefs? Fundamental value choices such as equality, equity, or adequacy? Market versus human service choices?

To help resolve the dilemmas there is a wealth of anecdotes, illustrations, and quotations as well as theories to help the reader—policy analyst or citizen—understand how choices can be made through human intelligence plus goodwill as well as by mechanical techniques. The author also includes his own criteria for effective social policy making in an open and diverse society."

Robert Morris, DSW
Emeritus Professor, Brandeis University;
Senior Associate, Gerontology Institute,
University of Massachusetts,
Boston

"**A**t present, when public support for social welfare programs is under attack, there is an urgent need to reexamine social welfare policy. This book provides a thorough analysis of the context in which social welfare policy is debated and formulated. The author demonstrates a thorough grasp of theoretical issues. But he is also 'street-smart.' He draws on his rich personal experience in working at high policy-making levels to develop viable social welfare programs. The book is valuable not only for the field of social work, but also for ethics courses dealing with social welfare policy in philosophy, religious studies, and theology. Where such courses do not exist, they ought to be created. Dr. Burch's book could well serve as their key resource."

George H. Crowell, ThD
Retired Associate Professor,
Social Ethics,
University of Windsor,
Ontario, Canada

Social Welfare Policy
Analysis and Choices

Social Welfare Policy Analysis and Choices

Hobart A. Burch, PhD

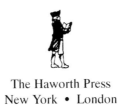

The Haworth Press
New York • London

The Haworth Press, Inc., 10 Alice Street, Binghamton, NY 13904-1580

Cover design by Marylouise E. Doyle.

Library of Congress Cataloging-in-Publication Data

Burch, Hobart A.
    Social welfare policy analysis and choices / Hobart A. Burch.
        p.   cm.
    Inclues bibliographical references and index.
    ISBN 0-7890-0603-0 (alk. paper).
    1. Social policy. 2. Public welfare. I. Title.
HV31.B79 1998
361—dc21
                                                                        98-8165
                                                                          CIP

CONTENTS

PART V: HUMAN SERVICE DELIVERY CHOICES

Chapter 14. Benefits: Broad or Begrudged?   251

Chapter 15. Rights or Alms?   271

Chapter 16. Public, Voluntary, or Commercial?   287

Chapter 17. Paying for It   307

ABOUT THE AUTHOR

Hobart A. Burch, PhD, is Professor in the School of Social Work at the University of Nebraska where, as Director of the School of Social Work (1976-1981), he rebuilt the school's program and was successful in securing reaccreditation after reorganizing, increasing financial support, upgrading faculty standards, and revising curriculum. Prior to teaching, Dr. Burch held national leadership positions in the government, church, and charities sectors, including an appointment as Assistant to the U.S. Commissioner on Welfare. He is widely published in the areas of social welfare and social policy and is the author of *The Whys of Social Policy.*

Preface

One problem with social welfare policy is that it doesn't stand still. We learn existing policies, and before we can turn around, they are no longer what we just learned. Political power shifts with an election. Interest groups gain and lose power due to technological change, economic consolidations, lobbying efforts and expenditures, or grassroots movements. Ideologies rise, repudiate "old truths," peak, and then decline as newer or more aggressive ones arise or in a nostalgic reaction to the "good old days" (none of which were as good as we fantasize).

Economic ups and downs anywhere in the world may change established beliefs and patterns within a few years or even a few months, as in the extreme cases of the OPEC oil crisis of the 1970s or the world depression of the 1930s. Security concerns go up, and liberties go down. "Yuppies" (and older urban professionals) go for the gold, with an ideology of competitive individualism at the expense of community and solidarity as a people.

Old flawed programs are discarded, to be replaced by new flawed programs, which may be better or worse than those they replace. Once abandoned programs and approaches reemerge as alleged innovations and new ideas.

As I write this preface, I am watching ocean waves rolling in to the shore; there is moderate white surf with an on-shore wind. Yesterday, there was a light offshore breeze, and the ocean was blue and gentle, with a quiet surf. The forecast for tomorrow is rain with intermittent violent thunderstorms that will bombard my little stretch of shoreline with powerful gray waves, which reach fifty feet beyond the normal tideline and erode the fragile dunes. The next day, the ocean may again be placid. Despite these daily changes, observed from an orbiting satellite, the ocean as a whole is relatively constant—"the ocean is always changing, yet always the same."

Similar to ocean waves, policy issues and choices are always changing, yet they always involve the same fundamental human/social needs, wants, and preferences—and similar conflicts between the needs, wants, and preferences of different individuals and groups within our larger community.

Current policy applications will soon be history, as they are replaced by new ones—different circumstances will require different solutions. Events of the past, and the circumstances in which they occurred, give us insight into the present but provide no blueprints to guide us.

The purpose of this book is to examine current social welfare policies, issues, and choices in historical (past-present-future) perspective—not organized in the traditional format of separate topical areas such as child welfare, sexism, health care, and income maintenance—and within a framework of basic human and societal issues that are relatively constant. These issues are illustrated by and applied to specific topical areas (which my students follow through the Internet, newspapers, and current journal articles).

Our aim is to understand what is, why it is the way it is, how it got there, and the beliefs, values, and interests that (explicitly, covertly, or unwittingly) are behind it.

With that insight, perhaps we can do a better job of *determining* social policies and programs using four different dictionary definitions of "determine":

1. *Understand* policies: to find out exactly; ascertain.
2. *Evaluate* policies: to reach a decision about, after thought and investigation.
3. *Guide* policies: to give definite aim or direction to.
4. *Impact* policies: to be the cause of; be the deciding or regulating factor in.

Another focus of the book relates to a primary concern in our society, shared by common folks and ironically by activists at both ends of our policy-position continuum—a growing malaise about an apparent erosion of traditional moral, ethical, and social values. People are disillusioned and cynical about directionless public leaders who seem to be guided more by special interests than by principle. A hunger for meaning, belonging, and purpose in our society is reemerging. In our down moments, of which there are many in social welfare policy, we ruminate with Shakespeare's Macbeth:

Tomorrow, and tomorrow, and tomorrow,
Creeps in this petty pace from day to day,
To the last syllable of recorded time;
And all our yesterdays have lighted fools
The way to dusty death. Out, out, brief candle!
Life's [policy] but a waking shadow, a poor player
That struts and frets his hour upon the stage
And then is heard no more: it is a tale
Told by an idiot, full of sound and fury,
Signifying nothing.

Macbeth, Act V, Scene V

This book provides frameworks for examining beliefs about human nature and about the nature of society, ways of thinking, values, the moral and ethical implications of those values, and roots of those values in religion, culture, historical traditions, myths, and rationalized self-interests. My own personal vantage points can probably be detected in these analyses, and I have tried neither to peddle nor to hide them. At the same time, I am hopeful that the method of presenting social-ethical choices, their origins, and their implications will enable you, the reader, (1) to determine what positions *you* choose to take on specific issues and why and (2) to ascertain where *others* are coming from so that you can better plan your strategies for relating to them.

Part I is an introduction to social policy analysis. Chapter 1 outlines policy sectors (public, organized private, and implicit), types of policy (de jure, de facto, and default), and the broad range of policies, program, and problems that fall within social policy. Chapter 2 examines the process of making choices, including ways of thinking, desirability, and feasibility; overt and covert intents; and manifest and unrecognized effects. Chapter 3 deals with intervention choices, including two public health models (host/agent/environment and primary/secondary/tertiary), and incremental reform versus radical change.

Part II lays the foundation for choice. Chapter 4 examines ways of thinking, including scientific and experiential approaches to "facts," a priori beliefs, and sorting out biases. Chapter 5 explores the interaction of values and interests and of the legitimate (and illegitimate?) competition among the values/interests of different groups. Chapter 6 covers a key area—our beliefs about human nature. Are we inherently good or bad? What is the value of each individual person? Are we self-determining captains of our souls or subject to "the slings and arrows of outrageous fortune"?

Part III discusses arguments for and against fundamental social choices that govern our specific policies. Chapter 7 discusses equality, equity, and adequacy as standards of fairness. Chapters 8 and 9 assess negative and positive freedom, their counterparts in passive equal opportunity and equalizing affirmative action, and their ideological bases in individualism and communality. Chapter 10 explores frameworks such as cost-benefit analysis, putting a dollar price on qualitative intangibles, welfare economics, and the Protestant work ethic that convert human policy into an economic calculation.

Parts IV and V move into specific mechanisms for social policies. Part IV takes a systemwide look at the economic market, examining how it works, its gaps and vulnerabilities, and measures taken to meet common human needs within a capitalist economy. Part V deals with how human service programs are provided.

Chapter 11 explains how the economic market operates in theory and identifies several common market variations in practice. Chapter 12 investigates two kinds of social state intervention: monetary and fiscal measures to enhance the economic market and minimize its cyclical problems and control, through regulation, of the potential abuses that can be expected in any system based on competitive self-interest. Chapter 13 considers social market programs that fill gaps which the economic market does not, and often cannot, meet, including private charity, public services, and social insurances. Ideologies, assets and liabilities, and affordability of the welfare state are discussed.

Chapter 14 explores different approaches to human services, such as institutional versus residual and universal versus selective, and different selective criteria such as means tests, diagnosis, compensation for diswelfares, deservedness, and investment payoff. Chapter

15 follows up with a discussion of moral and legal rights, including entitlements.

Chapter 16 analyzes the pros and cons of public, nonprofit, and commercial providers, with a special section on the First Amendment issue of church-related agencies and the state. Nowadays, the provider and payer are not necessarily even in the same sector. Chapter 17 discusses the methods of paying for services, including fees, charitable and public subsidies, and third-party purchase, as well as issues of pricing, cost control, and managed care, a rapidly growing and controversial structure of provision.

Chapter 18 returns to the broad issue of centralization versus decentralization, a complex of vertical (national/state/local) and horizontal (public/nonprofit/commercial) alternatives on both payer and provider sides. After an historical look at federalism, four other relatively successful approaches from around the world are discussed.

In closing, I will summarize two of the most important points supporting my own beliefs about social welfare policy.

First, the macroperspective: a society, *as* a society, has the moral imperative to promote the general welfare. Our society has the means, if it chooses. "Today we have the power to strike away the barriers to full participation in our society. HAVING THE POWER, WE HAVE THE DUTY."[1]

Second, its inescapable microcomponent: a social policy is no good in the abstract. "General Good is the Plea of the Scoundrel, the hypocrite, and flatterer."[2] A classic country music song pleads, "Hey, won't you play another somebody done somebody wrong song . . . so sad that it makes ev'rybody cry."[3] A good policy must be a "somebody done somebody *right*" song. The bottom-line question for every policy action is, "Who is better off? How? How much?"

Hobart Burch, PhD

---

1. President Lyndon B. Johnson, quoted in Report to the Secretary of U.S. Department of Health, Education, and Welfare, Washington, DC June 29, 1966.

2. William Blake, *Jerusalem* (1804-1820).

3. "Another Somebody Done Somebody Wrong Song" (1975). Words and music by Larry Butler and Chips Morgan. Nashville: Tree Publishing Company.

PART I:
POLICY CHOICE
AND INTERVENTION

Chapter 1

Social Welfare Policy: When and Where?

The pilot of the state who sets no hand to the best policy, but remains tongue-tied through some terror, seems vilest of men.

Sophocles, *Antigone*

This strategy represents our policy for all time. Until it's changed.

Marlin Fitzwater,
White House Spokesperson

Smoking tobacco is legal. One-quarter of us do. Three-quarters do not.

- Should smokers be permitted to deprive others of their freedom to work in a healthy atmosphere by imposing the unpleasantness and health risk of their secondhand smoke on co-workers? Can co-workers reasonably deprive smokers of their freedom to smoke comfortably eight hours per day?
- On the average, smokers have significantly higher health costs. Should nonsmokers be expected to subsidize the extra cost of smokers' habits through higher premiums on their group insurance? Should smokers, as with accident-prone drivers, be rele-

---

Note: Unless otherwise noted, definitions are from *The American College Dictionary* (1970, Random House) or *Webster's New 20th Century Dictionary of the English Language,* 2nd ed. (1971, World Publishing Company).

gated to a higher premium assigned risk pool? Should their emphysema in old age be treated at public expense through Medicare and Medicaid?
- If the numbers were reversed, with 75 percent of the population being smokers, should answers to these questions be different?

Mrs. Brown and Mrs. Green are single parents with school-age children. Mr. Brown died. Mr. Green just took off. Neither mom is employed; both receive government support.

"Welfare" and food stamps combine to give the Green family an income of half the official poverty line used by the Bureau of the Census. (In 1995, the poverty level for a family of four was $15,662 [Ambert, 1998].) To be eligible, Mrs. Green must seek, and take, a job regardless of the pay or working conditions. The Brown family receives triple that amount from Social Security. To be eligible, Mrs. Brown must *not* seek and take a job.

- Should these families be treated differently? Why?
- Should staying home to care for her children be required of one and forbidden to the other? Why?
- Does it "all depend"? If so, on what?

We buy our appliances in the open market. The electricity to run them is available only at a fixed price from a commercial monopoly in New York City and a government monopoly in Omaha.

- Is the public interest better served by monopolistic "public utilities" than by open competition? When? Why?
- Should utilities be socialistic, as in "conservative" Nebraska, capitalistic, as in "liberal" New York City, or nonprofit citizen co-ops, as in rural North Carolina? Why?

All of the above are social policy questions. This book does not answer them: it can't. As will be discussed in Chapters 4 and 5, before-the-fact vantage points have selected, defined, and colored both the perceived reality of what is and the vision of what ought to be. These vantage points vary among different classes, interest groups, subcultures, and sects in our society, and among individuals within each group.

This book does provide tools to help understand the facts required to answer those questions, by examining:

- the realities as you see them and what your perception is based on;
- the realities as others see them and why;
- key possible choices;
- the values and interests (whose?) affecting your choices;
- the professed rationales of opposing policy positions, the de facto values and interests upon which they are based, and their hidden agenda, if any;
- where special interests conflict, whose take priority, and/or how might they be balanced and why; and
- what is best for general welfare—and whether, in relation to the policy question, there is an unequivocal "general welfare" at all.

Social policy is a complex mixture of overlapping, inconsistent, and often contradictory intents and behaviors that affect different people in different ways. Our tools for understanding this complexity are concepts and frameworks that organize and distill key elements from the mass of detail. A *concept* is "a generalized idea of a class of objects." Concepts may be organized into a *framework*, "a structure serving to hold the parts of something together," or a *model*, "a representation of a social pattern."

These policy analysis tools are inherently selective and never exactly fit the disorderly reality with which you are dealing. You should neither accept the ones in this book as "the truth" nor reject them outright for their imperfections. Use these tools, but develop your own as well.

WHAT IS SOCIAL POLICY?

Policies are "courses of action, whether intended or unintended, that are deliberately adopted or can be shown to follow regular patterns over time" (Tropman, Dhuly, and Lind, 1981, p. xvi).

Social policies "have to do with human beings living together as a group in a situation requiring that they have dealings with each other" (Ibid.).

Welfare is "the state of being or doing well: the condition of health, prosperity, and happiness; well-being."

Social policies may be good or bad. Slavery was a bad policy; public education is a good one. What is the difference? The bottom line for every social policy is how it affects the welfare of human beings, collectively as a society and individually within that society.

Micro, Macro, and Mezzo Policy Levels

Edwin Chadwick compiled a macro-oriented report on poverty in 1842, *Report on the Sanitary Condition of the Labouring Population of Great Britain,* in which he concluded that "the amount of burthens produced [by "epidemics and all infectious diseases"] is frequently so great as to render it good economics on the part of administrators of the Poor Laws to incur the charges for preventing the evils that are ascribable to physical causes" (quoted by Fraser, 1973, p. 57). According to Trattner (1994, p. 142), "Probably no single document so profoundly affected the development of public health."

This was a remarkable turnaround from a micro-oriented report on poverty eight years earlier, *Report of His Majesty's Commissioners for Inquiring into the Administration and Practical Operation of the Poor Laws,* which placed total blame for poverty on individual victims and was the rationale for the punitive microinterventions of the 1834 British Poor Laws Reform Act—and for American public assistance during the past thirty years.

Policy may address micro, mezzo, or macro levels. Policy actions may strategically intervene at any or all levels. Analysis at one level commonly creates policy implications for the other two levels. For better or for worse, "it's all in one piece." Indeed, one can make a good case for *synergism*: "the simultaneous action of separate agencies which together have greater effect than the sum of their separate individual effects."

An illustration of this is the case of TV personality Kathy Lee Gifford. She was a longtime advocate and contributor at the *micro* policy level to direct services for needy children. Shocked to learn that her popular clothing line was manufactured in part by children for starvation wages under unsafe and abusive conditions, she moved to the *mezzo* (middle) policy level by demanding from the manufacturer that no garment bearing her name be made under such conditions. She also moved to a *macro* level by seeking to persuade the U.S. government to strengthen and enforce trade policies that prohibit imports manufactured abroad under inhumane conditions— even if that manufacturer is itself an American corporation.

In contrast, at about the same time, a basketball superstar was informed that a comparable situation existed in the manufacture of the line of sneakers that he promoted. He responded that he had nothing to do with that part of the business.

Often even effective microprograms do not by themselves cut the mustard. The 1960s' micro-oriented work and training programs appear to have been effective for hundreds of thousands of individuals and probably contributed to the largest short-term reduction of poverty in the history of the United States. Yet, it was also a period of great unrest—the urban "rebellions" or "riots," according to your ideological viewpoint. As the coordinator of NIMH (National Institutes of Mental Health) research on those riots, my conclusion coincided with those of Aaron Wildavsky:

> A recipe for violence: promise a lot, deliver a little. . . . Try a variety of small programs, each interesting but marginal in impact and severely underfinanced. Avoid any attempt at solutions remotely comparable in size to the dimensions of the problem you are trying to solve. (quoted in Dolgoff, Feldstein, and Skolnick, 1997, p. 97)

The Six P's

Policy does not exist in a vacuum. It is part and parcel of a collection of related activities, which we can call "the six P's."

Policy analysis (P1) develops an overall framework for *policy action* (P2), which works to get a policy adopted and carried out. The analysis incorporates such areas as beliefs and values, mission, existing circumstances, intents, directions, and boundaries. It addresses political, planning, program, and project factors that are likely to affect policy choices, particularly in relation to their feasibility for successful policy action.

Politics (P3), said Otto von Bismarck, is "the art of the possible." It is a give-and-take decision-making process, based on power and persuasion, that affects policy in several ways. First, in policy analysis, politics is a common process used to sort out the relative priority of stakeholders' conflicting interests and values. Second, it is a key feasibility process for testing what the traffic will bear. Third, it is a necessary policy action method to get the policy enacted, implemented, and accepted by those whom it will affect.

Planning (P4) is "any method of thinking out actions or purposes beforehand." It is concerned with determining how to get from here to where we want to be, developing a course of action that will do the job, and organizing a detailed strategy to carry it out. A "plan" itself is the road map for a chosen course of action, a draft or blueprint which reflects the results of a planning process up to that moment in time. As new input and perspectives based on data, experience, further reflection on values and priorities, and unexpected obstacles or opportunities are encountered, the original plan is revised and updated as appropriate.

A *program* (P5) is a tangible means for carrying out policy: "an outline of work to be done; a prearranged plan of procedure." Programming is a planning process to implement a policy. It develops clearly defined middle-range goals and the means to meet them. In administration, a program is an ongoing mechanism ("structure of delivery") to carry out a set of specific activities that deliver the product/result called for by the policy, be it universal health care, clean water, retirement benefits, treatment of clinical depression, or adoption of handicapped children.

A *project* (P6) is "a unique piece of work having a finite life and producing an identifiable product or achieving a specific aim on time and within specified resource limits" (Canadian Government, 1982, p. 82). Project planning is the nitty-gritty of achieving a limited concrete objective derived from a policy. Demonstration projects are often a stepping stone within a policy action plan. These projects test new approaches or methods on a small scale, in only one or a few specific settings.

THREE POLICY SECTORS

The Public Sector

Public social policies exist at the federal, state, and local levels. They are not difficult to identify. You can find them in the Bill of

Rights and in statutes that regulate the safety of workers, set up Social Security pensions, allow tax credits for day care expenses, etc. These policies are elaborated upon and applied by administrative regulations and guidelines. The public welfare agency I worked for had a foot-thick manual of directives and guidelines on exactly how the poor were to be aided.

When we disagree on what a public policy means or whether it is being properly carried out, our courts clarify the policy. Sometimes this can have a major social policy impact. Thousands of allegedly "separate but equal" schools had to integrate in 1954, when the Supreme Court ruled that segregation by race was inherently unequal treatment.

The Organized Private Sector

Private organizations, such as businesses, labor unions, charitable agencies, and professional societies, have social policies that apply within their particular realms. Examples of internal social policies include:

- a collective bargaining agreement with a union;
- admission standards in an Ivy League university;
- guidelines used by United Way to allocate contributions;
- refusal by a hospital to permit legal abortions within its facility; and
- a professional code of ethics requiring confidentiality.

In addition to affecting the well-being of persons within their jurisdiction, private organizations often have an impact on the larger society. In the 1990s, decisions by large private health insurance companies concerning what to reimburse and what to exclude from contracts significantly affected treatment of mental health and chemical dependency disorders by expanding less effective short-term intensive care at the expense of more successful long-term outpatient therapy and support approaches.

The organized private sector exerts considerable direct influence on public policy. Sometimes this is done through such formal associations as the Sierra Club, the Republican Party, the American Civil Liberties Union, and the National Rifle Association. In other instances, the organization is more informal, such as the "military industrial complex," whose influence concerned President Eisenhower.

The Implicit Sector

Have you ever moved from your "roots" to a new situation—college, job, larger or smaller community, another part of the country, different class or ethnic group—where "everybody" except you takes for granted many unspoken rules about what is okay and not okay and how things are done? In time, you learned these rules too. Then did you return "home" and notice, with new insight, what *you* had always taken for granted? If so, you are familiar with the implicit sector's nonorganized "courses of action" and "regular patterns over time." Classic portrayals of implicit policy include Sinclair Lewis's *Main Street* and Garrison Keillor's *Lake Wobegon* chronicles.

The implicit sector, also known as culture or tradition, is sometimes powerful enough to overcome even coercive de jure public policies: The traditional Russian peasant commitment to individualistic enterprise and reward subverted Stalin's collective farms. Prohibition was unable to overcome Americans' implicit alcohol use policy.

Implicit sector policy is the heart of institutionalized racism, sexism, and classism. While a boy whose parents were both college professors coasted with a B average into high school honors classes, his friend, the daughter of a blue-collar immigrant, was put into a secretarial track where the school said she "belonged," despite her straight-A average and her expressed desire to be a doctor. Eventually, facing a possible lawsuit supported by both sets of parents, the high school superintendent acknowledged an "error," pleading that "it wasn't personal" and "nobody meant any harm." He wasn't making excuses either; he was simply following suburban Mamaroneck's longtime implicit policy.

Because it is *not* organized, implicit sector policy is difficult, but not impossible, to change. In the 1940s, when New York passed the first fair employment practices law, its opponents, citing Prohibition, insisted that "you can't legislate morality." In fact, by creating minority opportunities, the law *did* change the implicit sector, which came to treat workplace integration as normal and routine. (However, it had little effect at that time on another implicit sector policy against residential and social integration.)

DE JURE, DE FACTO, AND DEFAULT POLICY

Policies may take the form of any one of the "three D's": de jure (official), de facto (informal), or default (the consequences of no recognized policy).

De Jure

De jure means "from the law." It is on paper and enforceable in court. Public de jure policy comes from statutes, regulations, and/or court decisions: Mandatory participation in Social Security is de jure by act of Congress. School integration is de jure by court interpretation of the Constitution.

De jure private sector policy is written in such documents as articles of incorporation, agency by-laws, board minutes, personnel policy manuals, university admission standards, and collective bargaining contracts.

De Facto

De facto means "from what is done." Such policy is unofficial but follows regular patterns over time.

Where no official policy exists, people use their own judgment, which in time evolves into traditional practices. Some of these evolve into de jure policy. As a river gradually builds up new land in a delta from silt that it has carried along, the courts gradually build common law from accumulated deposits of de facto policy.

De facto patterns can modify or subvert official policy. A supervisor's flexibility may permit workers to "bend" overly rigid rules in ways that increase their productiveness. A business that has an official policy of hiring and promoting on merit may de facto rely more on age, gender, ethnic origin, accent, dress, or manners than on job-related competence.

De facto policy can also change official policy. In the 1950s and 1960s, court decisions and new statutes guaranteed equal opportunity in employment and education, implemented firmly and vigorously by the executive and judicial branches. In the 1970s and 1980s, with a de facto policy shift toward "benign neglect," policy implementation staffs were reduced, enforcement agencies stopped initiating compliance reviews, and enforcement was limited to carefully documented individual complaints of specific direct discriminations, disregarding any subtle or implicit practices. Although the statutes were the same, public policy had changed dramatically.

When is a law not a law? De facto policy can subvert de jure policy: For many years, my local police treated spousal abuse as a noncriminal internal family affair, in effect legalizing criminal assault and battery. Before MADD's campaign, drunk drivers were often released by police and judges rather than punished.

A common policy dilemma is how to handle such discrepancies between formal and de facto policies. There are three basic responses: (1) conform the practice to the rules through honest enforcement as my local police now do regarding spousal abuse; (2) change the rules to legitimize the existing practice, as the repeal of Prohibition did; or (3) continue with deliberate ambiguity, keeping unenforced laws on the books to use on occasions when things "get out of hand," as my local police still do in regard to illegal gambling.

Default

Default means "failure to act." Default policy results, paradoxically, from absence of policy. Some default policies, such as deliberate nonregulation of a powerful special interest group's harmful practices, may be intentional. Others are unwitting results of indifference or ignorance. President Nixon called this "benign neglect." It may or may not be benign.

Default policy is difficult to confront or change because it tends to reinforce vested interests and the status quo. Until the 1960s, there was little or no policy regarding discrimination in housing. In this absence of policy, restrictive covenants against Jews and African Americans were frequently attached to deeds from the 1920s on. A famous 1950s' novel and movie, *Gentlemen's Agreement*, by Laura Hosbon, brought this practice into the open. Even then, the practices continued to be widespread until specific de jure public policies made housing discrimination illegal.

TYPES OF BENEFITS:
MATERIAL, THERAPEUTIC, OR OPPORTUNITY

A benefit is "anything that is good for a person." A social welfare benefit may have a material, therapeutic, or opportunity objective.

Material benefits relate to adequacy or equality of food, clothing, and shelter. Social Security, food stamps, and public housing are material programs.

Therapeutic benefits are intended to (1) cure personal problems through treatment, as in surgery, rehabilitation, marriage counseling, or remedial education, or (2) ameliorate them with supportive assistance, as in a hospice or a community support program for the mentally ill.

Opportunity benefits focus on helping people to succeed better in the world around them. One area is individual development, through such means as education, job training, or physical fitness. Related to this is empowerment of people to obtain rights and opportunities on their own, through assertiveness training, network building, political organizing, or community development. A third area is enabling access to existing rights and opportunities through such means as advocacy, legal aid, guidance counseling, employment services, and referral.

Benefits may be combined to accomplish multiple objectives. For instance, the Job Corps program provided financial aid, counseling, and vocational training in one package.

FORMS OF DELIVERY:
IN-KIND, CASH, OR VOUCHER

Social welfare benefits may be delivered as in-kind goods and services, cash, or vouchers.

In-kind benefits are the most controlled. The source of the benefit offers what it believes you need on a take-it-or-leave-it basis. Examples of in-kind goods include surplus government cheese, Christmas toys, soup kitchens, shelters, and public housing apartments. In-kind *services* include public schools, well-baby clinics, counseling in a United Way agency, treatment in state mental hospitals, and managed health care.

Cash benefits give the recipient market freedom. They may be based on specific determinations of need and clear indications on how the money should be spent. For example, welfare grants are supposed to be based on the cost of an adequate "package" of food, rent, utilities, clothing, etc. Pensions and Social Security are supposed to replace lost earnings to maintain a former standard of living. Family allowance programs and tax welfare deductions for dependents are meant to defray some of the cost of raising children. Nevertheless, the money received is legal tender that you can spend as you choose.

Vouchers are promises by a third party to pay for designated goods and services purchased from a choice of approved providers. In their traditional form, they are coupons, as in food stamps, or charge cards, as in Medicare. An increasingly popular variation is *tax credits,* which refund money spent for specified services such as day care.

Vouchers are a compromise between cash and kind. The authority may not trust the client enough to allow full freedom in spending. For example, food stamps permit free choice of: American-grown foods but cannot be used for shoes, booze, or buying the news. On the other hand, vouchers permit some flexibility within those limits. An example is traditional Medicare: although it can be used only for designated health services at designated prices, the patient may choose among competing doctors and hospitals.

Which method is best? Cash is most compatible with the ideologies of individual self-determination and minimum government influence. If social welfare cannot be avoided altogether, classical economists prefer cash because it is least disruptive to the free market system of buying and selling.

A pessimistic view of human nature may support in-kind benefits. If clients can't be trusted to make good decisions, we who know best will do it for them.

Vouchers are a compromise advocated by those who want to limit the product (benefit) choice while maximizing market freedom regarding providers.

Perhaps the method of provision should vary with the characteristics of the beneficiary, the environmental circumstances, and the objectives of the social program—if we could only agree on just what those characteristics, circumstances, and objectives are.

THE SCOPE OF SOCIAL POLICY

What does social policy include? Social policy affects the well-being of people within a society. Everyone agrees it includes direct health, education, and welfare programs. A more inclusive definition adds such areas as housing, employment, civil rights, consumer protection, environmental protection, and fiscal policy, each of which has a visible effect on individual well-being.

Dante's *Inferno* (1310) described hell as a series of concentric circles, with a progression from the lesser reprobates in outer circles to hard-core sinners at the center. Hopefully, without implying that "social policy is hell," we can use this model to examine the scope of social policy. We will move in the opposite direction from Dante, starting at the center with the most traditional direct service core and moving outward through progressively more indirect domains. Within this framework, you may define what you personally plan to address.

Circle 1: Direct Human Services—Public and Charitable

The innermost circle is direct benefits to individuals, free or below actual cost, provided through the two social welfare institutions that have been in the "business" for thousands of years—public welfare and charity. Benefits fall into two basic categories:

- *Material aid:* food, clothing, and shelter, such as surplus commodities and public housing developments, or the means to purchase them, such as food stamps and welfare grants.
- *Personal services and care:* medical treatment, rehabilitation, family counseling, psychotherapy, education, child care, etc. Services may be provided free, at cost, or on a sliding scale of ability to pay.

Public welfare is offered through such government agencies as local public school systems, state welfare departments, and the federal Veteran's Administration. Charitable services are dispensed by such nonprofit volunteer agencies as a family service agency, the Salvation Army, Girl Scouts, or a neighborhood settlement house. Many are sponsored by sectarian bodies and/or receive support from the United Way.

Circle 2: Mutual Assistance and Personal Welfare

Responding to the breakdown of feudalism, mutual assistance societies arose in the form of guilds, burial societies, and fraternal orders that took care of aged, widowed, and orphaned members. In the United States, this was a common nineteenth-century pattern among immigrants and other oppressed groups, for example, Hibernian societies, black churches, and Jewish community services. More recently, examples of mutual assistance may be found in union pension funds, credit unions, and co-op preschool programs.

Beginning in Europe at the turn of the century and in the United States in the 1930s, governments adopted mutual assistance programs on a large scale through public social insurance. Social Security, unemployment insurance, and Medicare are collectively paid for through payroll taxes by very large user groups. This contrasts with Circle 1 services, which are typically subsidized by nonmembers of the benefit group.

In Germany, as self-help social insurance became more formally organized and impersonal, a new generation of grassroots self-help associations offering personalized support services grew dramatically to complement the economic social insurances. They have tended to evolve, over time, into Circle 1 agencies with professional staffs (Clasen and Freeman, 1994, p. 104).

Also within the mutual assistance circle is probably the largest single social welfare sector of all, often overlooked because it is not formally organized—personal welfare, which meets human needs on a private person-to-person level. According to a 1997 AARP (American Association of Retired Persons) survey, 22.4 million families volunteered an average of eighteen hours per week of unpaid care to elderly friends or relatives. This totaled 21 billion hours, with a cash equivalent value (using an $8 per hour wage-plus-benefits rate) of $168 billion. In addition, these families spent $24 million per year in cash, for a total of $192 billion—just for personal welfare elder care (*USA Today*, 1997).

Add to this the expenditures of time and money on adult children and relatives for such things as room and board, college tuition, day care for their children, and help with buying homes and cars. Then throw in millions of instances every week of other cash, kind, and

service benefits, such as cakes and casseroles for ill or newly be-
reaved friends, blowing snow from the sidewalk and driveway of
the widow next door, groceries or a few dollars to help a friend or
relative over a rough spot, harvesting the crops for an injured farm
neighbor, and on and on. Cashed out, the total "budget" of this
sector of the population could well be pushing half a trillion dollars.

Although a general decline in neighborliness and extended family ties has occurred, the AARP survey found that the number of
caregivers to the elderly had tripled in the ten years since its last
survey.

Other terms for Circle 2 are solidarity, fellowship, community,
reciprocal altruism, and tribal socialism. The key concept may be
"we" in place of "I."

Circle 3: Occupational Welfare

A third direct service area is occupational welfare, benefits provided to employees. It dates back to Robert Owen's successful experiment in New Lanark in 1799. In its "classic" form, it has included paternalistic direct provision of housing, recreational
programs, and health clinics. Under attack from both the "right" and
the "left," it fell out of favor in America in the early part of the
twentieth century. One side accused it of "coddling" workers, while
the other side condemned it because it often went hand in hand with
low wages and repression of worker freedom in company towns.

In recent years, occupational welfare has reemerged in such areas
as day care, employee assistance programs (EAP), and fitness centers. Although such direct services may have an altruistic element,
they fall into Circle 3 instead of Circle 1 charitable services because
they are fundamentally enlightened self-interest investments, which
pay off indirectly in lower absenteeism, higher staff loyalty, and
increased productivity. Employers may engage in this on their own
initiative, as a result of bargaining with security-oriented unions or
as a strategy to avoid unionization.

Another direct occupational welfare benefit is the traditional company pension (which is actually deferred earnings, withheld explicitly or implicitly, to be paid after retirement). This includes civil service, teacher, and military pensions, which are often mistaken for

public welfare (Circle 1) or social insurance (Circle 2) because the employer who deferred the income was in the public sector.

Another, and larger, area of occupational welfare is health insurance and payments into equity retirement accounts not administered by the company itself. This has been "assigned" to Circle 5 because it purchases benefits instead of providing them directly.

Circle 4: Services for Profit

Not so many years ago, because they cost more than their users could pay, most human services were provided by subsidized public and charitable agencies, organized mutual assistance, and the individual charity of providers who gave free medical care and other services to disadvantaged people.

In the second half of the twentieth century, public and employer health insurance (Circle 5) developed as third-party payers for patient/client users. Lately, government has added additional service areas, such as corrections and child welfare, which were traditionally provided by the public and charitable sectors. This changed human services from a money loser to a potential profit center. In a free enterprise system, the natural response was a for-profit service industry, which by the end of the century was one of the most rapidly growing business enterprise fields in the United States.

A related response to the same forces has been the conversion of public and charitable hospitals and agencies into quasi-commercial businesses. They remain nonprofit in the sense that they do not distribute their earnings to owners or sponsors, but they have become self-supporting from sales (fees and charges), with little or no subsidy from taxes or charity. Similar to regular businesses, and for the same reasons, they tend to shun noncrisis patients who cannot pay.

Another development, public subsidy of private old-age pensions, as will be described in Circle 6, has fed a ballooning pension/investment management industry.

Circle 5: Purchase of Services to be Delivered by Others

In Circles 1 and 3, the cost of a service was traditionally borne by the consumer and/or the provider, the latter often subsidized from contributions or taxes. Increasingly, employers and government have found it easier to purchase services for their employees from outside suppliers than to operate their own clinics and pension plans. In Circle 5, the purchaser is neither of these two parties, hence the term, third-party payments.

Major public purchasers include Medicare, Medicaid, Vocational Rehabilitation, and Title XX (of the Social Security Act) social services. In the occupational welfare area, my university provides health insurance for its employees instead of treating them at the University Medical Center and makes payments into their equity accounts in an independent annuity fund in lieu of a company pension plan. On the personal welfare level, one of my neighbors preferred to buy nursing services for her ailing father rather than give up her career to care for him full time at home.

Among the popular vehicles for purchase of service are vouchers (as in national merit scholarships), credit cards (as in Medicare), coupons (as in food stamps), and contracts (as in capitation payments to a health maintenance organization [HMO]).

Circle 6: Tax Welfare

Let's say your sink clogs up, and you ask the landlord to fix it. The landlord says, "Call a plumber and subtract the cost from your rent." Next month, instead of $500, you send $425 and the plumber's receipt for $75. The net effect for you, the landlord, and the plumber is the same as if you had paid the full rent and the landlord had hired the plumber.

When the government tells you to buy day care and subtract the cost as a credit against taxes you owe, it is called a *tax expenditure*. When the government collects your complete tax bill first and they pay for the service, as in Medicare, it is called a *budget expenditure*. As with the clogged sink case, the net effect for the government's budget balancing, for you, and for the provider is the same. Because the expenditure is hidden in lower tax revenues, it looks "on paper" like less government spending. This seems to appeal particularly to politicians who want to support popular benefits while maintaining a "conservative" image.

There are three common forms of tax expenditures:

- After you have calculated your taxes, a *tax credit* is subtracted from what you owe. A $1,000 credit is a $1,000 benefit (provided you owe that much).
- A *tax deduction* reduces the taxable income *before* the tax is calculated. The size of the benefit varies with your tax rate. A $1,000 deduction is a $330 benefit, if you earn enough to be in a 33 percent bracket, $150 if your lower income puts you in a 15 percent bracket.
- *Tax deferral* is more complicated. Let's say you earn a nominal salary of $40,000, plus 5 percent ($2,000) which your employer deposits in your tax-deferred 401K private pension fund, along with 5 percent deducted from your paycheck. Your real pay is $42,000, of which $38,000 is taxable this year. Taxes on the $4,000 in savings are deferred until you withdraw it from the fund. If you had to pay taxes on it this year, in a federal 28 percent and state 7 percent bracket, your retirement account would have been $2,600 instead of $4,000. The deferred $1,400 accrues at a compounded annual rate of about 8 percent for the next twenty-five years, at which time it has grown to $10,000. You take it out and pay 35 percent tax on it, netting a $6,500 benefit due exclusively to the tax deferral—added to the after-tax $12,000 you earned on the other $2,600, which you would have had anyway without the tax break. That is for only this year's income; you can do it again next year.

Tax welfare typically funds benefits from middle- and upper-income welfare programs, which often parallel expenditure funding of similar programs for the poor.

- Head Start is public welfare. The day care credit for middle-income children is tax welfare.
- Rent vouchers subsidize low-income renters. Mortgage interest deductions subsidize middle- and upper-income homeowners.
- Retirement benefits paid by Social Security are budget expenditures. The 401k private pension supplement described previously is a tax expenditure benefit paid to middle- and upper-income persons.

Circle 7: Agents

The first six circles provide social welfare benefits directly to people. British sociologist Peter Townsend (1975) has said that this is not enough:

> Social policy is still conceived too narrowly. . . . Any worthwhile social objective—for example, educational equality, the elimination of overcrowding and squalor, the reduction of ill-health, and social integration—depends on the use and control of institutions like the fiscal system and the wage and fringe benefit systems of industry and not just the conventional group of public social services (education, health, social security, housing, and welfare). (Preface)

The focus of Circle 7 policies and programs is to get agents (see Chapter 3) to do less harm or more good to people: Affirmative action rules require employers to give equal opportunity to their employees. Environmental Protection Administration regulators and the police protect us from those who would do us harm. "Positive parenting" programs attempt to change child abusers into nurturing caregivers. Licensing restricts service provision to agents who meet high ethical and competence standards, and professional education is designed to supply persons who meet those standards.

Circle 8: Environmental Adjustments and Enhancements

There is a traditional story that describes a highway with a dangerous curve at which many accidents occurred. Victims often died before emergency medical aid arrived from, or en route back to, the city's only hospital on the far side of town. Concerned professionals were organizing a million-dollar campaign to build a new hospital next to the high-risk area (a good Circle 1 approach)—until a simple old soul asked, "Why dontcha just straighten the road?" This circle addresses the social environment.

- A key environmental factor is the *economic system:* the patterns of production and consumption, distribution and inequality, division of labor, and interplay among workers, employers, sellers, and buyers.

- A second one is *polity:* how the society handles democracy and authority, freedom and social control, centralization and decentralization.
- Closely related to both previous factors is *distribution of power*, which may be a mix of economic, social, political, ethnic, and gender factors.
- Other environmental factors include patterns of beliefs, values, cultural practices, climate, natural resources, and demography.

Interventions range from radical change through reform to enhancement. Radical change involves major departures from the existing system, such as abolishing slavery, collectivizing peasants' farms, moving from a centrally planned economy to a free-market system, or overthrowing an oppressive government.

Reform is "the improvement or amendment of what is wrong." It takes a more moderate and incremental approach to the social environment. We added to civil rights, by amending the Constitution to guarantee individual liberties (the Bill of Rights), ensure equal treatment under the law (Amendment XIV), and expand the vote to all citizens (Amendments XV and XIX). We have also reinterpreted the Constitution on segregation and supplemented it with specific laws, such as the Civil Rights Act of 1965.

Keynesian, monetarist, and supply-side government interventions, as well as international tariffs and quotas, are intended to enhance our nation's overall economy by tinkering with the law of supply and demand within our basic market system. Some critics believe that this is fundamental change rather than enhancement; others allege that it doesn't work and therefore is neither.

Circle 9: Corporate Welfare?

Is there one more circle? A social policy is one that affects the well-being of individuals within a society. By legal definition, a business corporation is an individual. Welfare benefits to corporate individuals may be either through tax expenditures (Circle 6) or through public budget subsidies (as in agriculture). There are also significant in-kind benefits, such as scientific and technological developments from government space, agricultural, and health research, that are made available to farmers and businesses for commercial development.

Because of the vast range of corporate welfare measures and the gray areas within them, there has been no comprehensive accounting of corporate welfare. Estimates begin at hundreds of billions of dollars per year.

Should corporate welfare be a circle within social policy? That depends on two questions: First, is "well-being of the individual" meant to include corporate individuals on the same basis as human individuals? If not, is selective corporate welfare still desirable within the agent and environment circles (7 and 8) when direct, traceable benefits to the well-being of *human* individuals in our society can be shown?

Chapter 2

Making Choices

No matter how qualified or deserving we are, we will never reach a better life until we can imagine it for ourselves and allow ourselves to have it.

Richard Bach, 1988

No choice is a choice.

Yiddish proverb

POLICY ANALYSIS

Normative and Empirical Dimensions

Policy analysis is the foundation for policy choices as well as for strategies to implement them as best we can. It involves a continuous interaction between two different perspectives, normative and empirical.

A norm is "a standard." *Normative* refers to determining norms and applying them to choices about what is desirable or not. Its sources include:

- our own personal values and beliefs,
- the traditions and culture in our society,
- existing laws and legal authority,
- the justifications by power elites of their vested interests, and
- the preferences of target groups.

Empirical refers to observed "facts" about the situation and inferences based on them. These facts relate to specific conditions,

25

what caused them, and what realistically can or cannot be done. In a good policy analysis, normative and empirical perspectives are blended, particularly in the following list of elements.

Area of Concern

"Policy" covers the universe. If you want to accomplish anything, you have to narrow it down to a policy (or cluster of policies), something you can grasp. What are the boundaries of *this* policy concern? What is the location—geographic, demographic, organizational? What is the specific need to be met, problem to be solved, potential to be realized? Who do we aim to benefit? What are their present circumstances?

The Existing Situation

In relation to your defined area of concern, what is the situation? You need information about the condition, how it came about, how it relates to the larger environment, and the effect of existing policies and programs. What are the particular circumstances—needs, resources, obstacles, opportunities? Who is affecting the situation now? How? Where is it heading if no change is made? Who besides your targets would be affected, for good or ill, by a change? Who are the key actors, for and against, on whom success will depend?

VIBES

Get in touch with your values, interests, beliefs, ethics, and slants (VIBES). Where are you coming from, both figuratively and literally? These characteristics ultimately determine your direction; they *will* operate—consciously or unwittingly. We are more in control if we know what they are.

Then analyze the VIBES of others. Who will you take into account—targets, other stakeholders, allies, opponents, other potential key actors? Where did they get their VIBES and how do theirs coincide or conflict with one another's and with yours? How do their VIBES affect what they see (and don't see) as facts, their opinions about what is desirable, and their choice of means to achieve their ends?

Nonbounded Rationality: The Desirable Situation

"The man who finds what he seeks as a rule has set his ambitions too low" (Anonymous). Before getting down to the nitty-gritty, start with nonbounded thinking, unlimited in advance by *any* presumed constraints. Rousseau is said to have observed that "The world of reality has it limits; the world of imagination is boundless." "Practical" politicians and bureaucrats write this off as "pie in the sky." When I worked for NIMH, we had a small branch devoted to non-bounded thinking about mental health. Colleagues wrote off members of this branch as "space cadets." Why waste time on that stuff? George Bernard Shaw gave us the reason why we should: "You see things; and you say, 'Why?' But I dream things that never were; and I say, 'Why not?'" (from *Back to Methusalah*).

Ideally, what situations/conditions should exist? The answer comes from your beliefs (and other VIBES) about what is good or bad and what is more or less important. It may be informed in part by your comparative study of actual situations, past and present, that are considered to be relatively "better" or "worse." Even if the ideal situation is not attainable, it is the standard against which you will compare available policy choices.

Bounded Rationality: What Can Be Done?

Nonbounded is well and good as far as it goes, but still, "if wishes were horses, then beggars would ride." Martin Luther King said, "I have been to the mountain," then he came back down and worked for specific civil rights policies and practices.

Bounded rationality operates within the confines of your informed assumptions about what can and cannot be done, given the existing mix of resources, politics, culture, ideology, power, and vested interests. What is the state of the art? How much existing support and acceptance is there? Where is it? How much power? The same holds regarding active and potential opposition. What would be the costs and negative side effects in comparison with the benefits? On whom would they fall? And overall, what will the traffic bear?

But don't be too cautious. It can't be done? Are you sure? A World War II Army Air Corps slogan was, "The difficult we do

immediately. The impossible takes a little longer." As my old literature professor used to say of the novel or poem we were studying at
the moment, "Let's walk around it one more time." If the best
policy is not feasible, what can be done to get part way? The trick is
to find the line that falls within the possible, yet transcends conventional wisdom.

MAKING POLICY CHOICES

Every realistic social policy choice is a compromise that balances
desirability, design, and feasibility.

Desirability

A policy may be desirable or undesirable. Some common sources
of undesirable are the following:

- *Bad purpose.* South Africa's policy of apartheid was deliberately designed to favor the interests of a minority at the expense of everyone else.
- *Other priorities.* In his 1854 veto of aid to mental health, President Pierce affirmed "the duty incumbent on us all as men
  and citizens, and as among the highest and holiest of our duties, to provide for those who, in the mysterious order of Prov-
  idence, are subject to want and to disease of body or
  mind"(Axinn and Levin, 1982, p. 75)—but not as high and
  holy as the antifederal position of a politician elected with
  Southern votes in the decade before the Civil War.
- *Ignorance.* President Hoover, a humanitarian who had led a
  hunger relief program credited with saving millions of lives in
  Communist Russia, took a hard line against hunger relief for
  his own American people in 1930-1932. Incredible as it may
  seem, he was so out of touch that he literally did not know how
  much they were suffering.
- *Inaccurate premises.* Historians Axinn and Levin (1982, p. 178)
  found a second contributing factor: "Trapped by the hope of
  his own prediction of an early return to economic normalcy . . .

Hoover was reluctant to have the federal government assume new responsibilities and powers."
- *Ideology.* According to a Social Darwinist, "Society is constantly excreting its unhealthy imbecile, slow, vacillating, faithless members to leave room for the deserving. A maudlin impulse to prolong the lives of the unfit stands in the way of this beneficent purging of the social organism" (Trattner, 1994, p. 91).

To make desirable policy choices, we must ask normative questions. In whose interest is a policy objective—your own, your peer group, a client group, some other target group, society as a whole? What values guide you in deciding whose interests take priority, what is good or bad for them, and what means are acceptable?

Design

Research uses the terms *necessary cause* and *sufficient cause.* Adapted to social policy, something is *necessary* if the objective cannot be achieved without it. Universal basic literacy is necessary for full employment, since nearly every job requires at least the ability to read instructions and signs. However, it is not sufficient because most jobs require other education and skills as well.

Something is *sufficient* if it can achieve the objective. In combating typhoid fever, either a clean water supply or vaccination may be sufficient. Either means-tested "relief" grants or universal old-age pensions, if adequate, could assure a guaranteed minimum income in old age. In such cases, you have a choice of options.

If no single intervention is sufficient, you may need to combine several. A highly skilled labor force is necessary for full employment. But if the jobs are not there, we also need economic development policies and perhaps a safety net, such as a public jobs program. Realistically, we had also better develop remedial training programs and a continuing education and retraining scheme to maintain worker competence as technology advances.

A senior citizen "does not live by bread alone." For quality of life in old age, you may want policies that provide:

1. a guaranteed minimum income program,
2. wage-related Social Security above the minimum,

3. tax incentives for private pensions,
4. full coverage Medicare,
5. meals-on-wheels and senior citizen centers,
6. medical research into Alzheimer's disease and arthritis, and
7. private sectarian services.

An ideal social policy design would incorporate all necessary elements in a package that is sufficient to fulfill the intent. Such packages are rare in the "real world." Yours is a good design if it is sufficient to meet a limited objective that contributes to—and does not preclude further progress toward—your long-range social policy goal.

Feasibility

A desirable intent plus a good design do not by themselves get the job done. You still must be able to carry them out. Intent and design must be adjusted to feasibility. Factors affecting feasibility include the following:

- *State of the art.* Can it be done at all? Can Niger guarantee an adequate income for its people under any circumstance? Can AIDS epidemics be ended by any existing means?
- *Resources.* Are the necessary funds attainable to support a program? If so, how can we ensure the availability of qualified staff to carry it out?
- *Motivation.* Will there be enough commitment to ensure implementation? There wasn't on the Eighteenth Amendment (Prohibition). There was on the Nineteenth Amendment (Women's Suffrage).
- *Politics.* What will the traffic bear with those who have to approve, provide resources, implement, accept, cooperate with, or use the policy or program? Are there special obstacles or opportunities? What kinds of environmental protection can be achieved within the context of lobbying by powerful commercial interests which make large political contributions?

In the United States, social policy decisions are seldom clear, decisive, and comprehensive. For better or for worse, most of our policy choices are imperfect compromises of intent and design with feasibility. With apologies to Tennyson, we might describe the charge of the "policy light brigade" as "Half a loaf, half a loaf, half a loaf onward."

INTENTS

The intent of a social policy may be self-serving, altruistic, or both. The food stamp program was both. Farmers were looking for a market for their chronic agricultural surpluses. Most customers were already buying as much as they needed. Where was there potential for increase? Answer: give to poor people who could not afford an adequate diet. Proposal: put food money in their pockets— but be sure it can be used only for American farm products. The agriculture lobby was joined, for entirely different reasons, by humanitarian liberals concerned with the well-being of the poor.

Manifest and Covert Intents

In the best of all possible worlds, intents would be *manifest:* "rational, explicit, open." As Flip Wilson used to say, "What you see is what you get." In reality, they are often hidden, ambiguous, or fuzzy. Policymakers may keep their intent *covert* (hidden, secret, concealed, disguised, deceitful) as a conflict tactic or because their purposes are less than noble. The simplest method is the Pearl Harbor approach: keep it secret until you are ready to strike so that the opposition will be caught unprepared.

A *hidden agenda* is more subtle. When psychologists in my state sought licensure restrictions on counseling and therapy, their stated intent was to protect clients. Although this was indeed one intent, another important intent was covert—increased income and competitive advantages for guild members.

In other cases, the stated intent is a *deliberate lie.* In the 1980s, lobbyists sought to replace progressive income tax brackets with a flat percentage rate for everyone. Their stated intent was simplification; their real aim was to lower their clients' tax rates at the expense of middle-income taxpayers. If simplification had been an honest intent, their proposed bill would not have also contained new tax exclusions and loopholes that would have increased the complexity of the tax law.

Misdirection is another strategy. In a football draw play, the quarterback, by pretending to set up for a pass, draws the defenders into rushing him, while handing the ball off covertly to a running back who slips through the hole the diversion creates. A head of state, intent on reducing the national role of social welfare, first reduced taxes, creating a large budget deficit, which "regrettably" made human service cuts "imperative." This strategy is reminiscent of the traditional illustration of chutzpah: a man on trial for murdering his parents asks for mercy on the grounds that he is an orphan.

In addition to raising ethical questions, covert strategies have practical liabilities:

- *Strategically*, if the deceit is discovered, a backlash may defeat the policy and destroy the deceiver's future credibility.
- *Substantively*, the policy may be poorer without the constructive criticism that overt scrutiny would have provided.
- *Procedurally*, covert behavior undermines the give-and-take essential to the health and stability of democratic systems.

On the other hand, are some ends important enough to satisfy the ethics and warrant the risk? Are there circumstances in which unjust misuses of power justify covert counterstrategies on behalf of oppressed groups?

Unrecognized Intents

Advocates and decision makers may be unaware of the real intent of their policies due to vagueness, self-deception, and/or internal disagreements.

Vague good intentions, "softhearted and softheaded," occur when advocates don't have a sound grasp of the existing situation or clarity about their values, interests, and ways of thinking. This lack of understanding leads to confusion and contradictions regarding the specific intent of particular policies.

Unawareness of one's intent can be a problem. In one local community, an intense emotional conflict developed between supporters and opponents of sex education. Each side mouthed its own catchwords and emotionally attacked the other side, yet both groups wanted healthier attitudes toward sex, less promiscuity, and fewer teen pregnancies. Perhaps if their real intents had been clearer, they could have worked together to find a mutually acceptable approach to their shared concerns.

Self-deception is a problem, particularly for righteous people, such as clergy, social workers, feminists, professors, and evangelical activists. We're all human. Self-interest is a normal element in the human condition, and there is usually some gain for us in altruistic behavior, often legitimate ("doing well by doing good"). When we believe ourselves to be morally superior to acting out of self-interest, our denial and rationalization skills flourish. Between the pious and the sinners, trust the sinners more; at least they *know* what they're doing. One of my old professors offered this advice: "Always hope that your opponents are evil, for in evil there is a strain of rationality and therefore the possibility of outthinking them. Good intentions randomize behavior. When good intentions are combined with stupidity, it is impossible to outthink them."

Differences of interpretation may go unperceived. In the Economic Opportunity Act of 1964 (War on Poverty), "community action" was interpreted in four distinct ways:

1. Social planners, impressed by the success of Ford Foundation "Gray Cities" projects, saw it as *reorganizing services* to aid the poor more effectively.
2. The President's top poverty aide, who had a collective bargaining background, stressed "maximum feasible *participation of the poor* " in decision-making structures that affected them.
3. Community organizers and civil rights leaders focused on *empowerment of oppressed groups.*
4. Mayors saw it as a vehicle to *strengthen city governments* in dealing with urban problems.

This ambiguity helped to pass the program but led to inconsistency and conflict in its implementation.

In a traditional or homogeneous setting, no one may even be aware that a choice has been made. Because it is not recognized at all, *mutually unperceived intent* carries an extra risk of being "bad" policy. In the 1960s, in the U.S. Welfare Administration, with its history of dynamic female leadership since the founding of the Children's Bureau a half century earlier, titles of address were the same for men and women. When I transferred from there to the National Institutes of Mental Health, which was then culturally identified with male-dominant psychiatry and clinical psychology, I encountered a de facto policy whereby men were formally addressed as "Dr. Jones," while their female peers were addressed on a first-name basis. When I raised the issue, the typical response from both male and female staff was a blank stare. Although this practice may seem to be only symbolic, it correlated with differences between the two agencies on gender equality in employment, promotion, rank, and power.

Behind the Intent: Facts, Interests, and Values

To understand the intent of a policy, you must learn where its supporters are "coming from."

First, what do they think the situation is? Where do the supporters' facts come from?

- *Empirical data:* What sources? How accurate? How complete?
- *Projection:* From what experiences are they projecting? Do projections coincide with other available information?
- *A priori:* What premises about reality do they take for granted? Are conclusions logically and consistently related to the premise? To what extent are they compatible with available data?

A common error is to treat an a priori belief or projection as if it were empirical data. The Welfare Reform Acts of 1834 (England), 1981, and 1996 were all based on the same a priori "certainty"—that paupers are inherently base, deficient, unmotivated, and of low human value (see Chapter 6 on human nature)—despite extensive documented empirical evidence of their eagerness to escape welfare when given the opportunity to gain the education and training that would enable them to obtain a decent job with an above-poverty-level wage.

Similar errors occur when empirical data are incorrect due to selection, biasing, and methodological error, or when personal experiences are inaccurately generalized to a group of people, the economic system, or society as a whole: "Anyone with gumption can . . ." "Profit-oriented entrepreneurs always . . ."

Second, what are their *interests*? Most policies that claim to promote the common good benefit some particular interest group more than others. Are they truly win-win, whereby advancing the interests of one group also benefits the larger society? Trickle-down benefits will raise the standard of living for workers, said the advocates of supply-side tax cuts. Did they? Humane social programs such as the post–World War II GI Bill, Vocational Rehabilitation, and Head Start create trickle-up benefits for the wealthy in the form of a more productive, gentler, and safer society, claim social workers. Do they?

Is the policy "zero sum," by which one's gain is another's loss? If so, who stands to gain the most? Do they especially need or deserve it? At whose expense? How well can the "losers" afford that cost?

Values also play a key role in intent. What are the stated values? Are they consistent with the de facto values inherent in the actual provisions and applications? If not, investigate further to discover why the discrepancy exists. Is it deliberate deceit? Hypocrisy? Self-deception? Does it stem from the ambiguity of a value conflict that has not been clearly resolved? A useful rule of thumb: "You will know them by their fruits. Are grapes gathered from thorns, or figs from thistles? So every sound tree bears good fruit, but the bad tree bears evil fruit" (Matthew 7:16-17).

Diversion of Intent

Implementation Processes

"There is many a slip 'twixt the cup and the lip" (Palladas, 400 B.C.). Original good intentions are usually compromised and watered down by the time they have run the gauntlet of legislative, political, and economic realities and are implemented by less-than-perfect agencies and individuals.

Good intentions may be reversed along the way. Patrick Moynihan, author of the Nixon Family Assistance Plan (FAP) to nationalize Aid to Families with Dependent Children (AFDC), proclaimed it an antipoverty program. However, after the White House had reworked it, administrative goals of uniformity, control, and cost reduction had taken priority over reduction of poverty. The original intent was further eroded when the Senate added punitive amendments and set the national aid standard 50 percent below the poverty line. The final plan, if implemented, would have made 75 percent of the recipients poorer.

Evaluation Processes

Social policy intent may also be diverted by technical tools. When the President of Ford Motor Company became Secretary of Defense in 1961, he brought with him a successful industrial efficiency approach called cost-benefit analysis, which converted all results (benefits) into dollars. Within five years, cost-benefit analysis had been adopted as the primary tool for evaluating social policy and program. The problem is that it is difficult to put a dollar price on self-esteem, satisfaction, physical and mental health, liberty, happiness, life itself—or Faust's soul.

Conversion to dollars gradually but inexorably displaces original intents. It works like this:

1. Unable to measure directly the individual well-being objective of rehabilitation, evaluators select earnings of rehabilitated persons as the indicator of well-being.
2. Since the indicator (future earnings), and not the actual intent (well-being), is what will be evaluated, administrators and staff naturally make earnings the basis for program decisions about what kinds of and to whom rehabilitative services are offered.
3. Eventually, policy and program people *forget the original intent* and begin to think exclusively in terms of the indicator. Meeting the needs of disabled individuals is subtly, but surely, displaced by a goal of maximized economic production. Investment return replaces need as the basis for selection. "Easier" cases that offer a bigger payoff at a lower cost are pre-

ferred. Those with the greatest need for rehabilitation become
the least desirable clients.

EFFECTS

*If a brother or sister is ill-clad and in lack of daily food, and
one of you says to them, "Go in peace, be warmed and filled,"
without giving them the things needed for the body, what does
it profit?*

James 2:16-17

Effects are the bottom line. In Don Quixote's words, "The proof
of the pudding is in the eating." To make policy choices, we must
predict their effects. Unfortunately, for a variety of reasons, the
effects may not be fully and accurately identified.

Manifest Effects

Manifest effects are those about which there is available, open,
and objective information and some basis for assuming a connection between the cause (policy) and the effect.

A manifest effect of Social Security predicted by its designers
was the reduction of poverty among retirees. The poverty rate for
the aged fell from an estimated 70 percent in 1935 to 25 percent in
1970 and 11.7 percent in 1994, lower than that of the general population. According to 1994 census figures, there were 3.6 million
persons over age sixty-five living in poverty and 18 million more
who would have been in poverty except for Social Security and
related railroad retirement pensions. This means that Social Security currently reduces the over-sixty-five poverty rate by five-sixths
(83 percent).

There may also be manifest *side effects.* The intent of Medicare
and Medicaid was to improve the welfare of patients. A predicted
by-product was to increase the income of physicians and hospitals
by reducing the incidence of unpaid bills and free service.

Some *unforeseen* effects become manifest only after the fact.
Based on the history of third-party purchase in child welfare, Medi-

care and Medicaid were expected to expand nonprofit health services in lieu of public services. No one predicted that over the long run they would be displaced by commercial health care providers. As it turned out, purchase of service for low-income and aged persons created a profit opportunity, which in turn led to displacement of nonprofits by aggressive business enterprises. (This is discussed further in Part V.)

Obscured Effects

To obscure is "to conceal from view; to hide; to make less conspicuous; to make less intelligible; to confuse." *Direct falsification* is one means of obscuring effects. Despite extensive documentary evidence from his own government agencies showing large increases in the poverty rate, an antiwelfare president proclaimed in a nationally broadcast speech, "There is no hunger in America."

The attempt to obscure may be more subtle. They say there are three kinds of lies: lies, damned lies, and statistics. In 1984, the government tried to reduce the reported poverty rate by counting as personal income of poor persons all fees paid to physicians and hospitals on their behalf. Thus, an elderly welfare recipient who had been hospitalized during the year was statistically middle income—while actually still living at the same poverty level as before.

Effects can also be obscured by *diverting attention.* One year my school board enacted an "economy" budget that eliminated the lunchroom, free textbooks, music, and extracurricular activities. By focusing public attention on tax savings of $100 per family, it obscured the much larger new costs that would be imposed on parents for books and supplies, higher-priced lunches in neighboring eateries, replacement private music lessons, and fees for their children to participate in self-financed school sports and clubs.

Another ploy is to *create confusion.* Faced with overwhelming evidence on the health hazards of smoking, the tobacco industry successfully delayed social policy changes for many years by using confusing technical criticisms of the research studies.

Deception about social policy effects may backfire sooner or later. Let's look at the illustrations given previously:

- The juxtaposition in time of highly visible unemployment and a homelessness crisis with the president's no-hunger statement aroused dramatic public rebuttals, reactivated social advocacy among unions, and stimulated a new wave of middle-class volunteers.
- Social scientists and others vociferously attacked the redefinition of poverty as misleading and invalid. The ensuing publicity about this ploy brought the actual increase in poverty to the attention of millions of Americans who usually ignored such statistics.
- After experiencing the actual cost of the school tax "savings," previously apathetic parents, now angered, elected a new school board that restored the old program.
- Passage of antismoking policies was accelerated by the tobacco lobby's loss of credibility, when exposure of internal correspondence showed that tobacco companies had privately accepted the truth of the allegations they were publicly challenging.

Some effects are obscured by *intervening variables*. The domestic economic policies of Presidents Nixon, Ford, and Carter appeared to cause inflation, while those of President Reagan seemed to lower it. However, the actual effects, if any, of their policies were obscured by the overwhelming effect of a dramatic rise in world oil prices in the 1970s and an equally dramatic decline in the early 1980s.

Some effects may not even be recognized at all. For instance, if iatrogenic illness (disorders caused by medical treatment) is a major health hazard, an effect of comprehensive national health care might be to *increase* certain health problems unawares.

Deliberate obscuring subverts democracy by keeping voters uninformed and reducing governmental accountability. Although there may well be a proper time and place for it, most obscuring is a tactic to cover up errors or promote special interests that could not survive the light of day. Exposing both intents and effects to public scrutiny improves social policies and programs in the long run; desirable ones can be supported and enhanced on their merits; ineffective or harmful ones can be revised or replaced.

When in doubt,
Bring it out.

Chapter 3

Policy Interventions

A man of words and not of deeds
Is like a garden full of weeds.

Benjamin Franklin

To sit in meditation is a policy without results.

Anatole France
Penguin Island, 1909

NO HIDING PLACE

A word processor offers two methods of selecting a format. You can set your own margins, type size, spacing, etc. If you don't, it automatically chooses a default format designed by someone else. Similarly, we don't have a choice about whether there will be social policy. There will! If *you* don't do anything, you have chosen *someone else's policy.*

Unfortunately, others' choices, whether de jure or de facto, may differ from what we believe in. They may promote advantaged special interests at the expense of less powerful groups or the general public. There may be important omissions or deficiencies. These are the areas of concern that beckon us. "We design our lives through the power of our choices. We feel most helpless when we've made choices by default, when we haven't designed our lives on our own" (Bach, 1988, p. 95).

We can't evade moral responsibility by not getting involved. "If you're not part of the solution, you're part of the problem." This 1960s slogan was not empty rhetoric: it addressed institutionalized racism, sexism, and classism which were so embedded in the fabric of society's beliefs, culture, relationships, statuses, and legal structure that they were being perpetuated, often unwittingly, by well-meaning fellow citizens in their everyday patterns of work and life.

A General Confession in the *Book of Common Prayer* recognizes this culpable default: "We have done those things which we ought not to have done *and we have left undone those things which we ought to have done*" (emphasis added). Social ethics theologian Reinhold Niebuhr accepted this view. Firmly devoted to Christian pacifism, he opposed all war under any circumstances, including U.S. entry into World War II. Later, as the incredible atrocities and suffering at the hands of the Axis Powers came to light, he supported the war effort because even the horrors of war were a lesser evil than the "sin of irresponsibility" in permitting such suffering to continue.

Personal accountability is not diminished by denying reality, minding our own business, washing our hands like Pilate, or retreating into private piety and micromoralism.

WHERE TO INTERVENE

During the building of the Panama Canal, health officers combating the scourge of yellow fever evolved an early systems model that identified three interacting elements as points for possible intervention:

1. *Hosts:* workers who became "hosts" to the virus—treat or immunize them.
2. *Agents:* carrier mosquitoes—kill them before they bite.
3. *Environment:* swamps in which mosquitoes hatched—drain them.

Adapting this to social policy, *hosts* are the ultimate *targets*, the victims or intended beneficiaries. These may be persons or populations with one of the following characteristics:

- *At need:* already have a problem, such as unemployed adults.
- *At risk:* may develop need, such as unmotivated students.
- *With potential:* candidate for enhanced well-being, such as low-income youth whose employment future could benefit greatly from a college education.

Agents are people and/or organizations that directly affect the hosts. Agents may be sources of problems, such as drug cartels and street pushers, or potential helpers, such as teachers and drug rehabilitation clinics.

The *environment* is the larger context in which the problem takes place. Related to the drug problem may be an affluent society, in which self-gratification has displaced traditional social values, or a poverty and racism setting, in which ghetto youth have little hope for a "respectable" future.

Social policies usually address one or a combination of these three areas. In social welfare, interventions with hosts are often called direct services and benefits, while those aimed at agents and the environment are known by such terms as indirect services, regulation, enforcement, and macroeconomics.

WHEN TO INTERVENE

The Medical Model

A traditional medical model addresses when to intervene by identifying three stages of prevention:

1. *Primary prevention:* keeping the problem from ever occurring.
2. *Secondary prevention:* early detection and treatment, when it is cheaper and more effective.
3. *Tertiary prevention:* treatment after the condition has become acute.

In regard to heart attacks, primary prevention might include a campaign against smoking. Routine screening for high cholesterol with follow-up steps to lower it would be secondary prevention. Triple bypass surgery is tertiary.

For child abuse, reaching out to high-risk potential future abusers, such as persons who were abused as children, is primary prevention. Training teachers to spot and report early signs of abuse in their students would be secondary. Tertiary interventions include public child protection services, medical treatment for abused children, and prosecution of abusers.

Maintenance

As desirable as prevention and cure are, medicine, as well as social policy, must deal with the sad fact of our inability to prevent or cure all problems. Maintenance is a logical fourth intervention. A permanently disabled heart attack victim may need long-term home health care and income maintenance. A child whose parents cannot be helped or punished into becoming nonabusive may need alternative long-term care.

Maintenance may stand by itself. There is no known cure for rheumatic arthritis, but a friend of mine has been kept in "remission" for nearly twenty years through maintenance doses of anti-inflammatories. In social policy, a retired person continues a satisfying life with the help of maintenance provisions such as Social Security and a company pension.

Maintenance may also be a complement to other interventions. A woman with limited education and skills and work habits related to a deprived childhood or adolescence needs tertiary interventions (education, training, counseling, support groups, employment assistance, day care) to become self-supporting, but that can't be done successfully if her children are hungry and she is slowed by malnutrition. Maintenance alone, particularly with hostile overtones, may mire her more deeply in dependency and low self-esteem. Combining tertiary intervention with maintenance achieves more than either alone. Ideally, we should add primary prevention environmental changes and secondary prevention individual services to keep other women from being in a similar situation.

Enhancement

The traditional medical model is limited to its negative definition of health as absence of ailments. This is fine as far as it goes, but it stops short of complete health and true well-being. The World Health Organization (WHO) defines health as "a state of complete physical, mental, and social well-being, and not merely the absence of disease and infirmity."

This calls for a fifth intervention stage, the purpose of which is not to prevent something bad but to create something good. I call this *enhancement*. Others call it a developmental approach. A good exercise program increases your energy level, stamina, and optimism. This is its principle purpose, but it may also contribute to primary prevention of any number of disorders and disabilities in the future. That is a bonus.

In regard to the "disorder" of being unemployed or among the working poor, a good high school education plus an occupationally oriented community college program should be ample prevention. Yet most of the readers of this book have chosen to go further—four years of college and perhaps a graduate degree besides. Why? Not because you have a problem that requires intervention, but because—to use the Army's recruiting slogan—you want to "be all that you can be." You are not, in this context, a *patient* ("one who is under treatment") nor a *client* ("one dependent upon the patronage or protection of another"), but a *student* (from the Latin for "busying oneself about a thing, zeal, applying oneself to learning").

DEGREES OF INTERVENTION

The Incremental Approach

There are two schools of thought about change. The incremental approach starts with what is, the status quo, and considers how it should be modified. Two common versions of the incremental approach are the problem-solving and developmental models. During the War on Poverty, the problem of a chronically unemployed and underemployed lower class was approached incrementally, with adult education, training, and work-experience programs targeted at the hosts. Such programs improved the lives of hundreds of thousands of individuals but did not change the circumstances that continued to create new disadvantaged workers to replace those who had moved on.

On the macro level, economic development programs have, from time to time, attempted to create incremental gains in the economies of depressed American regions and third world countries. Monetary maneuvers by the Federal Reserve Board have at times encouraged consumer spending and/or capital investment. Incremental economic development was pursued systematically and successfully over many years in building Japanese industry.

Social insurance programs of industrial nations reflect another incremental approach, the *supplemental* model. Their function is to ameliorate some of the gaps inherent in the economic market system, without radically changing it. In the United States, since their initiation in the 1930s, and despite periods of grand rhetoric in one direction or another, the actual policy trends in these programs have been incremental for sixty years—upward in coverage and adequacy the first half, downward the second.

Regulation is still another incremental approach. Like a comfortable pair of old jeans, we keep the fabric of business enterprise, with its patched holes and rips, rather than buying new pants.

The Goal-Oriented Approach

The other basic approach is to start with a goal, based on human needs and values. This is sometimes called *zero base* planning or budgeting or a *wellness* model, as distinct from the illness-focused medical model. Martin Luther King's civil rights crusade used a wellness model, as expressed in his famous "I have a dream" speech, about the kind of America both black and white citizens desire.

The wellness model goes to the root of the need or problem. Ideally, it may lead to a single "great leap forward." More often, it is blended with an analysis of politics, resources, culture, and other feasibility factors to develop a series of incremental steps toward the goal.

This synthesis of the two approaches differs from the purely incremental approach in two ways: First, rather than being fragmented and expedient, each small step contributes in a planned way toward the larger goal. Second, a purely incremental approach tends to get subverted or sidetracked in the unavoidable give-and-take of real-life policymaking. It may end up amended to the point where on balance it does more harm than good (see Chapter 2, "Diversion of Intent"). Although goal-oriented policy goes through the same political process, its supporters never lose sight of its purpose. Each compromise is weighed in the context of how it relates to the final goal. If, as is usually the case, the goal is not fully achieved, at least some progress has been made.

CHANGING THE SYSTEM

The great error of reformers and philanthropists is to nibble at the consequences of unjust power, instead of redressing the injustice itself.

John Stuart Mill, 1848

No existing society is perfect. Not all our businessmen are honest or our politicians wise. Our original Constitution permitted slavery and did not give voting rights to women or low-income men. In a nation that professes the ideal of equal opportunity, men on average are "more equal" than women, whites more than blacks, and affluent children more than poor children. Although our nation has one of the highest per capita incomes among industrial nations, it also has one of the highest poverty rates. We are, according to the Luxembourg Income Study, the second most unequal in income distribution of twenty-five industrial nations, exceeded only by Russia (Overberg, 1996).

Interventions may be desirable to improve our general economic, social, and political environments, as well as the behavior of agents within them. Even if all systems were A-OK, periodic adjustments would be needed as times changed.

Such interventions might involve either radical change or reform and enhancement. What's the difference? Let's apply it to lawn care. Mine is so-so; there are some lush spots, but mostly it is homely grass, thinning in spots like my hair and cohabiting with April dandelions and summer crabgrass. There are a few bare spots where the kids play catch. My annual spring *enhancement* is an application of "weed and feed," producing a rather nice yard in May and June.

Every few years, I embark on a series of *reforms*. I rent a roller, which aerates the lawn, scatter shade-grass seed in the front yard under the trees and plant grass seed in the backyard, put down chemicals that kill sod webworms and suppress germination of crabgrass, and fertilize. This yields incremental, semipermanent improvements.

My neighbor, Mr. Jones, burdened with a similar lawn, hired a landscape contractor two years ago to plow his whole yard under, lay fairway-quality turf throughout, and maintain it. Since his *radi-*

cal system change, none of the rest of us can keep up with the Joneses.

RADICAL CHANGE

When elephants fight, it is the grass which suffers.

Proverb

A radish is a root vegetable. From the same Latin origin, *radical* means "going to the root or origin, fundamental."

- A radical *political* system change was the move from representative democracy to dictatorship in Germany under Hitler—and another back to democracy after his fall.
- A radical *civil rights* change was the Thirteenth, Fourteenth, and Fifteenth Amendments that ended slavery and granted equal citizenship to former slaves.
- A radical *economic* change under Lenin was confiscating large estates and dividing the land among the peasants. Another, under Stalin, was confiscating the peasants' land and combining it into large estates (collective farms).

Many people are cautious about fundamental change. One issue is *feasibility*. Can both entrenched interests and public apathy be overcome? If a revolution succeeds, are the new leaders technically (and morally) competent to implement the "new order"? Another issue is *cost*. "You can't make an omelet without breaking eggs." The transition will inevitably disrupt the normal operation of life in that society. Many "innocent bystanders" will be hurt physically, materially, and/or psychologically.

The process involves risks. One is a *loss of freedom*. Radical change often meets heavy resistance. Some degree of coercive control is needed during a transition period to impose and consolidate the new system. This interim control may become permanent.

Another risk is *unplanned consequences*. In the best of circumstances, knowledge is incomplete and wisdom is defective. Every change creates economic, social, and/or cultural side effects. Small changes carry small risks. Big changes risk big mistakes. When radical changes are implemented by inexperienced leaders, the risks increase still more.

A third risk is *corruption*. The original noble goals of the change agents may be subverted by their own self-interests after they become the new "haves." For example, *The New York Times* observed that five years after the radical change from a command to a market economy, "Russians are angered by *new* economic inequities, including the windfall fortunes some of their countrymen made through the government's corrupt privatization program" (Editorial, 1996).

Given the costs and risks, why would anyone ever advocate radical change? The response is, "compared to what?" Fundamental changes may be necessary where untenable circumstances are so ingrained that adjustments simply won't do the job. Another argument for radical intervention is urgency: the existing situation is so harmful to so many people that we cannot afford the damage done while gradual reform takes its slow course. Of course, there is usually disagreement on what is "untenable" and how "urgent" the situation is.

Generally, the worse things are, the more attractive is radical change because there is less to lose and more to gain. "The proletarians have nothing to lose but their chains. They have a world to win." (Marx, 1848, in *Columbia Encyclopedia*, p. 435) Indeed, social radicals sometimes strategically oppose social reforms, lest the improved circumstances of "oppressed masses" make them reluctant to risk what they have in support of fundamental change.

Even "conservatives" favor some radical actions, such as the conversion of Eastern Europe from Marxism to capitalism and political democracy.

REFORM

We have seen that private enterprise is more efficient, innovative, and cost effective in providing goods and services. But the market, like seismic forces, is ethically blind. We don't expect morality from an earthquake.

Francis Underhill, 1996

The difference between radical change and moderate reform is *how far* it goes, *how fast*, and *how disruptive*. Reform means "to make better by correcting faults or defects." It tends to be problem oriented, following the medical model of diagnosis and treatment.

Whereas Marxist socialism was radical in its call for total system change, Britain's Fabian socialists were gradualist reformers. They took their name from Fabius Maximus, "the Delayer," the Roman general who defeated a far superior force under Hannibal by avoiding a pitched battle and instead wearing Hannibal's army down by attrition through selective small skirmishes. Fabians counseled *gradualism:* take a small step without disrupting the system, digest it, and evaluate the results before taking the next step.

When is reform not reform? When it does not "make better." While honest reformers believe that the change is for the better, there are also cynical "wolves in reform clothing." Supporters of 1996 welfare reform insisted that it was a correction of a discredited program. Critics agreed that "welfare as we know it" was unsatisfactory but feared that the reform replaced a bad program with a worse one, which mandated expulsion of families from even the meager allowance of AFDC if they failed to get a job within a set period of time, without taking steps to help them do so (education, vocational training, and initiatives to ensure that adequate jobs would be available).

Even the best of reforms will have articulate opponents who assert that it is not reform at all but rather subversion (undermining of existing good things) or regression (return to the bad old days). If you get into the reform business, you must be prepared to defend what you are correcting and how the reform makes it better.

RULES OF THE GAME

A popular reform method is to keep the basic system but to change the rules by which the game is played.

Professional football changes its rules periodically to make the game more attractive to the fans. When scoring was low, offensive linemen were allowed to more aggressively protect their quarterback. When scoring became too easy, pass defenders were given more latitude to bump receivers. The goal posts were moved forward ten yards to encourage field goals, and when these goals became too frequent, they were moved back again to discourage scoring. It's the same game, but each change affects strategies, scores, and styles of play.

Similarly, in social policy, rule changes affect the behavior of the players and sometimes the score. Rule changes may *further* already-established intents, *correct* ongoing faults, or *respond* to new problems.

Furthering Established Intents

According to Wilensky and Lebeaux (1965, p. 34), large and influential segments of the American people (not just businessmen) believe strongly that:

1. the individual should strive to be successful in competition with others, under the rules of the game;
2. these rules involve "fair play": (a) everyone should start with equal opportunity, and (b) no one should take unfair advantage through force, fraud, or "pull."

Because some people *do* try to take unfair advantage, we make rules and regulations to require fair play in such areas as financial transactions, labor standards, and consumer protection. Examples of social game referees are the Securities and Exchange Commission, the National Labor Relations Board, and the courts.

We periodically extend and update existing rules. In 1868, the Fourteenth Amendment guaranteed equal treatment "under the law." Originally it applied only to the legal system. The 1954 school desegregation decision updated it to include an array of public service programs established under the law that did not exist in 1868. Later this was extended to include private sector programs financed under the law through public grants, contracts, and/or tax welfare.

Rules of the game call for compensation for spillover costs or harms that befall "bystanders." This may kick in at any of the three stages of intervention. For example:

- A tertiary-level rule permits lawsuits for damages after the fact.
- A secondary-prevention rule mandates compensation when the damage occurs, such as requiring immediate reimbursement at

fair market value for private property confiscated to build an expressway.

- A primary-prevention rule requires an environmental impact study and approval *before* the development can be begun.

Equity law is a rule of the game safety net. It is defined as "(a) resort to general principles of fairness and justice whenever existing law is inadequate; (b) a system of rules and doctrines, as in the United States, supplementing common and statute law, and superseding such law when it proves inadequate for just settlements."

Responding to Change

Technology may create the need for adaptive policy reforms. The industrial revolution replaced small, diverse, personal employers with large, impersonal factories. The immense power advantage of the large-scale buyer of unskilled labor over individual sellers of that labor damaged the free labor market.

In contrast to Marxism's radical solution of replacing the market system with a central control economy, a reform response was the trade union movement, which attempted to restore parity between buyers and sellers of labor within the free-market system by collective bargaining, in which a single seller (the union) negotiated with a single buyer (the employer). The 1935 National Labor Relations Act set up "rules of the game" for collective bargaining. Since then, similar to the National Football League, the rules are changed periodically to maintain a proper balance (as viewed by the current rule makers) between employers and workers.

The rapid growth of communication satellites, portable cellular phones, and the information highway in the 1990s created a mini-crisis, in which we had to fumble for new rules to replace the obsolete "good old days" rules.

Growth by itself may create the need for new fair-play rules. In a once-quiet seaside community of 2,500 year-round residents, large resort-condominium developments led, at the height of the season, to chronic traffic gridlock and overflow sewage in the streets—and the summer population was projected to double again in the next decade. It seemed neither fair nor feasible for the mostly low-to-middle-income "natives" to foot most of the bill for the major capital investments required to meet the needs of these nonresident part-timers, so the city council enacted a new rule: impact fees were assigned to each new development equal to its projected share of the capital costs of widening roads, expanding the waterworks, and building a second waste treatment plant.

Correcting Inherent Faults

Rule changes are also made to correct faults in the original intent itself. A flaw in British "democracy" of the early 1800s was that it limited the vote to the upper classes. Thomas Carlyle, dismayed at the failure of Parliament to take into account the needs and interests of the working classes in the Reform Act of 1832, started the Chartist movement to gain them the vote. They finally got it a half century later, leading to their own political party and to policies more favorable to their interests.

It took longer to correct male-only democracy in the United States. In 1787, Abigail Adams urged her husband, John, to argue for women's rights, including the vote, at the original constitutional convention. He didn't. It took another 133 years, including nearly a century of work by women's suffrage movements, to correct this fault with the passage of the Nineteenth Amendment.

In each of these cases, the reforms did not update or extend an original intent: they changed it. The British power structure believed that only those who owned property should vote, and our Founding Fathers did not consider women competent to share in the government.

CHANGING AGENT BEHAVIOR

In the host-agent-environment model, some reform interventions are aimed at the environment itself; others seek to change the behavior of agents. Getting agents to do what you want is rarely a simple matter. Some variables that influence the effectiveness of this approach are the following:

- *Attitude* toward the behavior of those responsible to regulate or change it. Until MADD (Mothers Against Drunk Driving) got busy, police, prosecutors, and judges, many of whom drove after having "a few beers," tended to be indulgent toward drunk drivers.

- *Status of the agent.* Higher-status agents tend to be less compliant and to get away with more. While small-time thieves were serving prison terms, a leading brokerage firm that had defrauded millions from trusting associates and customers continued in business without prosecution.
- *Status of the hosts* whom the agent affects. The Environmental Protection Agency may be a bit more zealous on compliance with a company which pollutes the air in a Dallas suburb than one which does the same in a West Virginia mining town.
- *Agent's self-interest.* Unions have been more supportive of affirmative action when it is applied only to future hiring, without affecting the job security and seniority of any current member. Responses by health care providers to a possible policy change tend to coincide with its effect on their net revenue.

Coercion

An *external* approach to changing agents' behavior is coercion, "to effect by force, especially by legal authority."

The most extreme coercive measure is *eradication* of undesirable agents: exterminate mosquitoes, mass murderers, and terrorists; launch preemptive first strikes against security threats. A bit less extreme is to *block access* to the host: keep recidivist child molesters in indefinite protective custody; terminate parental rights of incorrigibly abusive parents.

Licensing is gentler coercion. Prevent undesirable agents by setting competence, performance, and ethical conditions for the privilege of engaging in certain endeavors, such as practicing a profession, offering day care, transporting travelers, or driving a car. If the agent is already in business, regulatory actions may be used to compel nonpollution, fair labor practices, pure food and drugs, or equal employment opportunity.

Coercion tends to be more effective in prohibiting clearly defined negative behavior than in motivating positive behaviors. If it is used, Theodore Caplow's tough advice to bosses may be worth considering:

What makes [a leader] feared is the reputation of acting decisively and ruthlessly. . . . The appropriate style is that punitive measures are imposed promptly and confidently, without any visible interest in the excuses of the offender. One or two harsh actions of this kind can make a leader more feared than a whole reign of terror conducted in a more capricious manner. The best policy to follow in developing a reputation for severity is to make all decisions . . . according to fixed principles announced in advance and applied so consistently that each application takes on a didactic character. (1976, pp. 10-11)

Gentle Persuasion

An *internalizing* approach is to persuade, "to cause someone to do something, especially by reasoning, urging, or inducement." The behavior of agents may be changed without coercion by appealing to emotions, values, relationships, facts, or logical argument. The Fabians called this approach *permeation*.

My varied experiences as a church social action leader, a federal poverty program planner, a corporate philanthropy consultant, and a university administrator suggest a common recipe for persuasion in any situation:

1. *Mutual respect.* Accept the "target" agents as honest and sincere despite issue differences. Conversely, earn credibility and respect by your behavior, value base, knowledge, and competence so that even if they disagree they trust you personally. Without these prerequisites, the opportunity to persuade rarely occurs.
2. *Rational argument.* People are seldom persuaded by rational argument, but at the same time, they are seldom open to change unless their rationales are understood. The key facts must be presented truthfully and accurately, whatever they may be, including those which may support the other side. Relate the target's own values and interests to the behavior sought. In the Church, I drew on biblical, creedal, and theological sources. In the government, I used economic cost-benefit analyses. In corporate philanthropy, I identified enlightened self-interest.

3. *An experiential element.* The previous two ingredients soften up the target (open a person to persuasion) but rarely change a person's feelings or social behaviors. When Wilbur Mills was chair of the House Ways and Means Committee, he listened intelligently to advocates for services to mentally retarded children but did not act. Then someone back home in Arkansas persuaded him to visit a state institution for retarded children, where he ended up holding and hugging them. The proposed program was funded soon afterward.

Incentives and Sanctions

A popular middle ground in social policy uses incentives (promised rewards) and sanctions (threatened punishment) that exert external pressure in the desired direction, while leaving some degree of free choice to the agent.

Incentives can be purely positive, such as tax deductions that encourage the wealthy to make generous charitable contributions. When the reward is needed or wanted enough, of course, incentives escalate to the level of an "offer you can't refuse." To receive federal grants, a university must practice gender equality. For my son, with a family to support and no money for tuition, it was, "If you join the Navy, we'll pay for medical school."

Many policies offer an explicit carrot-and-stick combination. Said Isaiah to Israel, "Come let us reason together, says the Lord. . . . If you are willing and obedient, you shall eat the good of the land; but if you refuse and rebel, you shall be devoured by the sword" (Isaiah 1:18-20). Environmental protection laws threaten polluters with fines should they continue to pollute but may offer direct or tax welfare subsidies to companies that cooperate.

The organized private sector may use incentives on agents too. When large California growers refused to bargain collectively with their farmworkers, many church, labor, and civil rights groups united in an effective consumer boycott of the growers' grapes and wine. Consequently, profits dropped. When the growers later agreed to bargain with the workers, they experienced their biggest ever consumption boom.

Incentives and sanctions are not always tangible. A common human need is the esteem of others. Public recognition and honor by religious bodies, United Ways, civic groups, and professional societies can stimulate a great deal of socially responsible behavior. Conversely, Senator William Proxmire's much-publicized "golden fleece awards" (for flagrant examples of fleecing the public) deterred many such notions by other federal officials and legislators.

Enhancement of Agents

A final method of affecting agents is simply to *help them.* Abusive parents may be dealt with coercively by separating them from their children or convicting and punishing them. For many, however, the most effective intervention may be helping them through counseling, therapy, and positive-parenting education.

Land-grant colleges of agriculture improve farming and conservation practices by providing education and technical assistance to already motivated future farmers. Similarly, an NIMH rural mental health grant to my program enabled us to do better what we were already committed to doing.

SUPPLEMENTING THE HOSTS

Another reform approach is to focus on the host rather than the agent or environment by providing compensatory benefits to offset the inherent omissions and deficiencies of the economic market system, without changing the system itself. This *social market* approach is discussed in Chapter 13.

SOCIAL POLICY AND THE COURTS

Theoretically, courts do not make social policy: they merely resolve disputes by finding the "true" intent and application of policies made by others. However, these decisions affect social policy in many ways:

- *Changing the operation of existing programs.* School segregation patterns were dramatically changed by a 1954 decision that separation based on race was inherently unequal.

- *Changing what is legal and illegal.* Abortion became legal and capital punishment became illegal for a period, because the Supreme Court found that existing laws didn't meet constitutional fairness tests.
- *Abolishing social programs.* In 1934 and 1935, much of Roosevelt's early New Deal was dismantled by a series of Supreme Court decisions that declared programs to aid farmers, businesses, and workers unconstitutional.

Wisdom and Politics: The Appointment of Judges

In theory, judges are selected exclusively for their ability to be wise and detached. They are given long-term, often lifetime, appointments to insulate them from political pressures and career temptations. A majority of judges work at being objective and fair according to their own perspectives. In practice, of course, they are products of their particular class and ethnic backgrounds, education, political affiliations, career and personal experiences, religious beliefs, and the prevailing social attitudes of their time and place in history.

All federal and many state judges are appointed by politicians, who naturally prefer judges who share their own ideologies and special interests. Roosevelt and Truman appointees moved the courts in social justice, pro-worker, and positive freedom directions. Eisenhower's "Warren Court" stressed negative freedom and civil liberties. Nixon and Reagan appointments redirected the courts back toward pre-Roosevelt positions on business and unions and pre-Eisenhower positions on civil liberty and civil rights.

Presidents Roosevelt and Reagan were particularly controversial in their attempts to change social policy through selective appointment of judges. After his 1934-1935 Supreme Court setbacks, Roosevelt, complaining about "nine old men" (appointed by his Republican predecessors), tried to "pack the court" by proposing a law that added a new justice to the Supreme Court for every one who was over age seventy. This would have given him six new appointees, enough to create a majority that leaned in his social policy direction. In the 1980s, President Reagan attempted to stack the court in the opposite direction through explicitly ideological choices.

Both were partially thwarted by Congress, which rejected Roosevelt's bill and Reagan's most extreme nominees. Even so, each still achieved long-term social policy reversals in the courts, through appointment of judges at all levels whose views coincided with their aims.

One way to change public social policy is to pass laws. Another is to control the administration of laws and programs through regulations and de facto practices. Obviously, a third way is to reinterpret laws and the Constitution through judicial appointments and test cases.

PART II:
FOUNDATIONS FOR CHOICE:
BELIEFS, VALUES, AND INTERESTS

Chapter 4

What's True? Facts and Beliefs

The man who is certain he is right is almost sure to be wrong and he has the additional misfortune of inevitably remaining so.

Michael Faraday, 1819

A tree's a tree. How many more do you need to look at?

Ronald Reagan

Journalist Gerald Johnson observed, "The past that influences our lives does not consist of what actually happened, but of what men believe happened" (Seldes, 1960, p. 715). To understand social policy, we must understand where those who make it or advocate it—including ourselves—are coming from in their beliefs, values, and ways of thinking:

- their *"facts"* about what is and why and assumptions about where various courses of action may lead,
- their *values* about what should be, and
- how they *process* their ideas.

BEING LOGICAL

Reason cannot save us and can even persecute us in the wrong hands; but we have no hope of salvation without reason.

Stephen Gould, 1991

Rational analysis involves *systematic reasoning* about *data,* guided by *logic.*

- *Reasoning* is "ability to think, form judgments, draw conclusions, etc."
- *Systematic* is "orderly, methodical."
- *Data* are "things known or assumed from which conclusions may be drawn."
- *Logic* is "the science of correct reasoning; valid induction and deduction." It starts with a *premise,* "a statement or assertion that serves as the basis for inferences."

Inductive and Deductive Thinking

Inference is "the process of deriving the strict logical consequences of assumed premises."

Inductive inferences abstract general conclusions from individual instances. An apple falling on his head may not have done the job alone, but Isaac Newton's law of gravity was inferred from many such observations. Diagnosis infers causes from examining results. For instance, observing that millions of lung cancer victims were also smokers and that relatively few nonsmokers became victims, clinicians inferred that smoking was a cause of cancer. Policymakers inductively generalize from specific cases. The base may be a single case, systematic analysis of many cases, experimental research, or millions of instances summarized in census reports and the like.

Deduction is "reasoning from the general to the specific, or from a premise to a logical conclusion." From an already-established general premise (which may be either an inductive conclusion from prior evidence or a before-the-fact a priori belief), deductive inferences derive specific standards and principles, which are applied to particular cases.

An old computer slogan is GIGO—"garbage in, garbage out." However faultless its circuitry, a computer can be only as accurate as its input (data and program). Deductive logic is a powerful tool for setting social policy directions, but as with the computer, it is only as good—or as bad—as its input (premises).

From his premises that (1) God controls everything and (2) there is a heaven and a hell, John Calvin deduced "predestination": God determines our destinations (heaven or hell) in advance. His Puritan descendants, deducing further that God would treat hell-bound persons badly in this life too, enacted social policies of harsh treatment for the (literally) damned poor.

Deists, from their premise of a benevolent, orderly Creator, deduced natural laws and natural rights, including "life, liberty, and the pursuit of happiness," and applied them to the civil liberty provisions of the Bill of Rights.

In their 1986 "Pastoral Letter on Catholic Social Teaching and the U.S. Economy," American bishops started with a premise, "We believe the person is sacred, the clearest expression of God among us." From this, they deduced a succession of progressively more specific inferences:

1. Human rights are the minimum conditions for life in community.
2. Society as a whole, acting through public and private institutions, has the moral responsibility to enhance human dignity and protect human rights.
3. These moral principles give an overview of the moral vision of economic life [which] must be translated into concrete measures. Our pastoral letter spells out some specific applications of Catholic moral principles . . . full employment . . . eradicate poverty . . . halt the loss of family farms . . . relieve the plight of poor nations . . . reaffirm rights of workers, collective bargaining, private property, subsidiarity, and equal opportunity. (National Conference of Catholic Bishops, 1986, pp. xi-xii)

In this book, we will continually go back and forth between abstract (general) and derivative (specific, applied) principles, as we seek to understand the basis for social policy choices and the implications of implementing them. In this process, a useful approach for moving from a social problem to a social policy might be adapted from the traditional homiletics model of preaching from a biblical text:

1. *Exegesis.* Start with the specific. Where did it come from? What did/does it mean in its particular context?

2. *Exposition.* Generalize from it (induction). What are its broader implications that transcend the original time, place, and incident?
3. *Application.* Return to specifics (deduction). What do these broader implications mean to us here and now? How do they affect our decisions and courses of action in this specific policy area?

Potential Errors

Social policy analysis has been susceptible to several errors in reasoning. One is to generalize from *inaccurate or incomplete data.* As noted in Chapter 2, President Hoover, a world-renowned humanitarian, ignored the plight of his own people because he never really knew how badly off they were.

A related error is for inductive conclusions to *exceed the data.* Herbert Spencer advocated a policy known as Social Darwinism that "the unfit must be eliminated as nature intended, for the principle of natural selection must not be violated by the artificial preservation of those least able to take care of themselves" (quoted in Trattner, 1994, pp. 90-91). Darwin's data related to genetic variables in different environments. They provided no empirical basis for generalizing to Victorian English society, in which the key variables were economic, social, and political, not genetic.

Another common problem is to *confuse a priori premises with empirical data.* President Hoover's economic policy responses to the Great Depression were ineffective in part because he thought the abstract closed-system, free-market model of classical economics was the real world, when in fact it had been undermined by corruption and fraud, nonproductive speculation, monopolistic practices, wars, and international mercantilism.

A reverse problem is *confusing empirical data with a priori values.* This often takes the form of "what is equals what should be." In medicine, some argue that the *fact* of technological ability to prolong physical life infers a blanket ethical obligation to do so in all cases. The fact itself does not. Such a conclusion requires two a priori premises that (1) put a supreme value on life and (2) define life exclusively as biological survival. If you change the second premise to define life holistically in relation to body, mind, and spirit, as most religions do, the technology becomes a resource to be employed selectively, with wisdom and compassion, to optimize full life. If you substitute an economic cost-benefit value for the first one, expensive new technology should *not* be used unless the patient will be economically productive after the treatment.

In making a policy choice, we properly draw upon both empirical data and a priori beliefs/values in a conscious, self-disciplined manner. Confusion between the two has often led to bad policy.

SCIENTIFIC AND NONSCIENTIFIC REASONING

The Scientific Method

Rational analysis is closely associated with *science*, "systematized knowledge of nature and the physical world derived from observation, study, and experimentation." The scientific method tests inferences about facts. Its general procedure is as follows:

1. Observe specific cases.
2. Infer theory from experience and observation (inductive).
3. From the theory, develop a hypothesis that predicts future specific cases (deductive).
4. Test the hypothesis by observing those cases, and compare the results observed with those predicted.
5. Revise the theory based on this new information, affirming and extending it where predictions were accurate and revising it where they were inaccurate (inductive).
6. Repeat steps 3 through 5 indefinitely to further refine and extend theory and application.

Assets and Pitfalls of the Scientific Method

Science is imperfect at best. However extensive and well-analyzed, gaps and distortions remain. Not all relevant information is available. From what is available, we necessarily slant our selection according to what we believe to be most important, our degree of comfort with the information, and how much we can afford to do. An important limitation on science for social policy purposes is its restriction to what can be measured and quantified. This automatically "deselects" everything else.

Science writer Stephen Gould (1991) warns:

> We have, on the one hand, "hard," or physical sciences that deal in numerical precision, prediction, and experiment. On the other hand, "soft" sciences that treat the complex objects of history in all their richness must trade these virtues for "mere" description without firm numbers in a confusing world where, at best, we can hope to explain what we cannot predict. (p. 496)

Another limitation is what Nobel physicist Werner Heisenberg called the Uncertainty Principle. It is impossible to measure precisely because the very act of collecting data always changes what you are trying to study. His insight came from studying electrons. A simpler physics illustration: "attempting to measure the temperature of hot water in a pot on the stove, the very insertion of a thermometer into the water changes the temperature—not by much, of course, but by enough to preclude exactitude" (Brennan, 1997, p. 164). If this is so for physics, how much more are social facts affected by studying them? Think of anthropologists living with primitive tribes.

In the process of assessing health needs, a survey changed what it was studying. Asking one set of questions about health problems and another about their use of available health care resources created new awareness ("felt need") and utilization of resources ("demand").

A common error is *pseudo* ("false, pretended") science. This scientific counterpart to dogmatic religion is easily spotted when practiced by charlatans. Its real danger comes from scientific and technical professionals who claim a level of accuracy and validity beyond the limits of their sources, models, and methods. Fallibility is unavoidable. "If a little knowledge is dangerous, where is the man who has so much as to be out of danger?" (Thomas Huxley).

For all its flaws, the empirical scientific method often gives us the best information available. Two simple practices will increase its value and lessen the pitfalls: One is to be open about its limits. The second is to check it against our intuition. William James asserted, "One has the right to reject a theory apparently confirmed by a very considerable number of objective facts solely because it does not respond to our interior preferences" (quoted in Lewis, 1991, p. 289).

I won't go quite that far. If scientific and intuitive conclusions differ, reexamine *both*.

Intuition

Not all good thinking is scientific and analytical. Many of the most important elements related to social policy are *intangible*, "not easily defined or formulated." We need perspective—how things fit together in the larger picture. We must make decisions based on limited, incomplete evidence, which is often fragmented and inconclusive. This calls for some nonscientific intellectual skills, such as the following:

- *Sensibility:* "keen intellectual perception; the capacity to respond intelligently and perceptively to intellectual, moral, aesthetic, or psychological events or values."
- *Insight:* "the faculty of seeing into inner character or underlying truth; the sudden grasping of a solution; configurational learning."
- *Intuition:* (from the Latin "to look at") "immediate knowing or learning of something without the conscious use of reasoning."
- *Considered judgment:* "experience-based insight."

Max Weber (1904) expressed a common attitude toward intuition: "The voluminous talk about intuition does nothing but conceal a lack of perspective toward the object." Ironically, Weber's own greatness was rooted in extraordinary intuition that he subsequently sought to document.

We are not exactly sure how intuition works. One view is that it is simply a faster-than-average rational analysis. A veteran policy/administration practitioner, accustomed to sizing up complex situations on several levels at once, making strategic decisions, and quickly elaborating a detailed course of action, moved into academia. In his first annual evaluation, his department chair faulted him for being "off the wall" in faculty meetings, coming in "over there" when the group was discussing "over here." The new professor responded, "In every case when asked, didn't I give you a logical step by step progression from 'here' A to 'there' G through steps B, C, D, E, and F?" The chair grudgingly admitted this was so.

In this vein, some say that intuition is *subconscious* rational analysis. We learn concepts and apply them self-consciously, adapting them to a wide variety of different cases. Gradually we assimilate all of this into our own customized "memory files," called "crystallized intelligence," and perform the process intuitively. (It is prudent to check the soundness of our intuition by periodically reconstructing it in a formal rational analytic format.)

The aforementioned professor was not quite honest with his linear-minded department chair. He had in fact been making intuitive jumps, which he skillfully *rationalized* ("to explain in a rationalistic manner") after the fact. This illustrates a different intuitive process called "right-brained" thinking, with holistic flashes of insight. Creative artists have this. A friend calls it "a glimpse." My wife, who meditates, calls it "visualizing." Whatever its nature, Einstein had it. So did Newton. So do many top administrators.

> There is a curious natural law in business that places a premium on managerial imagination—The Bigger the Problem, the Fewer the Facts. This law manifests itself in the necessary paradox of "scientific foreman and intuitive president." Many problems at the supervisor's level can be quantified, analyzed, and optimized down to the last few percent. . . . But most problems at the president's level involve such intangibles that any decision at all takes courage. (Mills, 1959, p. 1)

Intuition is scoffed at in some circles. Use it anyway, but learn to be "bilingual." Translate your insights into the language of your audience. Artists have their mind's picture, which they translate into pigments on a canvas. Skilled intuitive thinkers copy their mind's picture with analytic pigments onto a rationalistic canvas.

THREE SOURCES OF "FACTS"

In *Dragnet*, Sergeant Joe Friday used to say, "Just the facts, ma'am, just the facts." It's not that simple in real life.

In court, legal "facts" are whatever the jury thinks they are, which may or may not coincide with the actual truth. The facts that influence social policy are what each actor thinks they are. These facts may come from several sources: a priori beliefs, direct experience, and/or collected empirical data.

A Priori Beliefs: I Already Know

Stage hypnotists may tell their subjects that the next thing that touches them will be very hot. When touched with a cool object, the subjects react as if to a burn.

A priori means "prior to, and furnishing the basis of, experience." This includes perceptions about reality that color how we see the world. For example, I have three pairs of sunglasses, tinted green, blue gray, and yellow. The yellow pair is great on gloomy days because it makes them look sunny. The green pair is nice for driving, cutting the glare without diminishing the color of the trees and grass. The blue gray pair deepens the color of the ocean and sky on a too-bright beach day. They have other effects as well. The blue gray dulls the greenery and makes an ordinary day look like the Bronx in winter. The green destroys the azure of tropical sky and sea. The yellow obscures beautiful color contrasts. Perhaps I should get a fourth pair. They say rose-colored glasses make *everything* look good!

The problem is that because they are by definition before the fact a priori beliefs are inherently vulnerable to the fallibility of those who hold them. A seven-year-old ghetto child is reading poorly. Three people look at this fact: One sees genetic inferiority. Another sees a "culture of poverty." A third sees institutionalized racism. The teacher sees faulty parenting. The parents see faulty teaching. It reminds me of an old Fred Astaire–Ginger Rogers song, in which they go through a series of "you say . . . and I say" and conclude, "Let's call the whole thing off." (They don't, of course.)

Some a priori beliefs may be purely right. John Knox, founder of Presbyterianism, thought so when he asserted, "A man with God is always in the majority." The United States was founded on "self-evident" truths about our having been created equal with inherent rights. On the other hand, a priori "facts" have also justified slavery, subjugation of women, racism, terrorism, genocide, and blaming the victim.

To understand a social policy, we need to find out, and evaluate, the facts on which it is based. Some facts can be tested empirically.

If they are accurate, you should be able to predict future occurrences. Similarly, if your facts about causes (diagnoses) are correct, a treatment plan based on them should change future occurrences in a predictable way. If your predictions turn out to be incorrect, maybe your facts need to be reexamined. Unfortunately, however, even overwhelming empirical evidence may not convince a priori "true believers." Ask Galileo!

On the other hand, many beliefs, especially about values, are inherently beyond scientific proof or disproof and cannot be reliably measured by any objective criterion. A somewhat cynical rule of thumb for judging their credibility is the extent to which they conveniently coincide with the self-interest of the holder. Those which do may still be true but should be taken with an extra grain of salt.

Projection: My Own Experience Is Universal

A second major source of "facts" is projection from personal experience. We often generalize to the world from our limited personal experiences. This is exacerbated to the extent that a priori preconceptions have selected, slanted, and colored how we absorbed even that narrow information.

A look at recent history suggests that American presidents may have projected facts about poverty from their own personal experiences. Is it pure coincidence that at least three twentieth-century presidents from "humble origins" (Hoover, Nixon, Reagan) ignored the plight of the poor and blamed them for their condition? Did these self-made millionaires, proud of having risen from "poverty" by ambition and perseverance, generalize that anyone with gumption can do the same? (Note: their humble families *did* send them to private colleges.) Interestingly, a fourth president from humble origins (Truman), who did not get sent to college nor amass a fortune, gained a reputation as a champion of working people and civil rights.

Empirical Data: What Can We Find Out?

An antidote to the dangers of the first two kinds of truth is empirical data. Most professionals are more comfortable basing their beliefs about reality on objective facts, that is, systematically collected and processed *scientific* and *technical* data. As already discussed, the value of this source is immense—but also limited and flawed.

The limitations of objective facts can be hedged by using multiple sources. These can be as diverse as eyewitness reports, anecdotal accounts, newspaper articles, magazine features, census and other collected statistics, literature, biography, historical accounts, philosophical and ethical inquiries, clients' feelings, direct observation, and professional lore. All of these sources are selective and biased too, but generally the broader the foundation, the more stable the house.

Still, there is no guarantee that pooling the data will create an accurate picture. Neither can we be sure that by mixing colors we will achieve the rainbow. Comedian Allen Sherman, recalling the rinse water for his paintbrushes in school, described a committee as a place where everyone puts in a different color and it comes out gray.

Use Them All

Each type of source has its merits and its limitations. For social policy purposes, our best shot is to test all three against one another. How do objective facts compare with our a priori beliefs about human nature, society, and the world? How do both of these gibe with personal experiences? If all three don't come together, we explore further to figure out why the discrepancies exist and how to reconcile them.

The result is a hybrid truth that blends scientific and other evidence with common sense and intuitive insights. We do not accept what our leaders or opponents tell us on their authority alone. We test them against our imperfect but best available truth, with an important qualification—the humility to stand corrected when we encounter new insights or information.

BIASES AND HERMENEUTICS

Interests which we bring with us, and simply posit or take our stand upon, are the very flour out of which our mental dough is kneaded. Not a cognition occurs but feeling is there to comment upon it, to stamp it as of greater or lesser worth.

William James
Quoted in Lewis, 1991

How do we deal with the dilemma that all sources of information, including our own observations, are slanted, by a priori selective perception, perceived self-interest, what we think is important (as in a traditional focus of history on wars and upper-class male politics), and our degree of comfort with the information? A useful tool for handling these dilemmas is *hermeneutics*, "the science of interpretation."

Hermeneutics (named after Hermes, the Greek god who carried messages) emerged from the fields of art, literature, history, and Biblical scholarship, where scholars make their reputations by finding the "real" meanings in Shakespeare, Genesis, or Van Gogh. The outstanding thinker on this subject is Hans Georg Gadamer (1975). Hermeneutics seeks to correct the Age of Enlightenment delusion of objectivity, that one can know truth through pure reason that transcends individual bias or our cumulative cultural heritage.

At the same time, it avoids the opposite error of not generalizing at all. Eighteenth-century *classical empiricists* such as George Berkeley and David Hume believed that the only real knowledge is one's own subjective, sensory perceptions. We can't generalize reliably from these to the wider world. Relativists also reject generalizations because "it all depends," varying with the individual, time, and circumstances.

The synthesis: understanding is always *co-determined* by the subject (text, policy, circumstances, conditions) and the interpreter. Every interpreter, looking from a particular *vantage point*, will miss or ignore some of what is there and read into it some things that are not there. Tennyson saw a small flower poking out of a crack in a crannied wall and was moved to philosophical contemplation on the meaning of life. I would have passed it with the thought, "nice posy." If you are an amateur artist, you know that you can paint the same view ten times and produce ten pictures, each true to the view and yet each quite different.

If we are to understand the people we are working for, we have to discover *their* vantage points—what they believe and why, how they think, what they see and don't see, the tint of their lenses, what they care for most on both concrete and symbolic levels, what turns them off or on—in short, the world as *they* see it and want it to be. Too often those in power, even well-meaning ones, impose their particular vantage point on others "for their own good." Charity organization social workers did this to nineteenth-century immigrants, and sectarian activists today try to do it to our children by restricting content in public school textbooks to their particular vantage points.

To be effective in our social policy action, we need to study the vantage points of our allies, our opponents, and the "silent majority." Only then can we develop strategies to persuade, mobilize, convert, neutralize, or overcome them, as the case may be.

The following is a checklist of reference subjects that contribute to vantage points:

- Sociocultural background
- Demographic identification: gender, ethnicity, generation
- Relationship networks: family, friends, neighbors, co-workers
- Role models: mentors, parents, successful public figures
- Sources of ego affirmation: peers, family, higher status groups
- Occupational and professional socialization
- Information sources: their accuracy, completeness, slants, gaps
- Personal vested interests: career, financial, social, ego

Finally, we need to know our own vantage points. To be true to yourself, you must first know who you are and where you are coming from. If you are true to yourself, you can act with greater confidence and integrity, and you are less vulnerable to manipulations by those who would subvert—or divert—you. This is particularly important in the area of values and interests, as will be discussed in the next chapter.

The objective is not to become free from preconceptions. That is impossible. Says Gadamer (1975, p. 239), "The really critical question of hermeneutics is to separate true prejudices by which we understand from the false ones by which we misunderstand."

Chapter 5

What's Right?
Values and Interests

Strong convictions precede great actions.

Anonymous

I know your conscience always interferes except where your interest is concerned.

King George IV
to Lord Chancellor Eldon, 1820

VALUES

A value is an a priori belief about what is good, right, or desirable. Values are often rooted in beliefs about religion, natural law, and human rights: "We hold these truths to be self-evident . . . " They are installed by our culture of origin into our mental "programs" and subsequently customized through our particular experiences and circumstances. As the ultimate criteria for defining well-being and harm, gains and losses, benefits and costs, values have an overwhelming effect on policy.

You can analyze values rationally to be clear what they are. You can know where they came from by tracing them back step by step to a first premise. You can evaluate the consistency of an applied value with its professed premise. You can freely criticize other people's values against the standard of your own a priori beliefs. You can debate the merits of conflicting values. You can change them.

What you *can't* do is prove or disprove them empirically, for science can measure only that which is a physical substance. There may be an Absolute Truth. Some claim to possess it. (They don't.) Others say there is no such thing. Paul of Tarsus offered a middle ground. He claimed to be a carrier of "the light of knowledge . . . *but we have this treasure in jars of clay*" (II Corinthians 4:6-7, emphasis added).

We can create a fairly good working model of Truth and Good for our purposes by examining values with *bold humility*. The humility reminds us that we are only clay pots. G. K. Chesterton said, "Angels can fly because they take themselves lightly." The boldness enables us to go with the best treasure we have come up with so far. Whatever its deficiencies, it is better than blind groping, drawing straws, or cynical self-serving.

INTERESTS

What is "welfare" for some groups may be "illfare" for others.

Richard Titmuss, 1958

In finance, interest is the amount gained from lending money. More broadly, an interest is any gain or other advantage for a particular individual, organization, or collective group. All policies promote somebody's interest (and usually also harm someone else's interest, directly or as a side effect):

- The *public* interest is whatever is to the advantage or benefit of the society as a whole and of its individual members.
- *Private* interests favor a particular individual, organization, or group.
- A *vested* interest is an advantage already possessed, which the holders want to preserve and increase.
- *Self*-interest is "regard for one's own advantage or profit." Predators do so without regard to consequences for anyone else. *Enlightened* self-interest enhances one's actual long-run self-interest in a way which also benefits others.
- *Disinterest* is freedom from self-interest. *Altruists* have this quality. Judges should.

There are *perceived* interests (what we think is best for us) and *actual* interests (what is really best for us). What I want for dinner is steak and fries, but my doctor says beans and rice are actually in my best interest.

Paternalists believe that they know better than we what is best for us. Did your mother or father ever say "I'm only doing this for your own good"? (Sometimes they were even right, darn it!) This is the sincere view of the religious right and of various secular ideologists. Skeptics question both the wisdom and the altruism of those who presume to make such claims. At the other end of the continuum, libertarians stress self-determination based on one's own perceived interests, however wise or foolish they may be.

As we pursue policy choices, we need to identify the perceived interests of all stakeholders and key actors, discover to the best of our ability what is in their actual best interests, and give careful thought to how the differences can and should be handled. Then go with the best we know, in bold humility.

VALUES AND INTERESTS ENTWINED

Every society must produce an ideology which legitimates its inequities and thereby persuades those at the bottom to accept, and even reverse, their own inferiority.

Michael Harrington, 1980

Values and interests are so closely entwined as to be virtually inseparable. Values define *which* interests are more important. In your financial planning, you may have to decide between professional education or the down payment for a house. As a worker, is income, security, or intrinsic satisfaction more important? As a managed care administrator, do you value health or profits more?

Values guide decisions on *whose* interests take preference—Corporate stockholders or the people who work for them? Children or senior citizens? Suburban commuters or inner-city bus riders?

Interests influence value choices, sometimes consciously, sometimes unwittingly. This is illustrated in the long-running debate on whether the United States should ensure adequate health care for all citizens. Those who identify with the interests of 40,000,000 citizens who lack adequate health care cite such traditional values of our society as the worth of each individual and our common bonds as Americans. Those who identify with the interests of 40,000,000 citizens with above-average taxable incomes who already have excellent private health coverage stress another set of traditional American values related to individualism and economic freedom.

Saul Alinsky described the interaction of interests and values this way:

> The purpose of the Haves is to keep what they have. Therefore, the Haves want to maintain the status quo and the Have-Nots to change it. The Haves develop their own morality to justify their means of repression and all other means employed to maintain the status quo. The Haves usually establish laws and judges devoted to maintaining the status quo.
>
> Since any effective means of changing the status quo are usually illegal and/or unethical in the eyes of the establishment, Have-Nots, from the beginning of time, have been compelled to appeal to "a law higher than man-made law." Then, when the Have-Nots achieve success and become the Haves, they are in the position of trying to keep what they have, and their morality shifts with their change of location in the power pattern. Eight months after securing independence, the Indian national Congress outlawed passive resistance and made it a crime. (1972, pp. 42-43)

Much of the time, the impact of interests and values is obvious. Would you expect anyone to hire a trial lawyer who did *not* selectively slant everything possible, including values, toward the client's interest? As a consultant on philanthropy to a Fortune 500 company some years ago, I related every recommendation explicitly to enlightened self-interest. Self-interest was up-front in that commercial enterprise. You have to look for it more carefully when it is cloaked in hypocrisy—and even more so when it is denied by the good folk in self-righteous professions who deceive themselves.

Knowing what key actors' value-interests are and where they come from does not tell you whether they are right or wrong. However, knowing "where it's at" helps you make better choices and develop wiser strategies. Your chances for policy success are greatest when you can devise a proposal that appeals to the actors' altruistic expressed values and coincides with their enlightened self-interest. After forty years of squelching every major health plan, the physician lobby in 1965 accepted Medicare because (1) it was needed by deserving, suffering older people, and (2) it increased doctors' incomes.

Conflicting Value-Interests

It is rare not to have conflicts among values. Even as individuals we have internal value conflicts. I asked a friend of mine the other day why he looked so glum. He replied, "Last night I had an argument with myself—and I lost."

The most common source of conflicts is genuine competition among interests. You can't maximize all interests at once. In any policy choice, some will fare better than others.

There are also genuine value differences. My father-in-law, a Southern preacher whose father had been an alcoholic, was opposed to all drinking. He once quoted to me, "Wine is a mocker, strong drink a brawler; and whoever is led astray by it is not wise" (Proverbs 20:1). I saw no problem with moderate drinking and counter-quoted, "Use a little wine for the sake of your stomach," (I Timothy 5:23) and of course, the story of Jesus providing more than 100 gallons of wine for a wedding feast (John 2:1-12). This led us to a genuine social policy difference: he was for prohibition; I was for regulation.

A major source of value conflicts is tension between *substantive* values related to *outcomes* (reparation for damages, a generous supply of electricity, a secure old age, healthy babies) and *procedural* values related to how an outcome is pursued (due process in a lawsuit, nuclear power, mandatory pension deductions, free universal obstetric and pediatric care). This will be discussed further later in the chapter.

Finally we encounter a cluster of inconsistencies that cloud the picture. One is the discrepancy between what people *profess* and what they *practice*. The sources of this can be self-deception, hypocrisy, or a cynical con job, such as the one revealed by internal tobacco company papers in regard to promoting teenage smoking. So how do we sort out the real value-interest? My rule of thumb: "I can't hear what you are saying because what you are doing is shouting so loud."

A second common inconsistency is the us/them *double standards*, which will be discussed in Chapter 6.

A third is *compartmentalization*. The same person who is genuinely kind and caring in private life may have a very different value system at work. Historian Eugene Golob reported:

> The [Victorian] industrialist who worshipped gravely with his family on Sunday, contributed generously to charity, and condemned slavery was the man who spent his work in a single-minded search for profits and paid his workers little enough to make them objects of charity. . . . Nor was the hard-driving businessman a conscious hypocrite. The ideology of economic liberalism divorced economics from Christian ethics, and he could conveniently feel as righteous in his workday ethics as in his sober devotions on the Sabbath. (1954, p. 20)

It continues to be normal in such fields of endeavor as law, politics, and business. Alas, having been both a national church executive and a university administrator at various times in my checkered past, I can testify that compartmentalization is no stranger to those areas either.

Transcendent and Subordinate Value-Interests

When I was a young newlywed, my wife came home with a new hat and asked what I thought of it. I answered with painful honesty. She cried. I felt confused. Wasn't I supposed to be truthful? From this momentous occasion, I learned that in a given situation, one value (truthfulness) may conflict with another (kindness). How do we choose? By developing, consciously or not, a hierarchy of values in which one takes priority over another. (I learned quickly!)

Transcendent means "superior or supreme." Transcendent values and interests take precedence over *subordinate* ones, which we continue to follow to the extent that they are compatible with the higher one.

A transcendent value can be narrowly specific or broad. For both a national antiabortion organization staff member, interviewed by

Judith Hennessee in *Mademoiselle* (1986, p. 261), and her spiritual leaders "right to life" was supreme. However, the similarity ended there. Her value was restricted to life before birth. She did not advocate public policies to meet the special health, education, and welfare needs of fetuses after they were born, and she defended terrorist clinic bombings on the grounds of extenuating circumstances:

> I am not ready to spend the next twenty years in prison. But I don't condemn those who did. . . . But isn't this terrorism? What is the difference between bombing a clinic and blowing up U.S. Marines in Beirut? . . . They weren't killing [unborn] babies.

In contrast, the National Conference of Catholic Bishops (1986) defined their transcendent right-to-life value broadly. With the exception of a "just war," they opposed all taking of human life, from conception to natural death, including abortion, capital punishment, terrorism, euthanasia, and nuclear war. Further, their right-to-life value extended beyond biological survival to the economic, physical, emotional, and spiritual quality of those lives as well.

Value conflicts are not necessarily just between two values. There can be several levels. Although supporting law and order and opposing violence under normal circumstances, our Founding Fathers justified violent rebellion (the War of Independence) in defense of a transcendent value, human rights.

> Prudence, indeed, will dictate that Governments long established should not be changed for light and transient Causes. . . . But when a long Train of Abuses and Usurpations . . . evinces a Design to reduce them under absolute Despotism, it is their Right, it is their Duty, to throw off such Government . . . .They too have been deaf to the Voice of Justice. We must, therefore, acquiesce in the *Necessity* . . . [to] hold them . . . Enemies in War. (Declaration of Independence, emphasis added)

Martin Luther King agreed with Jefferson that human rights transcended loyalty to a legal authority that acted unjustly. But at this point he parted company, insisting that the resistance must be nonviolent and without malice. Why? Because of his religious values. Jesus said, "You have heard that it was said, 'You shall love your neighbor and hate your enemy.' But I say to you, Love your enemies and pray for those who persecute you" (Matthew, 5:43-44).

On a strict hierarchy of values basis, King's value of justice would have been subordinate to his value of love. But it needn't be just a matter of one value—interest superseding another as an either/or proposition. Our aim is to maximize all subordinate values to the fullest extent compatible with the transcendent one. The ideal is to find a "third way" in which all values may be salvaged, a win-win solution in which all interests come out ahead.

King found one that fully maintained both his nonviolence and his freedom/rights values: nonviolent civil disobedience. It took much more discipline to endure one-sided violence without either withdrawing or retaliating, but it worked.

As we look back, civil rights activists who used violence tended to further polarize the conflict and alienate "moderates." King's people, on the other hand, won the respect and attention of millions of white, middle Americans who were appalled at the actions of his persecutors. The results, while short of his "I have a dream" goals, were significant steps forward in voting, employment, public facilities, education, "community," and "brotherhood" compared to what had gone before.

This effort to maximize all values and interests, even subordinate ones, is called *optimizing*. It is the ideal of mediation and of much social policy.

Where full optimizing can't be achieved, it may still be possible to compromise for a lesser violation of the subordinate value or interest. In a class of social work students, all initially affirmed a powerful value against violence and killing. On probing, however, we discovered that every mother in the room would kill, if necessary, for a transcendent value—to save her children. For millions of Americans, the implication of this is to carry a handgun and shoot to kill. However, these women preferred the least violence necessary. Although willing to go as far as necessary, they entered into a lively sharing of effective nonlethal violent techniques, including martial arts, police techniques, dirty fighting moves, and pepper sprays.

A policy illustration: you have a transcendent value of adequate health care for all and a subordinate interest against increased taxes. By developing a universal health care system that is more cost-effective than the existing nonuniversal one, you minimize any tax increase (see Chapters 17 and 18).

Relativist Ideologies

Relativism as an ideology is "the theory of ethics of knowledge which maintains that the basis of judgment is relative, differing according to events, persons, etc."

Pluralism holds that no single universal truth exists. Said Henry David Thoreau, "If a man does not keep pace with his companions, perhaps it is because he hears a different drummer. Let him step to the music which he hears, however measured or far away" (1854, p. 345).

Classical empiricism carries this further, holding that the only reality is each individual's direct experience. *Nihilism* is the most extreme: it "denies the existence of any basis for knowledge or truth."

Skepticism believes "that the truth of all knowledge must always be in question and that all inquiry must be a process of doubting." John Stuart Mill (1859, p. 817) expressed it this way: "Mankind are not infallible . . . their truths for the most part are only half-truths . . . diversity [is] not an evil but a good until mankind are much more capable than at present of recognizing all sides of the truth."

Cynicism is "questioning the sincerity and goodness of people's motives; belief that people are motivated entirely by selfishness." Obviously, if this is so, any claim to highfalutin values is a con job.

ETHICS: ENDS AND MEANS

In the actions of men . . . the end justifies the means. Let a prince therefore aim at conquering and maintaining the state, and the means will always be judged honorable and praised by everyone, for the vulgar are always taken by appearances and the issue of the event.

Machiavelli, 1537

People who assert that the end justifies the means should keep in mind the limits of this rule by the rather simple truism, "except those means which undermine the goal itself."

Peter Lavrov
(Quoted in Golob, 1954)

Substantive versus Procedural Values

Substantive values relate to *ends*. Ends are about outcomes. In a proposed health care policy, who is covered? Is it only employees and their families? Selected population categories based on demographics, such as age, income, gender, geographic location? All citizens? All legal residents? All persons taken ill within the country, including visitors and illegal immigrants? What is covered? Acute conditions only? Primary and secondary prevention? Chronic care? "Heroic" efforts where there is little chance of recovery?

Procedural values relate to *means,* or how things are done. Given the goal of universal health services, should they be directly administered as in Britain or purchased from the private sector by a single public insurance program as in Canada? Should they be paid for by payroll taxes, general tax subsidies, patient co-insurance, or a combination? Should patients have free choice of physician and hospitals system or be required to join a prepaid managed care program?

Some major procedural areas are:

- the relative priority given to self-determination;
- how decisions get made: free market, collective bargaining, majority rule, consensus, direct exercise of power, technical analysis, elite experts, divine revelation, judicial due process, trial by combat; and
- how an end is achieved.

If a substantive end can be achieved by an accepted procedural means, there is no conflict. When neither of the countervalues is extremely strong, we can compromise each a bit. Even when it looks as if they are incompatible, there may be a creative alternative, such as King's nonviolent civil disobedience, which satisfied his values on both ends and means.

Does the End Justify the Means?

The tough question is how to balance substantive ends and procedural means when they do conflict. Does the end justify the means? The answers are yes, no, maybe, and who cares.

Yes, the end justifies the means. Terrorists, whether Palestinian, Irish, or American bombers, represent a sincere if frightening extreme. However, this also applies to less radical circumstances, as the otherwise antiviolence mothers in my class agreed when it came to protecting their children.

In the Iran-Contra Affair, White House officials sworn to uphold the Constitution, sold arms to declared enemies, misappropriated public funds for illegal purposes, flouted Congressional law, and then lied to Congress about their actions. There was no sense of guilt or remorse. They argued that national security ends took precedence over constitutional means. Acknowledging a series of illegal actions, one of them proudly called his criminal indictment "a badge of honor," claimed divine sanction, and ran for the Senate on this record.

No end can justify a wrong means. Certain principles are absolute and cannot be violated regardless of the end. Martin Luther King's movement rejected violence as a means no matter what the other side did. Somewhat less nobly, classical economists are so committed to the free-market process that the by-product effects on other fellow humans of inequality and deprivation are an acceptable "cost."

It all depends, say pragmatists. All things being equal, never use a bad means to promote a good end if it is reasonably avoidable. Such an approach is justified only when *all* of the following conditions apply:

- *The end is important enough* to warrant extraordinary means— not just any good purpose.
- *There is no available alternative* means that is less harmful or more ethical. It's "kaput" unless you use this bad means.
- *The cost does not exceed the benefit.* Will the long-term societal costs of a higher dropout rate due to a new "get tough" expulsion policy in a high school exceed the benefit of reducing disciplinary problems in the classroom?
- *The means do not subvert the end itself.* Can revolutionaries who overthrow an oppressor avoid becoming repressive themselves to stay in power against their defeated opponents? Can a bigger parent, by hitting/spanking his or her child, teach the child not to hit smaller kids?

Who cares? An *amoral* ("not concerned with moral standards") response is, "Hey, what's the big deal?"

> The *end* is what you want, and the *means* is how you get it. . . . The man of action views the issue of means and ends in pragmatic and strategic terms. He has no other problem; he thinks only of his actual resources and the possibilities of various choices of action. He asks of ends only whether they are achievable and worth the cost; of means, only whether they will work. (Alinsky, 1972, p. 24)

ETHICS: GRAY AREAS

There are few pure choices in real life situations. Legitimate interests and values are generally in conflict. No absolute resolution appears possible. In addition, choices are also influenced by each party's perceived facts about circumstances and expected consequences of alternative courses of action.

Proportionality

A traditional Catholic gray area principle is *proportionality*, a sort of moral cost-benefit analysis. Identify the positives, including side effects, of each available alternative, and do the same for the negatives. Project your best estimate of all probable consequences of each alternative. Weigh the good and the bad in each, and pick the one with the best proportion of good to bad.

Protestant Reinhold Niebuhr's variation on this was called *existential ethics*. Similar to proportionality, it recognized that real life choices are limited, that multiple values and interests are in conflict, and that no "pure" right is available. Make the best choice you can determine in that "existent" situation. Recognize your human fallibilities: limitations on knowledge, inability to predict the future with certainty, vantage point biases, and a penchant for rationalizing self-interest. Remain open to admitting errors and making corrective responses as you go along.

Double Effect

According to the Catholic principle of double effect, committing a sin is a bad effect, but if a greater good effect occurs as a result of the sin, there is a net gain in the double effect of the action, and the sin is erased. This is the rationale for a just war.

Niebuhr arrived at a similar position by a different route. As a pacifist he opposed World War II—until the extent of Nazi and Japanese atrocities came to light. Horrified, he shifted to support of the war effort on the grounds than even the massive sin of warfare was a *lesser evil* that the alternative *sin of omission*. To stand by and do nothing was to be a passive accessory in every one of those acts.

Double effect can legitimize Robin Hood. In social policy, although it may not be proper to take from the rich any of the wealth they have amassed or inherited to meet essential needs of less advantaged fellow citizens, the double effect principle can justify it as not only acceptable, but desirable.

Double effect is related to proportionality in that the asset of the second effect must outweigh the debit of the first effect. It supports the "it all depends" ends-means approach. Its biggest pitfall (shared with proportionality and utilitarianism) is that judgments are at best imperfect and can be abused as rationales for covert self-serving ends.

Utilitarian

Jeremy Bentham (1789) *utilitarianism* asserted that "the greatest happiness of the greatest number is the foundation of morals and legislation." Saul Alinsky (1972, p. 33) states, "To me ethics is doing what is best for the most." It is okay to trade off harm to some individuals for the sake of the general welfare.

This was Caiaphas's argument for crucifying Jesus after both the Roman governor and the religious council had found no capital offense: "If we let him go on like this, everyone will believe him, and then the Romans will come and take away both our place and our nation. You do not realize that it is better for you that one man die for the people than that the whole nation perish" (John 11:48-50). (The Roman Empire tolerated native religions and cultures so long as they posed no threat to the civil order but brutally crushed any sign of insurrection. A few decades later in 70 A.D. they crushed a Judean rebellion, razed Jerusalem, and plowed it under.)

Utilitarianism is discussed further in Chapter 10.

Triage: Relative Impact

Set your priorities according to the relative importance of each. On the French battlefields of World War I, faced with more casualties than they could handle at one time, doctors developed a priority approach which they called *triage*. Patients were divided into three groups: (1) those who would die despite treatment, (2) those who would live anyway even if treatment were delayed, and (3) those for whom immediate treatment meant the difference between life and death. Priority was given to the third group. Variations on triage continue to be a popular gray-area approach in making social policy choices.

Feasibility

A pragmatic yardstick is *feasibility*. "A bird in the hand is worth two in the bush." When faced with dilemmas of choice, go with what you know can be done. This is exemplified in the Alcoholics Anonymous prayer (in Niebuhr's original wording): "God give me the courage to change what can be changed, the serenity to accept what cannot be changed, and the wisdom to know *the one from the other*" (emphasis added).

Chapter 6

The Human Condition:
Jewels, Jackals, or Junk?

We are no other than a moving row of magic shadow: shapes that come and go.

Omar Khayyám

In the image of God He created him; male and female he created them.

Genesis 1:27

The natural man has only two primal passions: to get and to beget.

William Osler, 1904

How much are you worth? Is it all right to sacrifice you for broad national purposes? If you are in need, do you have a right to expect help from your fellow humans?

Are you innately good? If so, should social policy facilitate fulfillment of your potential? Are you a sinner? If so, should policy coerce and control you? Are you just a dumb animal? If so, should policy manipulate your instincts?

To what extent do you control your life? Should social policy shape your behavior, protect you, compensate for bad luck, or leave you alone?

Conflicting beliefs and values in such fundamental areas as individualism, social responsibility, freedom, equality, fairness, and basic human rights profoundly influence specific social policies. These will be discussed in subsequent chapters. Underlying all of these is something even more basic—our beliefs about human nature, the worth of individual persons, and the extent to which we are self-determining or subject to external circumstances.

WHAT IS A PERSON WORTH?

High: The Individual Is Sacred

> *All Men . . . are endowed by their Creator with certain unalienable Rights . . . Among these are Life, Liberty, and the Pursuit of Happiness.*
>
> U.S. Declaration of Independence

Western societies, influenced by Judeo-Christian beliefs, profess that the worth of each individual human being is extremely high. "Why even the hairs on your head are numbered" (Luke 12:16). To the extent that people are highly valued as individuals, social policies tend to support civil liberties, civil rights, social and economic justice, peace, antipoverty programs, quality of life, and other humanitarian objectives.

Low: Life Is Cheap

Despite rhetoric to the contrary, many economic, military, and political leaders have, de facto, put a low value on human worth. Some social philosophers have done so overtly. In 1798, Thomas Malthus warned that overpopulation would resolve itself in unpleasant ways. "Positive checks to population [include] all unwholesome occupations, severe labor and exposure to the seasons, extreme poverty, bad nursing of children, great towns, excesses of all kinds, the whole train of common diseases and epidemics, wars, plague, and famine" (p. 199).

His followers treated this gloomy prediction as a natural fact and put a cheap price on life. Among these followers were classical economists who accepted the misery and premature death of a majority of citizens as a routine cost of free enterprise. Later, Social

Darwinists carried it a step further, describing the wholesale suffering, hardship, and premature death of the poor as a "beneficent purging of the social organism" (Trattner, 1994, p. 91).

Salvation Army founder General Booth responded to policies based on these views with biting irony, when he proposed the "Cab Horse Charter . . . When [a draft horse] is down, he is helped up, and while he lives, he has food, shelter, and work. . . . [This] is beyond the reach of millions of workers" (quoted in Fraser, 1973, p. 122).

"Low worth" social policies comfortably sacrifice individuals for military goals (e.g., Hitler), political ideology (e.g., Lenin), the economic climate (e.g., 1981 U.S. anti-inflation measures that cost many millions of workers their jobs), or simply the self-interests of those in control. Where social welfare exists at all, it is an investment to be evaluated on the basis of its payoff in productivity, profit, or social control. According to Frances Piven and Richard Cloward, in *Regulating the Poor* (1971), this is the function of public assistance programs.

Conditional: "I Love You But . . . "

In the middle ground, individual worth is affirmed as a high value—except where a transcendent value takes precedence.

Some of these values are "noble," such as honor, patriotism, faith, or cause. Richard Lovelace (1649), forsaking human relationship while "to war and arms I fly," explained to his lover, Lucasta:

> I could not love thee, dear, so much
> Loved I not honour more.

Other "higher" values are as mundane as pelf. After Congress passed several laws to protect people by regulating environmental pollution, occupational safety and health, air traffic safety, etc., the U.S. Office of Budget and Management ordered enforcement agencies to subordinate human life to economic interests:

> In evaluating a new regulation, an agency will try to estimate how many lives it will save, what it will cost to adopt the rule, and thus *the cost per life saved. This cost is weighed against*

the [dollar] value of those lives as part of the "regulatory impact analysis" demanded by the Reagan Administration. (Keller, 1984, emphasis added)

Experts said that an airliner disaster killing hundreds of people in Dallas the following year would have been avoided if a planned new Doppler radar system at the airport had not been canceled after such a calculation.

Double Standards: Us and Them

Policymakers may apply different worth to different groups. Joseph Townsend differentiated by class in his *A Dissertation on the Poor Laws by a Well-Wisher to Mankind* (1786):

> It seems to be the law of nature that the poor should be to a certain degree improvident, that there may always be some to fulfill the most servile, the most sordid, and the most ignoble office in the community. The stock of human happiness is thereby much increased, whilst the more delicate are . . . relieved of drudgery and freed from those occasional employments which would make them miserable. As for the lowest of the poor, by custom they are reconciled to the meanest occupations, to the most laborious works, and the most hazardous pursuits; whilst the hope of their reward makes them cheerful in the midst of all their dangers and their toils.

Our Founding Fathers asserted their own unalienable rights—but denied them to women, Native Americans, and black slaves. Thomas Jefferson copied his Declaration of Independence statement of human rights for "*all* men" from a John Locke treatise that explicitly and unequivocally applied these principles against slavery. Later, as the Constitution was being framed, Jefferson wrote:

> The whole commerce between master and slave is a perpetual exercise of . . . the most unremitting despotism, on the one part, and degrading submission on the other. . . . The man must be a prodigy who can retain his manners and morals undepraved by such circumstances. . . . I tremble for my country

when I reflect that God is just; that his justice cannot sleep forever. (quoted in Johnson, 1991, p. 304)

Yet, Jefferson himself continued to expand as a slaveholder, and thirty-five years later owned 267 men, women, and children in bondage.

President James Madison told a British visitor, Harriet Martineau, that he wanted "all men of good will" to oppose slavery so that "we may destroy it, and save ourselves from reproaches and our posterity the imbecility ever-attendant on a country filled with slaves." Twenty years after his presidency, he sold sixteen slaves to a kinsman, and he also reneged on a promise in his will to free his slaves because he decided it would be financially undesirable for his widow (Ibid., p. 305).

The historical double standard for women is well documented. An example:

By marriage, the husband and wife are one person in law; that is, the very being and existence of the woman is suspended during the marriage, or at least incorporated and consolidated into that of the husband, under whose wing, protection, and cover, she performs everything. (Blackstone, *Commentaries on the Law of England*, 1791, quoted in Johnson, 1991, p. 474)

Distance may create double standards. When I was a national church official, I encountered *fifty-mile liberals*, who espoused civil rights in Mississippi, Washington, and South Africa—all more than fifty miles away—but resisted integration of their own Massachusetts neighborhoods. Robert Pinker calls this "the law of telescopic philanthropy . . . that the further away the object of our compassion lies, the more intense will be the feelings of concern and obligation which it evokes" (Pinker, 1979, p. 3).

Another set of our church members had an opposite double standard. These *caring conservatives* were generous and compassionate toward people they knew personally, while opposing social programs that extended comparable treatment to people they did not know.

Double standards on human worth can be found in "two-tier" approaches to social welfare, such as the segregated public school systems that were legal before 1954 or the different provision for Mrs. Brown and Mrs. Green (see Chapter 1).

NOBLE OR BASE?

Are human beings inherently noble and good or base and sinful? Or are they neither, just instinctive dumb animals? Social policies vary markedly according to the answer.

Noble and Good

Optimism about inherent goodness influenced the emphasis on liberty in the birth of our nation. The Psalmist (Psalms 8:5) carried it a step further when he exulted that we are "little less than divine beings."

Jean Jacques Rousseau, appalled by human behavior in Paris and nostalgic for his hometown in Switzerland, developed a "noble savage" perspective that preserved his optimism: man in a state of nature is *innately good* but is corrupted by modern urban society—a view shared by many of my Nebraska neighbors, as they view New York, California, and Washington, DC.

Protestant Liberalism in the late-nineteenth and early-twentieth centuries optimistically sought to reform society through the positive conversion of inherently good business and political leaders. My father called this "moving the movers" when he urged me to pursue my humanitarian vocation within "the establishment." Despite recent disillusionments, this continues to be a strong article of faith for millions of Americans.

A number of policy approaches make the "noble" assumption:

- *Decentralization* is based on a premise that those closest to the situation know and care more about the well-being of their neighbors.
- *Deregulation* assumes people don't have to be coerced into "playing fair."
- *Humanitarian opposition to public welfare* believes that private philanthropy and enlightened employers will voluntarily meet all human needs.

- *Democracy* expects voters and politicians to act in the best interests of all, not just their own narrow interests.
- *Populism* and other "power to the people" movements believe, with Rousseau, that even if the rich and powerful have become corrupt, the common folk are still innately good.

Base

Base means "morally low, without dignity of sentiment, mean-spirited, selfish."

The *sinful* version is that although we know better, "all have sinned and fallen short of the glory of God" (Romans 3:23).

The *brutish* version sees us as predatory animals following our natural instincts. Thomas Hobbes stated bluntly in his *Leviathan* (1651), "I put for a general inclination of all mankind, a perpetual restless desire of Power after Power, that closeth only in Death." His description of "man in the state of nature": "no arts, no letters, no society, and, which is worst of all, continual fear and danger of violent death, and the life of man solitary, poor, nasty, brutish, and short."

The brute animal view is not limited to cynics. It is also found in mainstream American ideology. Harold Wilensky and Charles Lebeaux described "great emphasis on the rational, acquisitive, self-interested individual" as being "of great importance to American capitalism":

> Individualism is both a theory of human behavior and a doctrine in justification of laissez faire. As theory, it tries to explain man's conduct in terms of a pleasure-pain calculus. Man, it is assumed, pursues his self-interest because of an acquisitive instinct or biological needs. Self-interest is seen in economic terms: he acquires and consumes material goods (pleasure); he avoids economic loss (pain). (1965, pp. 33-34)

Policies based on this pessimistic view of human nature apply social controls and sanctions to the first level of Maslow's (1954) hierarchy of human needs, physiological survival (an instinct shared with all other animals). They tend to overlook his three highest levels: social affiliation, esteem/recognition, self-actualization.

Poor law policy in nineteenth-century England and late-twentieth-century United States assumes that humans are by nature lazy freeloaders who won't work unless relief is made much more unpleasant than the worst job. Joseph Townsend (1786) expressed this premise succinctly: "What encouragement have the poor to be industrious and frugal . . . when they are assured that if by their indolence and extravagance, by their drunkenness and vices, they should be reduced to want, they shall be abundantly supplied [by the poor law dole]."

A different policy application is to protect us from the worst effects of normal base behavior through coercive regulation and control in such areas as consumer fraud, environmental damage, banking and finance, food and drugs, airline safety, labor standards, discrimination, and crime. Past experience with unregulated, laissez-faire practice in these areas has contributed to this pessimistic expectation.

A third policy response is to seek a *balance of power*, based on the assumption that "Power tends to corrupt and absolute power corrupts absolutely" (Lord Acton). This may include the following:

- *Empowerment* of disadvantaged groups, not as in the optimistic view because they are noble savages but rather to enable them to compete for their self-interests on equal terms with "establishment" groups.
- *Checks and balances* to keep any self-serving individual or group from gaining dominance, such as the American network of checks and balances among legislative, executive, and judicial branches, national and state governments, government and business, management and labor, etc. The capitalist ideal, premised on the brutish view of human nature noted by Wilensky and Lebeaux, relies on self-interested individual competition to balance conflicting interests.

A costly social consequence of the "base" view is the diversion of resources from social amenities to military security. During the cold war of the past few decades, the middle and lower classes of both the Soviet Union and the United States lost ground relative to their counterparts in countries that spent less for "protection" against an "evil empire." In recent years, although it is seldom publicized in relation to taxes, the skyrocketing populations in our prisons have caused a comparable effect.

FREE WILL OR DETERMINISM?

Are you master of your own fate? How much of your fate is determined by outside forces? What we believe about this guides our determination of who (or what) is to blame for social problems, what is "fair," and how we should intervene, if at all. American society is ambivalent.

Preordination

Medieval Christianity promulgated the belief that every person is born ("preordered") into his/her place, has God-given rights associated with it, and should not depart from that role. It is okay to be rich or poor, male or female, black or white, as long as you *know your place*. This was the moral foundation for feudalism, monarchy, aristocracy, and the Elizabethan Poor Laws.

Cecil Alexander celebrated this view in a familiar nineteenth-century hymn:

> All things bright and beautiful,
> All creatures great and small,
> All things wise and wonderful,
> The Lord God made them all . . .
> *The rich man in his castle,*
> *The poor man at his gate,*
> *God made them, high and lowly,*
> *And ordered their estate.* (emphasis added)

"The song is ended, but the melody lingers on." Many modern hymnals have deleted the rich-man/poor-man verse because pre-ordination is no longer respectable: it has rationalized American slavery, racial segregation, subjugation of women, and tracking of school children. Yet, it is alive and well today in such policies as inheritance, admission preferences for alumni children, and Social Security orphan pensions based on the former status of a father who no longer exists.

Although there is much upward, downward, and sideward mobility in America, a strong element of preordering remains in the implicit sector. My family has a four-generation tradition of being human service professionals (my grandmother, both parents, five siblings, my wife, and two of my three children). Some of my friends' families have comparable multigenerational ties to farming, plumbing, railroading, and banking.

Preordination offers stability and security at a price. The origins of both philanthropy and public welfare can be traced to its doctrine of *noblesse oblige*, that noble status carries with it a paternalistic responsibility for one's inferiors. On the other hand, it restricts self-determination and equal opportunity.

Interestingly, we appear to be on the threshold of a partial preordination revival, triggered by advances in genetic science. This may have a major impact on social policy in the early part of the twenty-first century. The implications and effects are not yet clear, but it has already become a hot topic in the medical and social ethics fields.

Predestination

The Calvinist doctrine of predestination emerged about the same time that medieval feudalism was giving way to an individualistic and competitive market economy. Believing that God had determined in advance each person's destination (the elect to heaven, the damned to hell), it inferred parallel divinely ordained differences in this life.

Preordination and predestination both rationalize inequality as God's will, but they differ in two important respects:

1. Preordination supports the status quo, for one's place in life passes from parents to children. Predestination legitimizes social mobility, for each individual's place in life is separately determined by God.
2. Preordination, theoretically, does not make moral distinctions about where your place happens to be. In predestination, poverty is divine punishment.

There are three social policy directions consistent with predestination:

- *Individualism.* Each person will find his/her own appropriate place in life. Let the chips fall as they may, without government interference.
- *Acceptance of inequality.* After all, it is a precursor of even greater inequalities in the next life.
- *Blame the victim.* The damned poor don't deserve help.

Although next-world predestination is out of fashion today, many of our national leaders continue to attribute a secular elect and damned status based on this-world wealth or poverty.

Capricious Determinism

Unlike the orderly determinism of preordination and predestination, *kismet* (fate) is a divine intervention that is either haphazard or unknowable. We call it luck, the roll of the dice. My daughter, after several years in Saudi Arabia, attributed that nation's reckless driving, such as passing on blind curves at high speed, to the drivers' belief that they are safe until their time comes, *Insh'Allah*, and when it does, there is nothing they can do to avoid it.

Although Americans profess not to believe in kismet, insurance companies and the popular press refer to seemingly capricious natural disasters as "acts of God." Combat troops fatalistically speak of "the bullet that has my name on it." Astrology, often only half believed, is a popular method of trying to second-guess fate.

American social policy responses to fatalism take two opposite directions:

- An individualistic approach has been *nonintervention.* Tough luck!
- A collective social responsibility approach has been to *provide for misfortune,* either through charity after the event or sharing anticipated risks through public and private insurance.

Secular Determinism

Determinism need not be divine. During the Depression, President Roosevelt attributed the suffering of individual unemployed persons to external economic forces beyond their control. He responded with a range of programs that included direct relief for current victims of circumstance, social insurance to compensate future victims, and economic assistance to businesses.

Environmental determinism is well established in the behavioral sciences: Analytical psychology focuses on early developmental experiences in one's family of origin. Anthropologists focus on subgroup cultures. Sociologists scan a broad psycho-socio-econo-cultural matrix. Epidemiology stresses environmental determinants of health and mental health.

Social policy positions differ according to what the determinist identifies as the external cause. In the 1960s, sociologists "discovered" a self-perpetuating culture of poverty, caused by a combination of social, economic, ethnic, and psychological environmental factors. Michael Sherraden (1990) countered that the cause is purely economic:

> Many behaviors labeled "culture of poverty" are better explained by financial inability to focus and specialize. Assets matter and people know it, and therefore, when they have assets, they pay attention [to opportunities, to plans, and to their own counterproductive behavior]. If they do not have assets, they do not pay attention. Indeed, in a sense, assets are the future. They are hope in concrete form.

The first view calls for an array of services to reprogram poor people to a middle-class lifestyle. The latter has a simpler conclusion: change their environment by lifting them out of poverty and let nature take its course.

Free Will: Self-Determination

> *I am the master of my fate; I am the captain of my soul.*
>
> William Henley
> "Invictus" (1888)

American democracy is a free-will ideology, based on John Locke's social compact assumption that only a government created by, and answerable to, the free choice of its citizens is valid. Individual self-determination is the cornerstone of John Stuart Mill's arguments for personal freedom in *On Liberty* (1859).

Social policy responses may be passive or activist. They should be passive, laissez-faire, say classical liberals Rowley and Peacock (1975, p. 80):

> We believe that mankind marks out its true distinction from the animal kingdom by exercising free will, by making choices and recognizing the responsibility that such choices imply. We are concerned therefore to assist in the development of a society that encourages individuals to exercise free will . . . and which confronts them with the responsibility for their decisions.

Another approach to self-determination is the go-getter view that "opportunity knocks but once."

> There is a tide in the affairs of men
> Which, taken at the flood, leads on to fortune;
> Omitted, all the voyage of their life
> Is bound in shallows and in miseries.

> Shakespeare
> *Julius Caesar,* Act IV, Scene III

Free will must be exercised aggressively or be lost by default. If the social order is not governed by a divine dictator or blind chance, then all social policy is the product of somebody's free-will choice. If you don't actively promote your interests, someone else will impose theirs at your expense, leaving you "bound in shallows and in miseries."

Organizers of the disadvantaged accept this as a fact of life. *Empowerment* has been a central theme of Alinsky's Industrial Areas Foundation, the civil rights movements, and the American Association of Retired Persons—as a prerequisite for achieving self-determination in the competitive policy arena.

Free Will Within Fixed Laws of Nature

Since Aristotle, natural law has been seen as divine principles of right reason that are independent of revelation. Because they are directly perceivable by reason, they are universal laws absolutely binding on all rational beings.

Emerging modern science "discovered" impersonal "laws of nature," which are "sequences of events that have been observed to occur with unvarying uniformity under the same conditions," notably Isaac Newton's laws of physics, such as gravity and motion, published in 1687.

From this physics model, social thinkers inferred a similar constancy in all spheres of life. You can make choices but only within the inexorable dynamics of a fixed natural pattern that cannot be evaded or changed. You choose—and reap the direct consequences. If you smoke, your heart and lungs will be damaged. If you drop out of school, you will suffer in the job market. As my mother used to tell me, "You can decide for yourself, but . . . " There are several different social policy responses to this worldview:

1. *Blame the victim.* Disclaim social responsibility for smokers, dropouts, and others who "brought it on themselves."
2. *Preventive education.* Help citizens avoid bad choices by warning them of the consequences.
3. *Protective controls.* Take away their freedom to make bad choices by banning tobacco and making education mandatory.

Some years after Newton, a physician-turned-economist, François Quesnay, applied his knowledge of physiology to social policy. The human organism is a self-regulating system that balances many internal and external elements. He observed that the medical interventions of his day did more harm than good, by disrupting the system's natural functioning. Calling himself a "physiocrat," he inferred that society, and specifically a free market, is a comparable self-regulating organism, integrating diverse, free-individual choices into an overall equilibrium that would be disrupted by "artificial" interference.

Quesnay reasoned that the proper public social policy was default. He called it *laissez-faire* ("let [people] do [as they please]"). Modern followers of this biological natural law model oppose regulation, monetary interventions, and welfare state services on the grounds that they subvert the natural functions of a presumably healthy social organism.

Free-Will Interventions Despite Determinist Beliefs

People who profess to believe in external determination often act in practice as if they really believe in free will:

- Puritans, who professed that God directly controlled every action and outcome, aggressively sought political and social control and enacted public policies to repress theoretically nonexistent freedom of choice.
- Karl Marx, after writing that historical determinism would inexorably bring down capitalism, spent his life exhorting workers to self-determining acts of revolution.
- Sigmund Freud, who attributed emotional problems to external causes (e.g., one's parents), developed therapies aimed at helping patients to achieve self-direction.
- The rhetoric of the 1960s War on Poverty was directed at social and economic causes of poverty, but most of its budget was spent for education and training programs to help poor individuals improve themselves.

How come? Two possible reasons for these apparent contradictions:

1. *Operating versus formal beliefs.* Perhaps Calvinists, Marx, and psychoanalysts intuitively leaned toward free will despite their intellectual ideologies. In Chapter 10, we will see how Calvinism evolved over time into the free-will Protestant work ethic.
2. *A mixed system.* It needn't be all or nothing. One may believe in powerful external determinism and also that there is an element of self-determination. Therapists and antipoverty workers, powerless to control those external causes, may focus on what they *can* do.

HUMAN NATURE AND THE CAUSES OF POVERTY

Beliefs about the causes of poverty lie at the root of many of our most important social welfare policies and programs. These, in turn, are derived more from the views of human nature contained in this chapter than from any other single source, including empirical data. They cluster into four categories: divine plan, moral deficiency, bad luck, and external forces.

Divine Plan

"The poor you will have with you always" (Mark 14:7). Poverty is a no-fault natural law. Shrug. *C'est la vie. Ain't my* problem.

Social Darwinism probably represents the most extreme version when it extrapolates, from a study of how plants and animals apparently adapted to different environments, a universal law that mandated callous disregard for human need and suffering.

Preordination affirms that the poor are an integral part of an unequal society, in which they faithfully serve their superiors, who in turn take care of them (at a poverty level). It differs from impersonal laws of nature in recognizing a responsibility of their "betters" to give the deserving poor (who know their place and perform their subordinate functions obediently) charity in time of old age, disability, or natural disaster.

Racism is a variant of preordination that categorizes certain ethnic groups as inherently superior or inferior (contrary to empirical evidence). Social policy tends to be harsher when a racial double standard is attributed to divine plan. Slavery involving Africans (in North America and the Caribbean) and indigenous peoples (in Latin America) was defended on the premise that they were created as lower species of humankind, of lesser ability and worth, to whom "natural" human rights did not apply. Through much of American history, even free Americans identified ethnically as African, Native American, or Asian were legally either ineligible for public health, education, and welfare services or entitled only to separate, inferior services.

Calvinism had a nonethnic double standard, based on God's differentiation between elect and damned individuals. Since the poor are assumed to be among the latter, there is no social responsibility for their well-being. However, for the sake of the social order, the elite must control the base tendencies of the poor in disciplinary and punitive ways.

Moral Deficiency

Moralism resembles Calvinism minus the predestination. If we have free will, aren't we responsible for our own condition? Those with a base view of human nature tend to interpret poverty as a just punishment for sinners who choose intemperance, indolence, and improvidence. "He made his own bed; let him lie in it."

Beginning in the 1970s, there has been a revival of the moral deficiency/low value view of human nature as a policy response to poverty. Under the 1960s "reform and remedial" approach, poverty declined. As the policy shifted to "benign neglect" in the 1970s, the numbers of poor people rose again. The moral deficiency response was a gradual escalation of punitive approaches, all of which were ineffective.

A different social policy response to the moral deficiency theory combines it with a higher value on each individual and a more optimistic view of the inherent goodness of the poor. Even though it's their fault, they are sheep who have gone astray and need to be brought back into the fold by a good shepherd. Our social responsibility is to help them fulfill their potential.

This was the rationale for the charity organization societies of the nineteenth century, which evolved into professional social work and a network of public and charitable rehabilitative services, such as therapy, counseling, adult education, job training, drug and alcohol treatment, and positive parenting groups for abusers. This second-chance opportunity approach, say moderate liberals and conservatives, is not just more humane; it is expedient, for it yields a better cost-benefit payoff to society than neglect or punishment.

Bad Luck

Although classical economics primarily embraces the moral deficiency theory, it admits that people do suffer unearned diswelfares in the form of natural disasters, and some (but not all), from ill health, disability, and accidents. Its policy response reflects low human value: "Let the loss lie where it falls."

On the other hand, when the bad luck view is linked with high human value, it fosters two complementary positive social policy responses.

Traditional charity and public welfare are *reactive*, providing needs-based special *assistance after the fact*. Victims of disaster receive emergency care and assistance in reestablishing themselves. The ill and disabled get medical care and rehabilitation. The impoverished receive food baskets and relief. Special education and child welfare services are rendered to those who, by an "accident of birth," have the unearned bad luck of genetic deficiencies or abusive families.

A second response is *anticipatory*, through private or social insurance. We predict that some of us will suffer illness, disability, widowhood, or loss of parents, but we don't know which of us it will be. As a precaution, we all contribute premiums and/or taxes to pay for care of the unfortunate ones among us on whom those "acts of God" happen to fall.

A related no-fault cause of poverty that is not technically bad luck is the effect of normal human life cycles. We tend to be more economically dependent at the beginning (before we are ready for employment) and end (after retirement) of our lives. Young couples at the bottom of their career ladders and with dependent children usually have a lower standard of living than they will twenty years later. This cause is generally approached in the same manner as bad luck, ideally through anticipatory universalistic and/or social insurance measures because it is so predictable. (In practice, our handling of it is often either reactive or benign neglect.)

External Environment

The fourth perceived cause of poverty views the poor as victims of circumstances beyond their control: The cause may be beyond anyone's control, such as technological unemployment. It may be the result of someone else's "base" behavior, such as an international oil embargo, racism, the longtime primary employer in a small community moving overseas for cheap labor, or an unscrupulous corporate takeover artist. It may be blamed on unwise decisions by leadership, such as the failure of an American industry to remain technologically competitive or government monetary policies that trigger a recession.

Combined with low value, the social policy response is the same as to bad luck: "That's the breaks, kid."

When external causation is combined with high value, social policy takes two directions: On a personal level, the focus is on *compensatory* measures, such as affirmative action, retraining, or unemployment insurance. On the macro level, policies are developed to *correct or enhance the environment itself,* through such approaches as economic development, full employment policies, federal tax and monetary interventions, regulation of business practices, and urban renewal.

All of the Above?

> *The lazy habit still prevails of tolerating [poverty] not only as an inevitable misfortune to be charitably patronized and relieved, but as a useful punishment for all sorts of misconduct and inefficiency that are not expressly punishable by law.*

George Bernard Shaw

The causes and the social policy responses may not be mutually exclusive. It is not unreasonable to believe that some instances of poverty are caused by a combination of the four. If so, no single policy response, however wise and effective in itself, will eliminate poverty.

A mix of policies may be needed. Perhaps a given individual's poverty is related to both the national unemployment rate and a personal decision to drop out of high school. The latter may require a "deficiency" intervention to make him or her employable. However, he or she will merely displace some other worker, unless "external" economic development interventions increase the number of full-time jobs with wages that enable all employable persons to earn a decent living.

PART III:
FUNDAMENTAL VALUE CHOICES

Chapter 7

Fairness:
Equality, Equity, or Adequacy?

Social and economic inequalities are to be arranged so that they are to the greatest benefit of the least advantaged.

John Rawls, 1971

Politicians or businessmen, about to cut back on social benefits or to close factories, always invoke fairness as part of their justification, along with such concepts as justice, rationalization, and efficiency. These mythological words come to replace thought.

John Saul, 1992

DISTRIBUTIVE JUSTICE: WHAT IS FAIR?

"Fair [fare] is what you get on the bus with." That is the only kind you can count on, says a friend who has the experience to back it up. Perhaps after considering the complications of determining fairness, setting your standards on what should be, and comparing them with what is, you may be tempted to agree with her.

Nevertheless, most Americans believe that there should be a "fair" distribution of income, wealth, rights, opportunity, status, and power. Social philosopher John Rawls said, "Justice is fairness . . . a proper balance between competing claims" (1971, p. 10). Right! But what *is* a proper balance?

The French Revolution answered clearly, *égalité!* If so, which kind of equality?

Individualists would substitute *equity*, what each person deserves. If so, what constitutes deservedness? Is it measured by effort, social contribution, or what somebody else is willing to pay you?

Humanitarians argue that the bottom line is *adequacy*, a minimum standard of living and quality of life to which every human being is entitled. The question is, how much is adequate?

Is there one universal guideline for all areas of social, economic, and political life? For example, might we advocate, at the same time:

- *equality* of opportunity, access, and due process;
- *adequacy* of income and essential services, a level below which no one falls; and, within these conditions,
- *equity* of earnings according to the market value of work performed.

In previous chapters, we have discussed beliefs and values as the basis for policy choices. The very idea of fairness assumes both high individual human worth and mutual responsibility of individuals in community.

There are other positions that reject or subordinate all of these competing ideas of fairness. Some of them will be discussed at the end of this chapter.

EQUALITY

Same or Equivalent?

If we want to treat each child in the family equally at Christmas, do we:

- give *identical* toys to a two-year-old and a ten-year-old?
- give toys that provide *equal pleasure*?
- give toys of *equal dollar value*?

Narrowly defined, "equal" is "the *same* quantity, size, number, value, degree, or intensity; having the *same* rights, privileges, ability, or rank." However, this does not allow for variations in circumstances and preferences, as in the case of the two children at Christmas.

We can solve this problem by broadening the definition to mean *equivalent*, "equal in value, quantity, force, power, effect, excellence, or meaning." To compare equivalence, we must have a common denominator for value. A good measure would be *utility*, "the power to satisfy the needs or wants of a person," our second toy option—it worked with my children.

In dealing with most adults, this isn't as easy. Try to define a unit of satisfaction on which everyone agrees! For this reason, we usually compromise on dollar price as a flawed, but measurable, indicator of equivalence.

The difference between *same* and *equivalent* can be significant for social policy. Most of us profess to believe in equal pay for equal work. However, a key social policy controversy rested on the definition used. In the 1965 civil rights law, "equal pay" referred narrowly to the *same* pay for the *same* work within the *same* company. This ignored widespread salary discrepancies, unrelated to the position's responsibility, difficulty, or contribution, between jobs predominantly held by males and those primarily occupied by females. The "equivalent" version, *comparable worth*, redefines the policy as equal pay for work of *equal value* in different jobs.

Input or Outcome?

Opposing policy positions may each claim to be based on the principle of equality. For example, take two parallel groups of diverse six-year-olds, some of whom are at a more advanced learning level than others due to home environment and social circumstances. Put all students in the first group in the same class with the same teacher and teach them the same subjects. At the end of the year, the advantaged children will continue to score higher on achievement tests than the disadvantaged ones. In the second group, give them all the same normal instruction but add special education supplements for the less advantaged ones to help them catch up with the others by the end of the year.

Which is an equality approach? Both! It depends on whether you are looking at what you put in or what results you get. *Equality of input* means everyone starts with the same materials but may end up unequal. *Equality of outcome* is the opposite. To achieve the same results, you make unequal contributionss to compensate for different circumstances.

The Declaration of Independence talks about *input* equality. We are born with an equal right to the *pursuit* of happiness—but don't necessarily end up equally happy. The basic Canadian Old Age Security program offers the same flat-rate pension input to all senior citizens. If you had no other income, you would live meagerly. If you were already well-off, it could pay for a trip south in the winter.

Group health insurance, on the other hand, seeks *outcome* equality. It spends more on group members who become ill in order to restore them, as much as possible, to the same condition as members blessed with "natural" good health.

Is one of these always the "correct" approach to equality? If not, on what basis would you decide which to use in each particular policy situation?

We might use both, at different times. Let's say our goal is equal opportunity for admission to a graduate program. The several roads to admission have been unequal due to "historical and social fortune" (Rawls, 1971, p. 74) and past discrimination in favor of or against applicants. In the first stage, preparation, we use outcome equality by helping the low-road travelers to catch up with those who had lucked onto the high road. For the second stage, selection, we use input equality, evaluating all applicants on exactly the same criteria, without reference to race, gender, age, place of origin, or relationship to alumni.

Vertical and Horizontal Equality

Another point at which people differ on equality is, "compared to what?" *Vertical* equality compares *all* people, whether anyone is higher or lower, better or worse off, than any other. According to the Constitution, Americans have vertical equality in voting and due process.

Horizontal equality compares only within peer subgroups that have similar circumstances or needs. Wage-based Social Security offers horizontal equality (you get the same as everyone else who made the same contributions) but not vertical equality (you get more than low-wage workers). Equity (discussed later in the chapter) is a horizontal equality concept.

Temporal Equality

Temporal equality compares the same person or group at different times. After interpreting the Pharaoh's dream of seven fat cows that were then eaten up by seven lean ones, Joseph in Egypt developed the first temporal equality social policy. He took grain from the people during seven good years and returned it to them to eat during the subsequent drought years. Unemployment insurance similarly reduces *cyclical* inequalities, using payroll taxes collected during high employment to replace income lost through worker layoffs during recessions.

Social Security contributes to *life-span* equality. Its taxes during working years pay for replacement of earnings during retirement years. Another temporal equality program in most industrial nations is the family allowance. Paid for by taxes over one's lifetime, it provides income supplements to help a family maintain a more level standard of living during both child-rearing and nonchild life stages.

British social welfare historian Howard Glennester calculated that "three-fourths of all the [social welfare–related] taxes that people pay come back to them individually but at different times in their lives. Only a quarter of the total goes to others, i.e., the lifetime poor" (1995, p. 227).

EQUITY

Some people's money is merited
And other people's is inherited.

Ogden Nash

Equality sounds good, but is it always fair? A hard working student turns in excellent papers and is rewarded with an A. A party-boy classmate is less conscientious and settles for a "gentleman's C." This is not equality. Should it be? Does the first student *deserve* a higher reward because he worked harder or because he produced more? This is the principle of equity; an equitable share is *proportional* to what you deserve. This part is easy. The tough part is figuring out what "deserving" is—and measuring it.

Social Contribution

The ideal measure is probably *social contribution.* Farmers, teachers, housewives, and ordinary employees tend to agree. The problem is that a viable social contribution equity system requires:

- a *common denominator* to measure dissimilar contributions,
- *agreement* on the specific value assigned to each contribution,
- reliable *measures*, honestly and impartially applied, and
- power to *enforce* the subsequent decisions.

"Realists" argue that the first two requirements are unachievable in a diverse society, and reliable measurement may be technically impossible. How do you measure the real effect of a pastor on human lives? Whom do you trust with the authority to do the measuring?—An elected politician? A bureaucrat? A technician? The winner of power struggles within your organization?

Merit pay systems are intended to provide outcome equity. However, they are frequently subverted by an inability to measure that output reliably and by de facto displacement of "deservedness" from actual work performance to personal qualities that please superiors. Educators, nurses, social workers, and other human service professionals, most of whom believe ideologically in equity rewards, end up bargaining collectively for egalitarian salary systems as a lesser unfairness than arbitrary and capricious *pseudo*-equity.

Market Equity

If we can't put a clear number on the social contribution itself, what *can* we measure? The market economics solution is to redefine social contribution as a product or commodity that someone else wants to buy. Its worth is whatever the market will pay. There are no troublesome social value issues, no arguments about whether the contribution is good for society or whether it is antisocial (harmful to people). Worth is purely an economic preference choice (see Chapter 10).

By this standard, a person who throws balls at a hoop is 1,000 times as productive as a teacher, for example:

> Michael Jordan got $30 million for one year*. . . . Christina Chase is a 30-year-old fifth grade teacher at the Jordan Elementary School in Mansfield, Mass. She earns just under $30,000 a year. . . . Calling [such a] contract "unfathomable," she says, "When you look at the payoff to society, it doesn't make any sense." (*USA Today*, 1996)

He makes money for his employers: she doesn't. Arenas sell out wherever he plays; more people watch his games on television, which means higher revenue from commercials; kids buy his brand of sneakers. Would you pay $50 to watch Ms. Chase teach? If her fifth-grade class was on TV, would you spend big bucks to buy advertising time to promote your beer? All she does is help her students to read, understand, think, write, and calculate better for the rest of their lives.

Is this fair? Sure! This is no conspiracy by "them." Advocates of market equity argue that for all its flaws, it is the best available system. It is a democratic decision: we have voted, one vote per dollar. It provides maximum work incentives because, in our society, the most effective reward is money. "Money isn't everything, but it's way ahead of whatever is in second place."

Not necessarily, say others. The strongest work incentives are self-fulfillment, satisfaction, and a sense of achievement. The materialistic preoccupation of commercial market equity undervalues and thereby subverts creative, artistic, and humanitarian contributions. Moreover, it diverts production from basic social needs to discretionary "luxuries." For instance, in a society in which millions of citizens are homeless or living in substandard housing, construction of luxury vacation homes is more rewarding under market equity than low-cost housing.

The "trickle down" theory argues that everyone ultimately benefits from a market equity approach because its incentives and rewards create a *meritocracy* in which the best rise to the top. There is some empirical support for this. There is also empirical evidence

---

*Not counting an estimated $40 million more for endorsements.

throughout history that (1) being at, or getting to, the top has had more to do with inheritance, class of origin, connections, and ruthlessness than ability to benefit others, and (2) in a majority of cases, benefits at the top did not trickle down to lower-income classes. Richard Titmuss (1967, pp. 358-359) warns, "History suggests that human nature is not strong enough to maintain itself in true community where great disparities of income and wealth preside."

Input Equity

Where there is no commercial measure (as in the case of the Jordan School fifth-grade teacher) and no consensus on how to quantify social contribution, what can we fairly use to define equity?

Military and civil service grades tend to fall back on what they *can* measure, *input*—the length of training, effort, stress, and level of responsibility that goes into a job—as the best available indicator of true worth. When I was in the government, bachelor's degrees started at GS7 or Second Lieutenant, master's degrees at GS9 or First Lieutenant, and doctorates at GS11 or Captain. Based on academic criteria, professional social workers earned the same as MBAs, and chaplains as much as lawyers.

If market equity is flawed because what the market pays is not necessarily a measure of real social contribution, input equity is flawed because it doesn't measure production at all. Still, its advocates point to the correlation of education, training, and experience with competence, of past educational and work achievements with discipline and effort, and of competence and effort with both quantity and quality of productivity, making it the best available indicator—and similar to price, it is measurable.

Comparable Worth

Comparable worth is an equity/horizontal equality approach that developed in response to patterns of discrimination in pay between male-dominated and female-denominated occupations.

In an appeals case, a federal judge (later appointed to the Supreme Court) voided a state comparable worth law on the grounds that it violated market equity. This rationale has subsequently been rebutted by substantial evidence. For instance, one of the most comprehensive research studies, *The Economics of Comparable Worth*, by Mark Aldrich and Robert Buchele (1986), concluded that "job evaluation as presently practiced is profoundly arbitrary" (p. 173).

Pay differences were not based on demonstrable economic principles but rather on a violation of them, due to traditional beliefs and practices regarding gender roles and relationships, i.e., *institutionalized sexism*.

One contributor to gender inequity has been the widespread opinion that women should be paid less because men are the primary family breadwinners. For instance, in 1975, one of my colleagues was offered a faculty position with a salary 30 percent below that of male faculty members with comparable credentials in the department. The department chair openly told her that she needed less because her husband was a full professor at that university. (Some years later, she led a successful effort that established comparable worth throughout the university system.)

Another dynamic was a discriminatory market, in which the normal supply-and-demand balance did not work. In a free market, all sellers have equal competitive access to all buyers, and all decisions are based solely on economic supply-and-demand forces. In this case, female sellers of labor did not have free-market access to all buyers (employers), for they were not readily accepted on equal terms with males in male-dominated occupations. Thus, the full pool of supply (women seeking jobs) had access to only a partial pool of jobs ("female" occupations). This created an excess of supply over demand in those occupational sectors, which lowers the market price of the item to be sold.

For the sake of measurability, most comparable worth proposals have used the input measure approach described previously, including such elements as education, training, licensure, skills, and years of prior job-related experience.

A more complex approach breaks each position into "job traits." One model uses a panel of mutually acceptable experts who rate each job on several predetermined factors in the following categories:

- *Knowledge* and *skills* required, both technical and interpersonal.
- *Mental demands*, the need to make, and amount of latitude for, independent judgment, decision making, and problem solving.

- *Accountability*, the extent to which the person is accountable for actions taken on the job and for results. For instance, as a national agency CEO, my contract specified that my annual pay adjustments would depend on how well the agency did, disregarding all extenuating circumstances, good or bad. As a teenage grocery stock clerk, I was accountable only for whether the right cans went onto the right shelves.
- *Working conditions*, with higher pay ratings for hazardous conditions, heavy physical demands, extreme stress, and discomfort. This, for instance, would raise the level of pay of police and firefighter jobs.

Comparable worth is no more nor less than equity. Its assets and problems are those of any equity-fairness system. With all its flaws, its advocates believe it is the best available alternative.

Equity and Equal Opportunity

A prerequisite for equity is what John Rawls calls *fair equality of opportunity*. "Once [equal liberty and equal opportunity] are satisfied, other inequalities are allowed to rise from men's voluntary actions in accordance with free association" (1971, p. 96). The problem is that this condition has never been met.

> No one deserves his place in the distribution of native endowments, any more than one deserves one's starting place in society. Thus, the more advantaged representative man cannot say he deserves and therefore has a right to a scheme of cooperation in which he is permitted to acquire benefits in ways that do not contribute to the welfare of others. There is no basis for making this claim. (Ibid., p. 104)

Given this limitation, if we want to use equity as a fairness guideline, the best we can do boils down to one or more of four choices:

- Settle for a less than fully fair equity; it's better than nothing.
- Equalize opportunity as best we can (see Chapter 9).
- Supplement flawed equity with social market transfers (see Chapter 13).
- Add a noblesse oblige trusteeship ethic (see Chapter 8).

ADEQUACY

In many social welfare programs, the first priority is adequacy. As a fairness principle, it means ensuring that people have "enough." If so, what is enough?

Barely Satisfactory or Fully Sufficient?

The dictionary gives two definitions of adequacy:

- Barely satisfactory (subsistence)
- Fully sufficient

Programs for the poor, the less powerful, and "them" (those with whom we share no close ties) tend to apply the bare subsistence definition. This was the approach in setting the "poverty line" adequacy standard. Department of Agriculture home economists constructed the lowest-cost monthly "food basket" that still met minimum nutritional standards—assuming the buyer has the expertise of a professional nutritionist and exceptional self-discipline (no Twinkies, potato chips, soda, or beer!). Based on census information which reported that poor people spent 25 percent of their income on food, social welfare researchers defined "barely satisfactory" as four times the food basket price.

Citro and Michael (1995) proposed that income used to measure adequacy be redefined as "disposable income," by subtracting from gross income one's payroll deductions, direct payments for medical care and/or health insurance, work-related expenses including day care, and child support payments (which, however, are added to the disposable income of the custodial parent).

Policies that involve middle- and upper-class interests or "us" tend to use a fully sufficient definition of adequacy, as in suburban public schools, interstate highways, and most national health systems.

In my local school system, the official standard of adequacy is not barely sufficient literacy (the ability to read simple workplace instructions and traffic signs) but rather a full high school education, verified by proficiency exams in English, social studies, math, and science.

Absolute or Relative?

Examining it from another angle, adequacy may be defined in absolute or relative terms. *Absolute* calculations are based on specifically defined objective standards, such as a particular food basket or a diploma.

Of course, the "absolute" list of necessities is itself relative, influenced by time, place, culture, the economy, and politics. When it was discovered that one-third of Americans were below the researcher's subsistence line, a politically unacceptable statistic to President Johnson, the official line was reset 25 percent lower. A British poverty line, the Deprivation Index, is more generous. Developed by Peter Townsend for his 1979 study, *Poverty in the United Kingdom: A Survey of Household Resources and Standards of Living*, it went beyond physical survival to include access to "basic goods and opportunities accepted as standard in a society," such as medical care, children's birthday parties, and television.

Relative standards for education have changed over the past century. In my father's day, fully sufficient educational adequacy standards for working-class Americans was the completion of eighth grade. In my day, it was tenth grade. In my children's day, it was twelfth grade. Based on current lifetime earning projections, the odds of earning an average salary are against you, without at least a community college education.

Relative adequacy also considers social and psychological factors, such as self-esteem, satisfaction, status, respect, and social integration. It defines adequacy in comparison to the "normal" level of a community, region, or nation. (An alternative definition of relative adequacy is 10 percent more than whatever you have now.)

While homesteading in northern Wisconsin, my mother's family lived well below any absolute poverty line but did not experience relative poverty because their income was on par with their neighbors and respected community leaders. By contrast, a recent president from modest middle-class origins who experienced a standard of living far higher than those homesteaders—or than what he proposed as adequate for AFDC children—described himself as "growing up poor." He was telling the truth. According to the relative definition of poverty, if he felt poor, he was poor.

Adequacy and Equality

Sometimes the standard for adequacy is *full equality.* According to the Fourteenth Amendment, nothing less than equal treatment under the law is adequate. The official policy objectives of most other industrial nations define "adequate" health care to include all essential health services for all citizens, regardless of income, wealth, or social status.

More often, adequacy programs *reduce inequality.* Although some private colleges do indeed offer special advantages, fully sufficient public universities have dramatically reduced the educational difference between the "upper" and "middle" classes. Even our below-poverty-line welfare grants redistribute *some* money from upper- and middle-income taxpayers to impoverished children.

MULTIPLE TIERS: ADEQUACY PLUS EQUITY

The Council of Europe (COE, 1993) reports two basic approaches to public old-age pensions. One, which it calls *universal,* follows the adequacy model—"guaranteed income maintenance at a basic level for the whole population" (p. 21). This is a priority in Britain, the Netherlands, and Switzerland. The other, called *professional,* uses an equity model (as well as temporal equality). Its intent is to "maintain an acquired standard of living for specific occupational groups" (Ibid.). This is the primary pattern in Germany, Austria, France, Belgium, Italy, and Spain.

Some countries, such as Canada and Sweden, have multiple tiers that include both models. This approach provides a floor but no ceiling. Most people seem to prefer some form of a multiple-tier system, on the grounds that if you earn or otherwise can afford something better you should not be held back, so long it does not deprive someone else of adequacy. Three types of multiple-tier systems may be identified using the "Burch ice cream cone model."

Standard and Premium Brands: Alternative Tiers

My father, from the dairy state of Wisconsin, was an ice cream aficionado. Early in life, I learned to distinguish between *standard* "store-bought" ice cream and *premium* hand-packed ice cream made by our local dairy. The standard brands were okay, but they couldn't compare with the ice cream Dad brought home: it's like the difference between tourist class and first class on an ocean liner.

Sometimes both tiers are public. When I lived in New York City, there were two tiers of public beaches. We took the subway to Coney Island, which was okay, but people who owned cars could drive to Jones Beach State Park, which was much nicer. Similarly, public schools were better in nearby suburbs than in The Bronx—provided you could afford to buy a house in Scarsdale.

Sometimes the premium brand is a private market alternative. Private school tuition may buy a premium that you value, such as personalized attention, a proper religious perspective, socialization to the upper class, enrichment for superior students, or special services for problem children.

Double-Dip Cones: Incremental Tiers

By the age of four, I had learned to ask for double-dip cones. They had more ice cream than regular ones. Incremental tiers let you keep the regular scoop and add a second dip besides, with an optional different flavor. The Council of Europe (COE, 1993, pp. 94-95) recommends three scoops for old-age security, which it calls the "three-pillar model":

1. *state* social insurance to carry primary responsibility for the basic guaranteed minimum (adequacy),
2. *compulsory occupational welfare* to guarantee a retirement standard of living comparable to what you had while you were working (temporal equality), and
3. incentives for *individual retirement savings* (equity: you benefit from your meritorious prudence).

Swedish retirees often have four scoops:

1. The Basic Pension System provides a flat-rate benefit at age sixty-five. One hundred percent of retirees receive this (Circle 1 in Chapter 1).

2. The National Superannuation Pension provides a Social Security–type of wage-related pension to all employed persons. Most retirees qualify (Circle 2).
3. Most unionized workers have collective bargaining contracts for employer-financed pensions administered by a private insurance company. Maybe half of retirees receive these benefits (Circle 3).
4. Private personal pensions (similar to our Individual Retirement Accounts) grew rapidly after the government began to subsidize them in the 1980s with favorable tax rules (Circle 6).

During World War II, ice cream scoops became smaller. We had to buy two scoops to get what used to be in one. This has happened more recently to senior citizens. Originally, Medicare was intended as a single scoop to meet most of their health care needs. As inflation and political decisions eroded it, they had to add a second tier of private "medigap" insurance. Actually, the Social Security Administration recommends three scoops to each new retiree: (1) Part A, universal hospitalization benefits; (2) Part B, medical insurance for which retirees pay a monthly premium to the government, and (3) Part C, commercial "medigap" insurance for a range of medical services not covered under Part B.

Ice Milk: The Safety Net

One sad day, I encountered ice milk. It looked like ice cream, but it wasn't creamy and smooth: it was thin and watery. The premium and double-dip methods offer a standard level with optional supplements *above* them. The "safety net" goes the other way. In America, it is assumed that normal people should be able to "make it on their own." For those who fail, there is a thin ice-milk tier (the poorhouse, relief agencies, some state mental hospitals) *below* that standard level. Alfred Kahn has noted, "Services designed for poor people tend to be poor services" (1979, p. 79).

William Beveridge, credited with being the "father" of the modern welfare state, wrote, "In establishing the national minimum, [the state] should leave room for voluntary actions by each individual to provide more than the minimum for himself and his family" (1942, p. 17). Some ice-milk tiers offer the opportunity to add an equity scoop. This was the policy of the AFDC work-incentive programs of the 1960s and 1970s, in which a recipient who went to work could deduct work-related expenses and then keep the first $30 per month of net earnings, plus one-third of the remainder, and maintain Medicaid coverage. If you did the math, the benefits phased out, in most states, at about the poverty line. This ice-milk-plus incentive was eliminated in 1981.

Opposition to multiple tiers in general is based on *equality* arguments:

- Unequal opportunity is perpetuated when the privileged classes buy special advantages for their children.
- More lucrative second tiers may attract personnel who would otherwise be teaching and healing "ordinary folk" in the first tier.
- Private alternatives weaken support for basic programs. In communities in which wealthy children go to public school, support for quality public education is much stronger than in those in which such children go to private schools.

NONFAIRNESS DOCTRINES

Social policies are not necessarily based on any of the three fairness criteria (equality, equity, adequacy). Nonfairness doctrines should be distinguished from unfairness: the latter violates accepted fairness criteria. Nonfairness does not accept their validity, and it may stem from several different ideological bases.

Preordination affirmed a nonequity inequality built upon inherited wealth, status, and other advantages. A variation is the ancient idea of intergenerational personhood, that you live on through your "seed." If this is true, you enjoy the fruits of your labor when your children inherit advantages from you.

> Who is the man that fears the Lord?
> Him will He instruct in the way that he should choose.
> He himself shall abide in prosperity,
> And his children shall possess the land. (Psalm 25:12-13)

A less ideological variation is a cynical justification for passing on wealth and advantages to your children, which brings us back to "fair [fare] is something you get on the bus with." All that idealism about equity and being born equal is fine, but that isn't how it operates out there. Equal opportunity is a myth. If you naively refrain from seeking every possible competitive edge for your children, someone less scrupulous than you will take advantage of them. In the hierarchy of values, taking care of "me and mine" claims precedence over abstract equality and equity concepts.

Predestination legitimized both inequality and inadequacy. Inadequacy was hardly an inappropriate condition for someone destined for the ultimate state of inadequacy, eternal damnation.

Racism justified subhuman treatment of black slaves and Native Americans on the grounds that they were inferior species.

Social Darwinism, believing that the poor were genetically inferior, sought to improve the human race by letting poor children live below the subsistence level and die before reproducing a new generation of inferiors.

Collectivism doesn't accept high individual worth. The interest of the whole takes precedence over its parts (persons, families, groups). This includes Communism, as practiced in the twentieth century, and it also includes welfare economics (see Chapter 10), which subordinates the well-being of individual citizens to the aggregate economy. In its hierarchy of value-interests, issues of equality, equity, and adequacy don't exist. The 1980s' and 1990s' paradox of substantial growth in aggregate wealth in tandem with a declining standard of living for half the population is related, at least in part, to policies based on this viewpoint.

This relates to the doctrine of *less eligibility* (see Chapter 10). For nearly two centuries, this doctrine has taken precedence over adequacy as the basis for aid to the destitute. A healthy economy requires a pool of low-wage laborers; this can be maintained by making sure that "the pauper class is placed in its proper position below the condition of the independent laborer of the lowest class" (Chadwick, 1833, quoted in Schweinitz, 1961, p. 228). Although the term is archaic, the principle was the explicit rationale for the terms of the 1996 Welfare Reform Act.

Amorality takes a different perspective: it dismisses moral standards as irrelevant. I call this the *pyrite** rule: "Do unto others what

---

*Iron disulfide, commonly known as "fool's gold."

they would do unto you if they got the chance." Sometimes it is openly *predatory*. Powerful interests cynically pursue their own ends at the expense of the majority. In other cases, vested interests are claimed to coincide with the collective good. In 1952, CEO George Wilson, who later became Secretary of Defense, was unequivocal: "What's good for General Motors is good for America." Still others profess to espouse the "ideal" of adequacy in income, housing, health, education, etc.—but regretfully "we" cannot afford it or "they" are unwilling to support our efforts.

Property rights as a transcendent value means that any consideration of distribution must be in the context of the existing property status quo—whatever it is and however it may have been arrived at—as a nonnegotiable given. This argument is often also extended to unearned income resulting from ownership of property (e.g., capital gains).

A different rationale for disregarding distributional justice concepts such as equality, equity is libertarianism's absolute priority on negative freedom (see Chapter 8). The only limitation is that the exercise of your freedom may not deprive another of his or her freedom.

INEQUALITY AND REDISTRIBUTION

There's nothing surer, the rich get rich and the poor get poorer,
In the meantime, in between time, ain't we got fun.

"Ain't We Got Fun"
1921 song by Richard Whiting

Distribution is *who gets what* within the society. Although it may be applied to anything of value, including freedom, power, status, esteem, and opportunity, it usually refers to income (what you receive) and/or wealth (what you have accumulated). The terminology for distribution and redistribution uses an equality standard:

• *Progressive* redistribution reduces inequality.
• *Regressive* redistribution increases inequality.

How Much Equality?

Most Americans place a high value on equality. However, if pressed, we hedge. We strongly advocate horizontal equality, equal rewards (or treatment) within subgroups that have "like circumstances"—except of course where we ourselves have an advantage. We don't really want the same as everyone else. Like Garrison Keillor's Lake Wobegon, where "all the children are above average," we all aspire to do better than average.

The stated social policy of most nations is not precise equality but a limit on the degree of inequality:

> Modern industrial life, with its many demands, depends in large part on citizens' believing that they are being treated fairly in the distribution of a nation's resources. This equity . . . does not necessarily mean equality in incomes but some understandable relationship between income and contribution to society, which translates into a reasonable gradation between income classes at the bottom and at the top of the ladder. Reducing disparities in income among classes of workers, or between workers and the helpless . . . or redistributing income, are common ends and objectives. (Morris, 1988, p. 14)

Distribution and Inequalities

Historically, private sector economic market distribution has tended to increase the disparity between rich and poor in most times and places. One twentieth-century approach to counterbalance this is to *regulate distribution*. This may be done marginally through "rules of the game" that limit predatory, fraudulent, and exploitative practices or more extensively through central control of wages, prices, and profits.

In the United States from the 1930s to about 1970, market forces moved distribution moderately toward greater inequality. This was somewhat offset by the effects of (1) government regulation in the interests of equity (such as the Fair Labor Standards Act, the National Labor Relations Act, and minimum wage legislation) and (2) redistribution through progressive taxation and tax-supported health, education, and welfare programs.

As the 1970s and 1980s unfolded, changes in policy direction affected this balance. For example, collective bargaining rules permitted workers to strike if they and management could not agree: workers lost wages; the company lost profits. This was an incentive for both sides to find a mutually satisfactory compromise. Then, policy changes enabled companies to fire striking workers and hire hard-up new workers, often recent immigrants, at low wages. The balance of power shifted dramatically to employers, especially in semiskilled occupations. Workers faced two choices: accept less pay or be replaced. The employer gained either way.

Wage reductions in existing jobs were only part of the trend toward lower pay for half the workforce. Higher-paying industrial, technical, and administrative jobs were eliminated, many due to technological progress, while lower-paid service sector jobs expanded. Further, employers reported a trend toward replacing permanent full-time employees, having higher pay and benefits, with part-time and temporary workers at lower wages and no benefits.

As a result, in constant dollars, earnings of the top 10 percent of full-time workers rose more than 10 percent between 1980 and 1995, while the median wage of all workers fell $3^1/_2$ percent and the earnings of the lowest 10 percent of workers declined 10 percent (Reich, 1997).

The increase in inequality was even more dramatic when the salaries of average corporate employees were compared with those of their bosses. In 1960, the average after-tax income for large corporation chief executives was twelve times greater than their *lowest* paid workers. By 1994, their salary and bonuses added up to 117 times that of their *average* workers (Yates, 1995). In 1996, while Fortune 500 companies averaged an increase of 23 percent in profits and 54 percent in top executive pay, their workers averaged a 3 percent increase—just enough to match inflation. The CEO-to-worker income ratio had nearly doubled again, to 209. By comparison, European and Japanese CEOs earn twenty to thirty times as much as workers, not 200 times as much (Sklar, 1997).

Regressive fiscal policy changes further widened after-tax income disparities. The 1981 Tax Reform Act lowered income tax rates for corporations and upper-bracket individuals by about 40 percent (later reduced to about 25 percent), while raising the Social Security tax rate paid by wage earners. This was accompanied by an increase in tax welfare benefits for corporations and investors (see Chapter 1, Circle 9). Meanwhile, redistributive public health, education, and welfare programs were cut back, particularly those that served lower-income groups.

Overall, income inequality increased, especially at the top and the bottom. "Between 1979 and 1995, the inflation-adjusted income of the richest fifth of families grew by 26 percent while the income of the poorest fifth fell by 9 percent" (Reich, 1997, p. 27).

The effects of this trend appear in worldwide comparisons. In the mid-1990s, the top 1 percent of families had 42 percent of American wealth, twice their 1972 share. In 1994, the top fifth of households received 47 percent of all income, about eleven times the share of the lowest fifth's 4.2 percent, the widest disparity in a half century.

Consequently, the United States became one of the most unequal countries in the world, along with Brazil, Britain, and Guatemala, in each of which the poorest fifth survive on less than one-quarter of national per capita income. By comparison, the gap is only half as great in such countries as Japan and The Netherlands (United Nations, 1996).

Redistribution and Equalizing

There are three public policy methods to reduce inequality. One is to equalize individual opportunity through universal and/or compensatory development programs, such as a quality public education, and to minimize the incidence and severity of debilitating conditions, particularly at the primary and secondary prevention stages, through universal health programs.

A second is to ensure market honesty and fairness to workers, consumers, and businesses in such areas as antitrust provisions, honesty in advertising, consumer product standards, fair labor standards, equal opportunity employment, and banking regulation (see Chapter 12).

The third is a progressive second-round *re*allocation to offset some of the effects of a regressive private sector dynamic. A "redistribution transfer" is "a payment from one to another that does not arise from current productive activity" (Jacobs, 1993, p. 90). Redistribution may be horizontal among peers, through private or public insurance, temporal, through pension plans that return in "lean" retirement years what they took out in "fat cow" working years, or vertical, through taxing "haves" to pay for services to "have-nots."

Taxes are progressive when the wealthy pay a higher *percentage* of their income than do the less affluent. In the United States, personal income taxes are progressive (but less so than many of its European peers), as are business profits taxes, the costs of which tend to be "shifted backward" to wealthy stockholders in the form of reduced dividends. A potentially progressive tax is inheritance taxes, as in the United States, where a large amount is exempt, after which the tax rate progresses steeply.

Taxes that take a higher percentage from lower incomes are regressive. The most common one is the sales tax and its cousin, the value-added tax (VAT), the costs of which are "shifted forward" to consumers in the form of higher prices. Low-income families spend much of their income immediately on taxed *goods*. Wealthy families can afford to save some of their income and spend more of the rest on *services*, which are taxed less often. Because they spend a smaller percentage of their income on taxable items, their sales tax "rate" is lower. The 1981 tax reforms mentioned earlier were regressive because they lowered the percentage of income paid as taxes by the wealthy, while slightly increasing the percentage paid by the poorest taxpayers.

Social Security wage taxes are flat (same percentage for incomes of all levels) among lower- and middle-income workers but regressive as a percentage of total income between middle- and upper-income groups. The latter pay a smaller percentage of their income because they do not pay the tax on wages above a certain amount (about $70,000 at the time of this writing) nor on their often considerable "unearned" income from investments.

Government spending that tends to benefit lower-income persons, such as Medicaid, welfare, public housing, and food stamps, is progressive redistribution. Tax welfare such as mortgage deductions and corporate welfare are regressive, as are expressways that primarily serve suburban commuters because they redistribute benefits toward higher-income persons. Some benefits are difficult to classify. For instance, who gains the most from Medicaid, the low-income patients who receive the service or the upper-income physicians and health corporation investors who receive the money for services rendered?

The bottom line on redistribution is the net effect of taxation and expenditure combined. Means-tested welfare programs, financed from progressive taxes and paying benefits only to low-income people, are very progressive. Public education is less progressive, benefiting all income levels but at more cost to wealthier property owners. Government matching of gifts to private universities and the arts through tax deductions, however desirable, is doubly regressive because it lowers the taxes of upper-income people, and the services thus subsidized also tend to benefit the upper-class group.

Rationale for Redistribution

According to Social philosopher Leslie Jacobs, redistribution is an application of the principle of *comparative justice:*

> Comparative justice suggests that the burden of helping the needy should fall more heavily on those with more resources at hand because, as the resource-based approach implies, they are likely to have fewer unmet needs in comparison with other individuals against whom this right is held. The practical force of this point is that it shows why a state is justified to implement a progressive taxation system for funding its actions designed to help the needy. (1993, p. 179)

S. M. Miller and Charles Collins (1996) view redistribution in the context of equity-fairness and democracy:

> One reason for direct redistribution is that the burden of social change should be borne by all groups in society. When the costs of social change are ignored, the vulnerable and poorly off largely pay the bill rather than those who can more easily absorb these costs and often are its principal beneficiaries. . . . They are gaining from the new economy but do not do their bit to reduce the burdens on the rest of us. . . . Perhaps the greatest distortion resulting from the concentration of income and wealth is that it results in a concentration of political power. Money shapes politics and extracts policy decisions at all governmental levels. . . . Concentration undermines democratic practice. (p. 8)

Chapter 8

Negative Freedom and Individualism

Every man, as long as he does not violate the laws of justice, is left perfectly free to pursue his own interest his own way, and to bring both his industry and capital into competition with those of any other man or order of men.

Adam Smith, 1776

This is a free country. I can do as I please! Is it? Can I? Should I be able to? How does doing what I please affect other people? How does their exercise of freedom affect me?

Liberty is "freedom to choose." There are two dimensions to liberty and two corollary dimensions of justice. *Negative freedom* is the *absence* of external interference in making individual choices. *Negative justice* is, in the spirit of the Ten Commandments, to *refrain* from direct hurtful actions (steal, kill, defraud, violate a contractual agreement), but there is, on the other hand, no obligation to take any positive actions. If I fall into deep water, you may freely ignore my cry for help.

Positive freedom is the *presence* of means to exercise the choice that negative freedom theoretically permits. *Positive justice* goes beyond refraining from direct harm to affirmative actions that protect and promote the well-being of others. It is the basis for civil rights (beyond the narrower sphere of civil liberty), equalization of opportunity, humanitarian programs, charitable activities, and response to need. Positive justice requires that if I fall into deep water, you should help me to the fullest extent you reasonably can. (Ethics philosophers argue on where the line of "reasonable" stops.)

FOUR KINDS OF "LIBERAL"

In his successful 1988 presidential campaign, George Bush scored major political gains, when he implied a vaguely subversive un-Americanism to his opponent by accusing him of "the L word" ("liberal") and ridiculed him as "a card-carrying liberal."

This is amusing—and confusing. We call antigovernment champions of individualism, such as Rowley and Peacock (1975) and Milton Friedman, economic guru to the Reagan Administration, "conservatives." Yet, Rowley and Peacock proudly present themselves as spokespersons for a Liberal Party ideology, and Friedman (1962, p. 12) summarized his market economics ideology with the assertion that "as liberals we take freedom of the individual . . . as our ultimate goal in judging social arrangements."

This illustrates the confusion about the meaning of *liberal*. Derived from the Latin word for free, it is used to describe four applications of "free": (1) negative freedom, (2) open-mindedness, (3) sharing and caring, and (4) positive freedom. A given person may be "liberal" in one or all of these ways.

Classical liberals embrace *negative freedom*. The British Liberal Party, formed by nineteenth-century capitalists, remains a champion of free-market economics with a minimum of government intervention. The American Civil Liberties Union, often ironically mislabeled by opponents as leftist, exists solely to defend individual freedoms, particularly those spelled out in the Bill of Rights.

Liberal thinkers are creative and open to new ideas. The liberal arts are committed to the *free flow of ideas*. This overlaps into negative freedom in the spirit of Voltaire, who reportedly said, "I disapprove of what you say, but I will defend to the death your right to say it."

Humanitarian liberals are committed to individual well-being through *giving freely*. Private philanthropy, neighborliness, and volunteer service are expressions of this value, as are tax-supported public health and welfare services.

Social justice liberals emphasize *positive freedom*, equalizing the opportunity of each American to exercise her or his freedom in practice. This has been a theme of labor unions, civil rights and feminist groups, the settlement house movement, Catholic and Protestant social ministries, and Jewish communal organizations. It was the rationale for establishing public schools and later for desegregating them.

NEGATIVE FREEDOM

In the tradition of John Locke, Patrick Henry, John Stuart Mill, and the Bill of Rights, classical liberals define liberty as the absence of outside interference with an individual's choice. In addition to government, this principle refers to intrusion by employers, "moral majorities" who presume to prescribe what you can and cannot do in your private life, and predators (both legal and illegal) who deprive you of choice for their private gain. This is called negative freedom. Economist Friedrich von Hayek (1960, p.19) gives the term an upbeat spin:

> It is often objected that our concept of liberty is merely negative. This is true in the sense that peace is also a negative concept . . . it describes the absence of a particular obstacle—coercion by other men. It becomes positive only through what we make of it. It does not assure us of any particular opportunities, but leaves it to us to decide what use we shall make of the circumstances in which we find ourselves.

Classical liberals have three social policy priorities, according to Rowley and Peacock (1975, pp. 86-90). The first is intellectual and moral freedom, without which "the notions of political and economic freedom may be rendered meaningless, however wide they may seem to be in a superficial sense."

- Freedom of *religion* and *conscience* permit us to worship as we please or not at all and to refuse to do what we believe to be wrong.
- *Speech, press,* and *academic* freedom permit us to speak and hear, read and write, study and teach, without censorship or reprisals.
- Freedom of *privacy* and *nonconformity* permit us to conduct our private lives as we choose, regardless of the prevailing orthodoxy.

A *second* priority is to prevent "concentrations of political and economic power, whether in the hands of the State, of bureaucrats, of firms or of private citizens" because of the "difficulty of eliminating discretionary power and its abuses once established" (Rowley and Peacock, 1975, pp. 86-90). *Political* liberty is derived from John Locke's (1690) social-compact theory that government is a voluntary creation of free individuals for the sole purpose of protecting their lives, liberty, and property.

- Freedom of *assembly* and *coalition* permits citizens to meet on any subject or issue and to combine with others for common purposes.
- Freedom to *vote* (by secret ballot) and run for office enables citizens to select and guide their government without intimidation.
- Freedom of *revolution*, says the Declaration of Independence (but not the Constitution), means that when a government deviates from the social compact, "it is the right of the people to alter or to abolish it and to institute a new government."

Economic freedoms are rooted in Adam Smith's (1776) economic theories:

- *Market* freedom is the right to buy and sell both goods and labor at a price agreeable to all parties. This includes freedom of consumption and of contract (to enter into binding agreements).
- Freedom of *occupation* and *enterprise* permit unrestricted entry and open competition with others in all employment and business areas.
- Included in the previous two is freedom of *travel* and *migration* in pursuit of economic and social goals.

The *third* priority is *procedural protections,* especially "due process" and "equal treatment under the law," as expressed in the original Constitution, Bill of Rights, and Fourteenth Amendment.

LIMITING FREEDOM

Liberty as a Default Value

Negative freedom is a default value in our society: it automatically applies unless there is a compelling reason to the contrary. This position was effectively put forth in an official British statement on homosexuality:

> [Law's] function, as we see it, is to preserve public order and decency, to protect the citizen from what is offensive or injurious and to provide sufficient safeguards against exploitation and corruption of others. . . . It is not, in our view, the function of law to intervene in the private lives of citizens or to seek to enforce any particular pattern of behavior, further than is necessary to carry out the purposes we have outlined. (Wolfenden Report, 1957, paragraphs 13-14; as quoted in Glennester, 1995, p. 155)

Each Other's Freedom

John Stuart Mill set one limit: "The liberty of the individual must be thus far limited; he must not make himself a nuisance to other people" (1859, p. 817). When the freedoms of two parties are mutually exclusive, something has to give. A recurring policy dilemma is whose freedom takes precedence—and why?

- Does freedom of the press justify violation of an individual's freedom of privacy in the area of consenting sexual behavior? Does the priority change if that individual is a celebrity or a politician?
- May residents of a retirement community exercise their freedom of contract by entering into restrictive covenants that deny market freedom to families with children?
- To protect the market freedom of customers and competitors, can government restrict freedom of enterprise by prohibiting monopolies and "sharp" practices?
- To protect the occupational freedom of women and minorities, may an owner be denied the freedom to hire whom he or she pleases, for whatever reason he or she chooses?

Protection from Others

To what extent is it desirable to exchange freedom for well-being? How much and for what? John Locke (1690) described "man in the state of nature" as free but in constant danger from predatory fellow men. His social compact defined a minimum *trade-off of freedom for security:*

> The great and chief end, therefore, of men uniting into commonwealths, and putting themselves under government, is the *preservation of their property;* to which in the state of nature there are many things wanting. *Firstly,* there wants an established, settled, known law, received and allowed by common consent to be the standard of right and wrong, and the common measure to decide all controversies between them. . . . *Secondly* in the state of nature there wants a known and indifferent judge, with authority to determine all differences according to the established law. . . . *Thirdly,* in the state of nature there often wants power to back and support the sentence when right, and to give it due execution. (pp. 806-807)

The Preamble to the Constitution emphasizes the protective role of government: establish justice, ensure the domestic tranquility, provide for the common defense, secure the blessings of liberty. We go well beyond Locke's basic police protection and due process: Libel laws limit the use of free speech to hurt others. National security laws deny freedom of the press for information that might "give aid and comfort to our enemies." Consumer protection regulations restrict free enterprise.

Protection from Ourselves

Mill said, "The only purpose for which power can be rightfully exercised over any member of a civilized society against his will is to prevent harm to others. He cannot rightfully be compelled to do so or forebear because it will be better for him, because it will make him happy, or because in the opinion of others to do so would be wise or even right" (1859, p. 810).

By those criteria, we would accept limits on our freedom to hurt others but not to protect us from ourselves. Laws might restrict my freedom to push drugs but not my freedom to smoke pot and even cultivate a marijuana patch for personal consumption. Laws might keep me from driving drunk but not from refusing to wear a helmet when motorcycling.

Every nation does enact "for your own good" policies. Our dilemma: in the conflict between freedom and protection, what is important enough to control? When is the process of freedom more important than the consequences? Are there general guidelines?

In the United States, we are divided and inconsistent about where to draw the line. We restrict "downers" in pill form but permit unlimited consumption of alcohol. We outlaw marijuana and subsidize tobacco.

In another "for your own good area," involuntary commitment of mentally ill persons judged to be a danger to themselves is well accepted—but we want due process to protect us from the Soviet practice of using this device to incarcerate sane political dissidents who had committed no crime.

Our "for your own good" policies are not all negative. A "positive" restriction of freedom is compulsory education. We hedge this requirement in ways intended to minimize the external interference with freedom of choice. Some parents believe that education must be provided within the context of their specific religious beliefs. Others want to give their children better schooling than their local school provides. Our policies offer free public education but also permit alternative private and home schooling, so long as parents provide the education the child will need when he or she grows up. The latter is done through minimum learning standards, which can be met in one of two ways: accreditation of the private school or annual exams taken by individual students.

We need to watch "for your own good" rationales in a society that relies so heavily on cost-benefit analysis. Is a decision to deny the freedom to smoke really for the smoker's sake or to save society billions of dollars annually in medical care? Do we support a freedom to die policy for the patient's sake or because it may save us $100,000 for his or her terminal care? Do we require education for the individual's benefit or for economic development payoffs? The ulterior motive may also be a good reason for limiting negative freedom, but if so, deal with it where it belongs—in the individual freedom versus general welfare dilemma area (to be discussed in the following material).

Clients with Impairments

Presumably, we must make exceptions for people who are unable to make all of their own free choices. Young children, psychotics, and Alzheimer's patients have conditions that render them dependent. Others have lesser physical, mental, emotional, educational, or social disabilities. It would be convenient to draw a line and say, "These people need a protective and controlling level of care; these do not." However, disabilities vary not only in degree, but in kind. A person who is physically dependent may be fully competent and highly productive mentally.

In each situation, several policy questions must be addressed:

- What level of control is *unavoidable?* Are you sure? Why?
- What level of control is *best for that individual?* Why?
- What level of control is *best for society?* Why?
- What are the *civil rights and liberties* of persons judged by society to be dependent? To what extent does a mentally ill patient being institutionalized or a twelve-year-old being placed in foster care have a right to due process?

In recent years, a consensus among libertarians, humanitarians, and fiscal conservatives has focused on the concept of *normalization*, the least restrictive setting possible in each case. Where effective community support systems have been developed, this approach may successfully blend the values of negative freedom, client well-being, and cost reduction. However, in other instances, the inadequacy of community supports (too much "freedom") has been harmful to the patient and costly to society in the long run.

The General Welfare

In an article on computerized invasion of privacy, titled "Why fear data rape?", Amatai Etzioni (1996) asked, "Will all these new kinds of knowledge techniques lead to a police state as civil libertarians constantly warn us?" His answer was, "Giving up some measure of privacy is exacctly what the community requires." His criteria were (1) a compelling need, (2) no alternative way to meet the need, and (3) safeguards against abuse and undesirable side effects.

His list of "compelling" needs to invade our privacy included fingerprinting all schoolteachers, child care workers, welfare recipients, and unemployment insurance applicants, "to catch the few frauds"; collection and sale of personal credit information by commercial businesses, without the consent of the individuals; information that one's neighbor was convicted of pederasty; and firing of public employees who default on their college loans or child support payments.

The Constitution commits the government to provide for the general welfare. Health, education, and welfare services are financed by mandatory taxes that reduce our economic freedom to spend part of what we earn as we see fit. Although most people agree that some of this trade-off of freedom for well-being is desirable, they disagree among themselves on what and how much. Even the nearly unanimous commitment to universal public education has been undermined by taxpayer revolts, often led by childless taxpayers or older citizens whose children are already educated.

It gets confusing when the same people who argue strongly for freedom in one situation are intensely against it in another. For instance, many who object to mandatory Social Security as an invasion of their personal freedom are eager to deny personal body freedom to women. Two concepts discussed in earlier chapters offer possible explanations. One is hierarchy of value-interests. Embryonic life may be a transcendent value, while life in old age is given low value. Thus, the former transcends freedom, while the latter is not important enough to do so. The other concept is double standard. People may cry foul at any policy which conflicts with their preferences, while taking a cavalier attitude toward ones which coincide with what they had already chosen to do.

Economic Freedom: Property Rights

Under strict negative freedom, I have the right to buy, own, use, and sell property as I choose. A standard limitation is that the property cannot be acquired at the expense of any other person's property, such as by theft, extortion, or fraud.

Another widely accepted restriction is that I can't use my property in a way which lowers your property's value. Can I divert water from a river flowing through my land to the extent that it deprives farmers and cities downstream of water on which they depend? No? Then how about just enough water to irrigate my crops? Can I build a lard-rendering plant on your residential block? No? Then how about an apartment complex?

Another question is whether there are different kinds of property with different rules. Lesley Jacobs makes a useful distinction between two kinds of property, personal and fungible (impersonal). In a hierarchy of values, the first is given high priority as an extension of the person and therefore subject to the stricter standards of personal negative freedom. The second carries a lower value, subordinate to human values and the general welfare, and therefore may be compromised within reason on behalf of the general welfare.

> *Personal property* is property we closely associate with our personal identity . . . a wedding ring, a family heirloom or a home. Because personal property is so closely linked to our personal identity it cannot be completely replaced by money or some other commodity. *Fungible property* is, in contrast, completely commodifiable . . . money or some other commodity can be substituted for that property without a loss. Its ownership is not intrinsic to one's personal identity. . . . The point then is that there can be full liberal rights of ownership in private property but not in fungible property. Thus, taxation of fungible private property would not involve the violation of rights. (1993, p. 81)

Exploitation

All examples given so far are freedom restrictions that the advocates truly believe are best for our society. Controls may also be imposed in bad faith for exploitative reasons, as in slavery, dictatorships, or the oppression of workers by the old "robber baron capitalists."

CLASSICAL INDIVIDUALISM

> *From each according to what he chooses; to each according to what he makes for himself.*

> Robert Nozick, 1974

In a community regulated by the laws of demand and supply,
the persons who become rich are, generally speaking, indus-
trious, resolute, proud, prompt, methodical, sensible, unimagi-
native, insensitive, covetous, and ignorant.

John Ruskin

An ape was seen pacing his cage with a Bible under one arm and
Darwin's *Origin of the Species* under his other. The keeper came
closer and heard him mumbling, "Am I my brother's keeper or my
keeper's brother?" If you believe in both creationism and individualism, the answer is "none of the above."

In Genesis, when God asked Cain about his younger brother
Abel, whom Cain had killed, Cain defiantly replied, "Am I my
brother's keeper?" Was he? Are you? To what extent?

Charles Murray in *Losing Ground* gives as unequivocal answer:
"Why should one person give *anything* to a stranger whose only
claim to his help is common citizenship?" (1984, p. 197).

David Harriman of the Ayn Rand Institute rejects the idea of
social responsibility as the antithesis of liberty. Each citizen "is an
end in himself, not a means to the ends of society. His highest
purpose is the pursuit of his own happiness. The benefits we enjoy
in America were created . . . by individuals selfishly pursuing their
own ends" (1997).

The dictionary defines individualism as "the pursuit of individual
rather than common or collective interests." It "emphasizes the right-
ness of individual self-seeking, the individual's voluntary selection of
goals and objectives, the ownership and transfer of property . . . and
the obligation that individuals provide for the material welfare of themselves and their dependents" (Kuenne, 1993, p. 56).

In economics, the "justice as freedom" perspective was developed by Friedrich von Hayek's "Austrian School" and Milton
Friedman's "Chicago School." Kuenne summarizes it as "egoistic
free choice," without the principles of "social corrective" (governmental regulation) or "social compassion" (services to the disadvantaged) (Ibid., p. 56). Its influence is observable in the policies of
the United States, Switzerland, and Austria, in contrast with those
of nations with a stronger tradition of common identity, such as

Sweden, Germany, and Japan. This difference appears in a comparison between our social welfare policies and theirs.

The ethics of individualism say that, although you can't actively harm your brother, you don't have to help him. In the parable of the Good Samaritan, individualism would affirm the priest and the Levite who walked around the victim. (The Good Samaritan is okay too because his helping was an individual preference. The ethic doesn't say you cannot, only that you need not.)

Arthur Clough, a contemporary of John Stuart Mill, satirized the individualism ethic in *The Latest Decalogue* (1862):

> Thou shalt not kill but needst not strive
> Officiously to keep alive . . .
> Thou shalt not covet; but tradition
> Approves all forms of competition.

Martin Hewitt (1992, p. 39) summarizes individualism's social policy position: "The state which privileges the rights of the deprived over others . . . leads to an unjust hierarchy of values and a false ideology of social justice, rights, and needs." This policy viewpoint appears to be based on three premises about the human condition:

1. Individuals can control their lives by exercising their free will.
2. Everyone has roughly equal opportunity to "get ahead."
3. The basic human right is a hunting license ("pursuit of happiness"), as distinct from the Catholic bishops' belief (quoted in Chapter 4) that "society as a whole, acting through public and private institutions, has the moral responsibility to enhance human dignity and protect human rights."

This view has many thoughtful critics. Arthur Dyck examines historical origins of these beliefs: "The key problem with Hobbes is that he equates rights with egoistic, asocial, individual wants and whereas he regards these as primary and natural, he regards obligations and communities as artificial, attained only by force" (1994, p. 36).

Carol Gilligan (1982, p. 155) gives it a modern, psychology spin: "There seems to be a line of development missing from current depictions of adult development, a failure to describe the progress of relationship toward a maturity of interdependence." Fellow parents, is she recalling, as I do, the "terrible twos" period in our children's development?

Robert Goodin is more blunt. Describing individualism in much the same way as Hobbes, he concludes, "such behavior is blatantly immoral" (1986, p. 166).

John Tropman considers the price we must pay for individualism from another angle: "'Struggle for such things as liberty, one's own job, and the goods of life generally is a constant in life. One can never relax . . . because of the possibility of erosion" (1989, p. 98).

Optimistic and Pessimistic Rationales

Individualism has been justified by both high and low beliefs about human nature. An optimistic rationale for individualism, based on the "natural law" of classical economics, assumes that "the good of all will best be served if each individual pursues his self-interest with minimal interference . . . unhampered by government restriction, unchallenged by labor organizations" (Wilensky and Lebeaux, 1965, p. 34).

Andrew Carnegie expressed this view in *The Gospel of Wealth* (1900).

> The "good old times" were not good old times. Neither master nor servant was as well situated then as today. A relapse to old conditions would be disastrous to both—not the least to him who serves. . . . The poor enjoy what the rich could not before afford. What were the luxuries have become the necessaries of life. The laborer has now more comforts than the farmer had a few generations ago. The farmer has more luxuries than the landlord had, and is more richly clad and better housed. . . . Individualism, Private Property, the Law of Accumulation of Wealth, and the Law of Competition; these are the highest result of human experience, the soil in which society, so far, has produced the best fruits. (pp. 618, 619, 621)

Vic George and Paul Wilding report that human-nature *pessimists* espouse competitive individualism for a different reason, namely as a bulwark against a greater danger—centralized power in the hands of a corrupt and fallible few:

> Individualism prefers to view man not as highly rational and intelligent but as a very irrational and fallible being, whose individual errors are corrected only in the course of a social process. For this reason no one can have a panoramic view of society and can know what ought or ought not to be done on a grand scale. . . . The spontaneous network of individual checks and counterchecks is enough to eliminate excessive demands, unworkable plans and so on by particular individuals. Any serious interference with this process by the State is bound to produce more harm than good. Competition even by imperfect and irrational men is the ideal road to progress. (1976, p. 8)

Individualism and Personal Prospects

In an earlier chapter, we noted that interests influence values. This correlates with Tropman's observation on who espouses an individualism ideology as opposed to the positive freedom/fraternité vantage point:

> Our society prefers self to group advancement. Part of our preference, however, may relate to our perception of whether times are good or bad. If we perceived that times are good and the resources for individual gain are available and even plentiful, we opt for self gain. If, on the other hand, times are bad or resources are limited or even receding, then we may opt for group gain (spreading the misery or group loss). (1989, pp. 71-72)

INDIVIDUALISM AND TRUSTEESHIP

The bread that you store up belongs to the hungry; the cloak that lies in your chest belongs to the naked; and the gold that you have hidden in the ground belongs to the poor.

St. Basil

A trust is:

- something received and the responsibility or obligation resulting from this (moral), or
- nominal ownership of property which one is to keep, use, or administer for another's benefit (legal).

Andrew Carnegie made it big, from poor immigrant to one of the richest men in the world. He didn't get there by being Mr. Nice Guy. He played hardball with his competitors, ruthlessly oppressed his workers, and exploited his customers through monopolistic price-fixing. He believed that this fierce individualism was not only in his best interests, but also best for society. He projected that such practices would lead to a meritocracy, for the ablest would rise to the top of the power and wealth ladder.

Deeply religious according to his lights, he developed his "gospel of wealth," which adapted the idea of noblesse oblige to individualistic meritocracy. He believed that God specially blessed people such as himself—but that they held this wealth as a trust from God to be used for the common weal:

> Thus is the problem of rich and poor to be solved. The laws of accumulation will be left free. . . . Individualism will continue, but the millionaire will be but a trustee for the poor . . . entrusted for a season with a great part of the wealth of the community, but administering it for the community better than it could or would have done for itself. . . . There is no mode of disposing of surplus wealth creditable to thoughtful and earnest men into whose hands it flows, save by using it year by year for the general good. . . . The man who dies rich thus dies disgraced. (Carnegie, 1900, pp. 624-625)

The Carnegie Foundation today is a legal trust, operated by trustees who disburse the funds in the interest of literacy and world peace.

Social Catholicism, strong in Europe since the late-nineteenth century, was a major factor in the development of Germany's postwar, private sector–oriented social state (discussed in later chapters). It expected each worker to be honest, cooperative, industrious, and loyal. Each employer must have the same qualities, "but in addition ensure to the best of his ability that his workers live as well and as morally as possible on the job and off" (Golob, 1954, p. 549).

This carries trusteeship beyond Carnegie's focus on money, to the way in which an entrepreneur relates to people who are subject to his or her power. At this point, we are still on the private enterprise/individualism side of the line, but we are beginning to move toward the subject of the next chapter, positive freedom and fraternité.

Chapter 9

Positive Freedom and Fraternité

The world has never had a good definition of "liberty," and the people just now are much in want of one. We all declare for liberty; but using the same word we do not all mean the same thing.

Abraham Lincoln, 1864

The love of liberty is the love of others; the love of power is the love of ourselves.

William Hazlitt

By fraternité only will liberté be saved.

Victor Hugo

POSITIVE FREEDOM

Negative freedom is the *absence* of external interference in making individual choices. Positive freedom is the *presence* of means to exercise the choice that negative freedom theoretically permits. Academic freedom isn't worth much if you can't read and write. Market freedom is useless if you are broke. Occupational freedom was a mockery in 1931, when one-third of the workforce couldn't find *any* jobs.

The first requisite for positive freedom is negative freedom. This is illustrated by the dual objectives of the civil rights movement: Its first task was to achieve negative freedoms by removing external discriminatory barriers in such areas as voting, occupation, public accommodations, and housing. Then the task shifted to equalizing ability to exercise the newly won freedoms, by restoring positive freedoms that had been subverted by institutionalized racism, sexism, and classism.

Four key social policy areas affect positive freedom:

1. *Economic adequacy and security.* Lord Beveridge (1945), architect of the British welfare state, pointed out, "Liberty means more than freedom from the arbitrary power of governments. It means freedom from economic servitude to Want and Squalor and other social evils" (p. 9). Franklin Roosevelt, observing Nazi Germany and Fascist Italy, warned, "Democracy has disappeared in several other great nations because the people of those nations had grown tired of unemployment and insecurity. . . . In desperation they chose to sacrifice liberty in the hope of getting something to eat" (quoted in Trattner, 1994, p. 288).

2. *Relative equality*—social, economic, and political. "Freedom rests on equality because if there are major inequalities of resources or power, some men are in bondage to others. The fundamental ideal of liberty . . . is power to control the condition of one's own life—and this means equality" (George and Wilding, 1976, p. 66).

3. *Participation* in collective decisions affecting one's life. "Economic freedom means that men should have a voice in the conditions of their work, that they should be recognized as possessing certain rights in relation to it, that no one should be in a position to exercise arbitrary power of regulation or dismissal over them" (Ibid.). Collective bargaining, social development, organizing for political action, and "maximum feasible participation" of consumers and employees on governing boards are positive freedom strategies.

4. *Personal resources,* such as physical and mental health, knowledge and skills, aspirations, self-esteem, and confidence. Among programs that contribute to this are universal health care, prenatal services, mental health, rehabilitation, and perhaps most important of all, education. The United Negro College Fund high-

lighted positive freedom with its long-running slogan, "A mind is a terrible thing to waste."

Those who have suffered inequality, deprivation, or disability appreciate the importance of positive freedom. Those who already have the positive resources listed previously tend to think of liberty only in terms of negative freedom, for freedom from outside intervention is all *they* need. Rowley and Peacock express this comfortable viewpoint.

> [To] advocates of positive freedom . . . the demand for freedom is the demand for power to be attained and protected by legislation. . . . This is the philosophy of "bastard" liberalism as currently preached in the United States. The granting of this effective power brings with it the power of coercion for some individuals to wield over others and this is the negation of freedom. (1975, p. 85)

So they said. Yet, later in their discussion, they called for government to use its power to preserve their negative market freedom through coercive antitrust measures against competitors too powerful for them to handle. It would appear that the real issue after all is not whether to intervene for positive freedom but rather where, how, and for whom.

PROCEDURAL JUSTICE

A key positive freedom area is procedural justice, also known as equal employment opportunity or EEO, which can be represented by a three-legged stool. The first leg is negative freedom to apply; the second is an equity selection system; the third leg is a "level playing field," on which no competitor is given an advantage or a handicap.

Passive EEO—Pure Procedural Justice

John Rawls (1971) advocated the negative freedom side of equal opportunity, which he called "pure" procedural justice. "Those who

(1) are at the same level of talent and ability and (2) have the same willingness to use them, should have the same prospects of success, regardless of their initial place in the social system; that is, irrespective of the income class into which they are born" (p. 74).

This is *as-is equal opportunity*. It is pure negative freedom, eliminating all direct discriminations, whether against (as in racism and sexism) or in favor (as in "connections"). Candidates are evaluated on their merit *at that moment,* based on traditionally accepted measures, such as standardized tests, degrees, experience, and credentials. "The great advantage of pure procedural justice is that it is no longer necessary in meeting the demands of justice to keep track of the endless variety of circumstances and the changing relative positions of particular persons" (Ibid., p. 87).

This is also its great weakness. It disregards any advantage, related to inherited privilege or deprivation, past discriminations for or against, or institutionalized racism, sexism, and classism factors in our society that gave one candidate an advantage over another one of equal caliber.

As-is equal opportunity is sufficient for applicants whose only barrier is direct discrimination. When I was a student at Princeton, which was located within sixty miles of a majority community of all Jewish Americans, it had a reported 10 percent quota for Jews and admitted no women regardless of their ability. After adopting as-is equal opportunity, the university accepted my daughter into a class that was half female and perhaps a third Jewish. All these two groups had needed was pure procedural justice.

The second leg of the stool, selection on merit, can be enhanced by *correcting measurement biases.* My academic program used the Millers Analogy Test (MAT), in which you tell whether a given item is most analogous to A, B, C, or D, as a predictor of academic ability. On review, it turned out that high scores did correlate with high performance, but low scorers varied across the spectrum from low to high performance. I asked those students with low scores but high performance levels about their test experience. The consistent answer: "Doing the analogies was easy except that on a lot of the questions I wasn't familiar with the items being compared." These students came from a variety of nonmainstream backgrounds: rural, inner-city, low-income, English as a second language, a minority subculture, or a combination.

The test measured three things: vocabulary, mainstream American culture, *and* reasoning ability. Low scores indicated a deficit in any one of the three, two of which did not predict academic potential. It is therefore an error to use the MAT as a universal equal employment opportunity measure. (However, since high scores are reliable positive indicators, it is an appropriate EEO tool for applicants who had low GPA scores from undergraduate years, to submit for consideration as evidence of here-and-now academic readiness.)

Full Procedural Justice: Positive Freedom of Opportunity

By happenstance, some of us were born into an affluent, stable, professional family, which offered many social and educational advantages. Others with comparable potential experienced severe poverty, racism, sexism, and other diswelfares. Although tribulation can be overcome, and privilege may be dissipated, pure procedural justice gives some of us an unearned competitive advantage due to what Rawls (1971) calls "historical and social fortune."

This reality was confirmed by a University of Chicago study, which tracked 25,000 teenagers over six years, beginning in the eighth grade, "that focused on potential barriers to choice and access in higher education." This study reported that "74 percent of those in the most affluent quarter of the group attended four-year schools [while] only 37 percent in the lowest income quarter attended four year institutions" (*The New York Times,* 1996)

Full procedural justice calls for *positive freedom* to actualize the theoretical potentials of negative freedom. The "like circumstances" cohort group must be broadened to include all players, not just the winners of the historical and social fortune sweepstakes. This requires some form of corrective action to equalize opportunity in the pursuit of life, liberty, and property. The question is how best to do this.

There are several basic approaches, which are not mutually exclusive. One is to *reduce advantages.* Elimination of private prep schools, for example, would narrow inequalities by lowering the ceiling.

In his *Intelligent Women's Guide to Socialism,* George Bernard Shaw proposed the opposite tack, *reduce disadvantages:* "Instead of sympathizing with the poor and abolishing the rich, we must ruthlessly abolish the poor—by raising their standard of life."

Strategies for this include universalistic programs that provide high quality services and benefits to all citizens. Rawls wrote, "Chances to acquire cultural knowledge and skills should not depend upon one's class position, and so the school system, whether public or private, should be designed to even out class barriers" (1971, p. 73). In our present job market, this may need to include post–high school education and training. Other universalistic programs that reduce disadvantages in many nations include health care, family allowances, free school lunches, and housing developments.

Disadvantages can also be reduced through *enhancements* of the social system, such as economic development, countercyclical fiscal and monetary interventions, full employment initiatives, collective bargaining rights, minimum wage laws, and community organization for mutual assistance and/or political action.

AFFIRMATIVE ACTION

Given the inherent inequalities of a market economy, a legacy of institutionalized racism, sexism, and classism in most societies, and the limitations (or absence) of policies and programs that prevent them, disadvantages from past inequities are a fact of life. After touring East Harlem with Don Benedict, cofounder of the East Harlem Protestant Parish, world-famous theologian Paul Tillich returned in shock, mumbling, "Cumulative evil! Cumulative evil!"

Accumulated inequities need to be corrected by *compensatory* interventions to *equalize* opportunity: this is called *affirmative* action. These positive interventions can be external, internal, or both.

Internal Compensatory Development

Compensatory development involves extra input in such areas as education, training, confidence building, and mentoring, which enable diswelfared persons to gain parity with the advantaged members of their cohorts.

The Goodrich Program at my university does just this; it takes in disadvantaged students who give evidence of high potential. During their first two years of college, they attend enrichment courses and receive tutoring, counseling, and other support services in addition to financial aid. In their last two years, they are on their own within their respective departments across the campus, with only financial aid and the informal social support of Goodrich friendships. They have a higher graduation rate than the rest of the student body.

Historically, compensatory development has been featured by the Settlement House Movement since the 1880s and by 1964 Economic Opportunity Act programs such as Head Start, Upward Bound, the Job Corps, and the Neighborhood Youth Corps.

External Compensatory Preference

Compensatory preference aims to equalize disparities between privileged and diswelfared groups in current job and training markets. That is, it uses selection preferences to increase the proportion of the disadvantaged in the workforce to what it would have been if there had not been past inequities.

- *Quotas systems* are temporary devices to create opportunities for groups disadvantaged by past discrimination (overt or de facto) in a given setting to catch up to what their numbers would otherwise have been. For instance, at one time, the Alabama Highway Patrol was under a court order to reserve 50 percent of new positions and promotions for the underrepresented group, *until* such time as the makeup of the force approximated the ethnic makeup of the state's population.
- *Bonus points.* On civil service exams, World War II veterans were given five extra points to offset career development advantages enjoyed by competitors who had stayed home, ten points if disabled. For example, let us say a civilian scored 87 points on the exam for a certain position, a veteran 84 points, and a disabled veteran 81. The adjusted scores would be civilian, still 87, veteran, 89, and disabled veteran, 91. The latter would get the job.
- *Preference among qualifiers.* First, all fully qualified "as-is" candidates are identified. Within that pool, preference is given

to applicants from underrepresented groups. Often a two-tier approach is used. Outstanding candidates are accepted first, on pure as-is merit. Within the larger pool of fairly comparable satisfactory, but not exceptional, candidates, target group members get preference.

• *Double standard,* also called *reverse discrimination,* is the most controversial. I once worked in a graduate program that required a 3.0 GPA minimum for admission, except for minorities, who needed only a 2.5. The system succeeded in integrating the program at a crucial time. Because as-is evaluations are fallible for reasons given previously, some students whom we would otherwise have rejected proved to be outstanding. Most of the others, with courage and "true grit," developed into able and respected professionals in the community.

On the other hand, there was a price. A number of persons admitted on the lower standard did less well academically, creating a general impression among other students that minorities were inferior. Further, the self-esteem of minority students who had exceeded the admissions standards was damaged. Many of them came to me privately over the years, seeking reassurance that they were really "okay, not a token."

Without taking an absolute pro or con position on any particular compensatory preference strategy, I will be absolute on one thing: do not use compensatory preference without a follow-up plan for compensatory development to enable the persons selected to become as fully qualified as their cohorts. This obviously benefits both the employee and the employer. The latter gets better productivity, and the former is now in a position to pursue his or her future career under as-is negative freedom conditions.

FRATERNITÉ

The French Revolution slogan was, "liberté, égalité, fraternité." We have already discussed liberté and égalité. The third standard, fraternité, treats us as brothers and sisters within one family. There are a number of synonyms that can be used as readily:

- *Community*—"a society of people having common rights and privileges and common interests," and *commonality,* an ethos of community with others in a society.
- *Solidarity*—"social sharing; a common sense of community and an equitable distribution of the command of resources" (COE, 1993, p. 96).
- *Fellowship*—"a mutual sharing; partnership."
- *Cohesion*—"sticking together."
- *Mutuality*—"reciprocity; interchange."

Fraternité affirms that all members of a society (or a community or the world) are one family, with mutual responsibility for one another. "No man is an island, entire of itself; every man is a piece of the continent, a part of the main; . . . any man's death diminishes me, because I am involved in mankind; and therefore never send to know for whom the bell tolls; it tolls for thee" (Donne, 1624).

The applications of social responsibility are briefly touched upon next. They are discussed in greater detail in Chapter 3 and the remainder of this book.

Benevolent Control

One approach to social responsibility has been *collectivist,* which stresses the overall best interests of the society as a whole rather than the interests of individual citizens. This is the approach of such ideological disparate actors as Communist China and the U.S. Federal Reserve Board.

Plato, disillusioned with the demagoguery in Athenian democracy, believed that the greatest common good would be achieved not by individual self-determination and democracy, but by the rule of a "philosopher king" who operated with consistent wisdom and goodness. One of his protegés actually applied this model, in consultation with Plato, as ruler of Syracuse around 350 B.C. Unfortunately, he was assassinated by a trusted friend who became a tyrant (Plutarch's *Lives,* "Dion").

Skeptics doubt that any central authority could ever achieve the level of competence required. Human-nature pessimists add that even if it did, it would soon be subverted by controllers who misuse their power to advance their own interests at the expense of the common good. Based on Dion's experience, perhaps they are right.

Nevertheless, most people prefer *some* social control, subject to checks and balances and democratic accountability. The issue is when and how?

Voluntary Responsibility

An anticontrol approach to social responsibility trusts the voluntary actions of individuals. Whereas social contract theory assumes that the predatory nature of humans requires a trade-off of some freedom for welfare and security, "voluntaryism" assumes the inherent goodness of people.

This takes many forms. One is the type of nonorganized mutual caring and assistance described in Circle 2 of Chapter 1. Another is the vast network of nonprofit charitable programs and voluntary service in the "organized private sector," for which the United States is noted.

A combination of altruism and freedom with responsibility is the rationale for philanthropy:

> There remains, then, only one mode of using great fortunes; but in this we have the true antidote for the temporary unequal distribution of wealth, the reconciliation of the rich and the poor—a reign of harmony. . . . Under its sway, we shall have an ideal State, in which the surplus wealth of the few will become, in the best sense, the property of the many, because administered for the common good. (Carnegie, 1900, p. 623)

A third area is occupational welfare. In the United States, one can debate the extent to which this is voluntary responsibility. Much of it is the result of market negotiations with sellers of labor (collective bargaining) or a shrewd investment/profit move to enhance and maintain employee loyalty and productivity. I prefer to think that some corporate leaders also have a social responsibility motive.

The most extreme application of the anticontrol approach may be anarchism. Derived from the philosophy of Zeno, it became a nineteenth-century political ideology "that formal government of any kind is unnecessary and wrong in principle." Free association of individuals and groups on the basis of equality and fellowship can and should replace both economic and political authority. Marx believed (incorrectly, it turns out) that Communism would evolve into this. Anarchism has been practiced with mixed results on a small scale in communes of nineteenth-century utopians and twentieth-century hippies.

Interdependence

A more pragmatic approach to social responsibility builds on commonality. Recognizing that they are all in the same boat, people find it in their mutual best interest to join voluntarily into cooperatives such as kibbutzim, farmer co-ops, condominiums, and credit unions. When human nature falls short of the ideal, these collaborations may experience internal divisiveness or evolve into fairly standard businesses, yet they usually retain a significant residual fraternité ethos. Cooperatives have proven to be viable in both a capitalist nation such as the United States and a mainline Communist nation such as China.

Interdependence is also the basis of social insurances. Vehicles for the sharing of risk run the gamut of commercial (Aetna), mutual (Omaha), nonprofit (Blue Cross, historically), tax-funded public (Medicare Part A), and premium-funded public (National Flood Insurance). All share the same bottom-line rationale: "Bad things happen. They fall upon us unevenly, and we don't know what or on whom. Rather than risk being wiped out, let's pool the risk and make it both safe and affordable for all of us."

Social policy and programs in several European countries are rooted in cultures with a strong sense of common identity. Germany, for instance, has a complex pattern of interrelationship that involves federal government, state government, employers, unions, voluntary mutual assistance organizations, nonprofit human service agencies (often church-related), nonprofit insurance companies, and professional societies, with a funding mix which includes employer, employee, state and federal contributions. To an individualistic American, this is all but incomprehensible, but it makes holistic sense from the vantage point of a solidarity *weltanschauung* (worldview).

MIXED REALITY

No major society today is a "pure" example of benevolent control, voluntary responsibility, or individualism. Complete social control by fallible leaders would be as untenable as the unrestrained individualism of Hobbes's state of nature. In the United States, individualism is in conflict with social responsibility on an uneasy, ambivalent middle ground. Competitive individualism is softened by a frontier legacy of mutual assistance, a tradition of noblesse oblige, and a potpourri of human service programs. Benevolent control, through regulation, is kept in balance by judicial review, democratic elections, and division of power between the public and private sectors. Our policy dilemma is twofold.

First, how do negative freedom and egoistic self-interest stack up against humanitarian and community values? What is the place of altruism? Does it even exist? If so, is it the highest human achievement or a sucker's game? We need a hierarchy of values to sort out our priorities and resolve the inevitable conflicts—or at least some sort of framework to guide us.

Second, even when we get our values straight, there are still many "ifs, ands, and buts" involved in specific applications. As illustrated in relation to limitations on negative freedom, we have to accomplish the imperfect and fallible task of making *specific* policies that deal with the messy realities of life in our society. Then, we have to negotiate with others who have different legitimate interests and viewpoints (as well as other forces whose interests and viewpoints may not be so legitimate).

Chapter 10

Economic Animals?

Insofar as the free market society denies morality, law, culture, and religion, it agrees with Marxism by reducing man to the sphere of economics and the satisfaction of material needs.

Pope John Paul II, 1991

Numbers are an excellent aid to reasoning, but it's an increasingly common error to use only the numbers available and to fail to quantify the rest of the situation.

Marilyn Vos Savant, 1997

Humans are economic animals. According to historian Eugene Golob, in *The Isms: A History and Evaluation,* the following has been the working premise of mainstream economic theory for more than two centuries:

> Every individual acting in the economic sphere was thought to operate in a purely rational way. His object was profit, and the means to this end he chose through a rational analysis of his own self-interest. No other considerations entered into his decision; ethics and psychology were as rigidly excluded from the science of economics as they were from the science of physics. (1954, p. 9)

This premise is so deeply rooted that even the economic policy goals of religio-political movements that decry "secular humanism" appear to be more in tune with this secular ideology than the teachings of their religion's founder, who declared, "Do not store up for yourselves treasure on earth. . . . Store up treasure in heaven . . . for where your treasure is, there will be your heart. . . . You cannot serve God and Money" (Matthew 6:19-24).

Similarly, Marxism, champion of the common people, reduced them to economic creatures, ignoring emotional, social, aesthetic, psychological, spiritual, ethnic, cultural, religious, family, and self-identity elements. This may have been a major factor in the ultimate breakdown of the Soviet Union as an economic system and political body.

ECONOMIC REDUCTIONISM

Real life is more complex than we can handle. Wouldn't it be nice if we could explain it by manageable formulas. A common technique in social policy is to reduce all social values to *economic utility*.

A central principle in social ethics today, *utilitarianism* is "the ethical doctrine that virtue is based on utility and that conduct should be directed toward promoting the greatest happiness for the greatest number." The challenge has been to quantify happiness, using a common denominator that could be measured "scientifically."

Economics offered a solution. First it reduced utility from happiness to "satisfaction of a human want or need." Then it limited satisfaction to *commodities*, "things which can be bought and sold." The next logical step was to substitute purchasing power for the commodities themselves. A sign of this process can be seen in the shift from "life, liberty, and the pursuit of *happiness*," in the Declaration of Independence, to "life, liberty, or *property*" a century later, in the Fourteenth Amendment. Another century later, according to one observer, "Rights are reduced to calculation of gains and losses on a balance sheet" (Jacobs, 1993, p. 14).

Money becomes the ultimate measure of value, to which all other measures must be converted or be left out. Its policy advantage is simplicity. Its biggest *pitfall* is the other side of that same coin: what you leave out diminishes your accuracy.

One dilemma is how to translate complexity into a simple model, without falling into the trap of mistaking the model for the reality itself. There is no sure way to avoid reductionist mistakes, but the surest way to guarantee them is an arrogant belief in the infallibility of one's technology.

Social policies reflecting economic reductionism tend to focus on financial gains and losses, not only in the private economic market sector, but also in such public human service areas as education, health care, and vocational rehabilitation. Economic reductionism is also the a priori premise of *privatization:* a profit motive is the surest guarantee of quality and cost-effective health and human services. However, a National Academy of Sciences study, which tested this premise, concluded, "There is no evidence to support the common belief that investor-owned organizations are less costly or more efficient than not-for-profit organizations" (Gray and McNerney, 1986, p. 1525).

Although altruism and charity have no place in this belief system, selected public and private human services can be justified as enlightened self-interest, if they show promise of enhancing someone's economic productivity. Britain's first step toward national health care, the 1911 National Insurance Act, was advertised as an investment. As such, it covered male breadwinners but not their wives. The government's official justification: "Married women living with their husbands need not be included, since where the unit is a family, it is the husband's and not the wife's good health which is important to insure" (quoted in Fraser, 1973, p. 155).

COST-BENEFIT ANALYSIS

Cost-benefit analysis is as old as commerce: it involves investment and profit. Profit is sales revenue minus the money invested in producing and marketing the product. Ford CEO Robert McNamara brought Ford's version to the public sector as PPBS (program planning budgeting system) when he became Secretary of Defense in 1961. Within five years, the system spread to federal social programs and, through their grant programs, to the nonprofit sector.

The concept is simple. Figure the dollar cost of doing something and the dollar value of its results (benefits). By comparing the two, you can evaluate its payoff. There are two basic concepts: One is *profit.* Will the results be worth more than the cost of doing something? The other is *opportunity cost.* There's no free lunch. It costs something (in time, materials, facilities, cash, etc.) to achieve any objective. If you use it to do this, you can't do that. For example, you have money to invest so you can (1) buy a house that will appreciate in value, (2) buy bonds and collect annual interest, or (3) pay tuition for a master's degree, which will increase your future earnings. However, you can do only one of them. The opportunity cost of each is what you could have gained from one of the others. The best opportunity cost choice is the one with the best payoff.

Officially, this cost-benefit analysis is the primary basis for government social policy decisions. Not quite, says Michael Hill: "[Economists] bring a naivete about the political processes which actually determine policy. Their naivete consists in a belief that the consideration of efficiency and effectiveness will dominate the political decision-making process" (1990, p. 9). Nevertheless, it is enough of a factor that you should do cost-benefit analyses wherever feasible and use them both in clarifying your own thinking and in persuading others.

The key elements of cost-benefit analysis are:

1. a program accounting system that separately identifies and prices all input for each product or intended client outcome; and
2. a basis for putting a price on every product, whether it be a refrigerator or a high school diploma.

Advantages

Because everything is reduced to one measure—money—virtually anything can be compared with everything else. The results are neat, clean, and statistical.

Cost-benefit analysis can show whether something is worth doing. Add up the benefit dollars; subtract the cost dollars. Voila! If the *bottom line* is a gain, the plan is worth doing. If it costs more than the result is worth, beware.

It can go further and tell you *how profitable.* This enables you to select, from among several positive choices, the one with the best payoff. Simply divide the benefit by the cost to get the *benefit-cost ratio.* If choice 1 offers a $110 benefit for a $100 cost, your 110 ÷ 100 ratio equals 1.1, a reasonable 10 percent profit, but not as good as choice 2, with a $200 benefit for the $100 cost, a 2.0 ratio.

If you are a purist, the benefit-to-cost ratio dictates the choice: "The basic premise of cost benefit theory is that alternatives should be selected according to a systematic comparison of the advantages and disadvantages that result from the estimated consequences of choice" (Merkhofer, 1987, p. 60).

Limitations

There are other considerations, such as ethics—who wins and who loses—and social values. The overall most profitable course may also be the most damaging to vulnerable bystanders. The intensity of a client's need, or quality-of-life intangibles, may be more important than economic profit. As such, even if it is clearly the right choice in the abstract, it may be impossible to overcome opposition from powerful vested interests.

No one who works with cost-benefit analysis should fail to read Jonathan Swift's devastating satire concerning it (before it was officially invented), *A Modest Proposal for Preventing the Children of the Poor People of Ireland from Being a Burden to Their Parents or Country, and for Making Them Beneficial to the Public* (1729). In this work, he develops a detailed program for selling year-old Irish babies to British aristocrats to be eaten like suckling pigs. This solves the problems of Irish overpopulation and poverty at the same time, as well as providing a new taste treat for jaded British palates.

Edward Mishan makes the same point in a more pedestrian way:

> Cost benefit analysis as traditionally practiced is no more than a useful technique in the service of social decisions. The outcome of a cost benefit analysis alone is not socially decisive. A cost benefit analysis neglects distributional effects. It neglects equity. It may have to ignore spillover effects. . . . In summary, a cost benefit study can be only a part, though an important part, of the data necessary for informed collective decisions. (1976, pp. 412-413)

Use cost-benefit analysis with two qualifications. First of all, use it as one of *multiple* inputs to the decision. By itself, "we see meanminded and heartless bureaucrats thinking like computers" (Merkhofer, 1987, p. 177). Blended with qualitative perspectives, it helps produce a "combination of a cool head and a warm heart . . . [shielded from] sentimentality on the one hand and indifference on the other" (Howard, 1980).

Second, use it as a servant, not a master. Identify your values explicitly and be sure that the pricing reflects those values as nearly as possible.

ALTERNATIVES:
COST UTILITY AND COST-EFFECTIVENESS

Cost-benefit analysis requires economic reductionism. Two variations of this permit us to address noneconomic benefits.

Cost Utility

Cost-utility outcomes don't have to be measured in pounds and pence; they can be based on any common denominator of human satisfaction on which key actors agree. I call utility units "goody points."

Cost utility is most desirable in specific situations where dollars simply won't cut the mustard. Can you measure with dollars the comparative educational or quality-of-life worth of majoring in accounting versus music? That's similar to my asking you which painting you like best and you tell me what each sold for. Where qualitative or subject values are involved, even a crude utility measure may be better than a precise answer to the wrong question.

A transplant team turned to utility when faced with decisions on who would get organs, when only one out of three of those in need could be served. They rejected a market criterion (the highest bidder) and a cost-benefit standard (future earning power). What they used was a utility scale called "health years," an index of relative expected posttransplant health level times age-based life expectancy.

Utility is used less often than effectiveness for two reasons: it is more difficult to quantify precisely, and it is difficult to obtain voluntary agreement on the utility point criteria. The previous transplant utility illustration may be vulnerable to both these problems. Try it out in any diverse group to see if you can you get them to agree on this scale or any other!

The size and nature of the group makes a difference. Utility works best when the decisions makers are part of a small, homogeneous group, such as a family, close colleagues, a small agency board, or the inner circle of a larger body. It is least feasible in large, diverse, politicized settings.

Cost-Effectiveness

Cost-effectiveness, alias *efficiency,* can't compare the relative merits of buying apples or oranges. It operates only after the objective has already been chosen. Effectiveness is the ability to achieve the desired result; cost-effectiveness is the ability to do so in the least expensive way.

Cost-effectiveness uses quantitative, but usually noneconomic, outcome measures. At the simplest level, this can be a yes-or-no category: Was the handicapped child adopted or not? A more sophisticated scale may use indicators that differentiate the degree of success. In a remedial reading program, the students are given a standardized reading test before and after completing the course. A unit of success would be each point gained on the "after" score.

This method can also be used to compare different ways of achieving the objective. In the reading program, you might experiment with three approaches: using individual tutoring with one set of children, group learning methods with the second, and a computerized program with the third. For each set, (1) calculate the total cost of the instruction, (2) add up the total number of points gained by the set, and (3) divide the dollars by the points. The most cost-effective approach is the one with the lowest dollars per point.

What cost-effectiveness can do is tell you which method of improving reading is the best buy; what it can't do is tell you the relative merit of putting the money into a reading program rather than a new gym.

PUTTING A PRICE ON INTANGIBLES

Indicators in General

If you can't measure a qualitative element, does it correlate with something that you *can* measure? If so, you use that as an indicator to represent the unmeasurable element. In professional licensure, we are not equipped to measure your actual competence so we measure instead your ability to answer exam questions about practice.

An indicator needs two things to be useful. One is its *consistency* in measurements (numbers); the other is *correlation*. An indicator is *valid* to the extent that it accurately represents the real thing. Exams can be valid measures of *knowledge* (but don't differentiate well between short-term, crammed memory and long-term, absorbed memory). Are they equally valid as measures of future *practice* competence?

It's nearly impossible to have perfect correlation between an intangible quality and its numerical indicator. We accept deviation within tolerable limits. What is a tolerable limit? There is no set guideline. How could you *ever* be sure, since the reason for the indicator in the first place is inability to precisely measure the entity itself? We have to use our best judgment on whether the imperfect indicator is better than none. Many are; some are not. An inaccurate indicator that misdirects policy is worse than none at all.

An indicator is *reliable* to the extent that it *varies at the same rate* as the entity. Obviously, a valid indicator is also reliable. However, invalid measures may sometimes be reliable anyway. My humidity gauge is always wrong: it reads ninety when the humidity is seventy-five, and sixty-five when it is fifty. However, it is reliable, because it varies consistently with the real humidity. All I have to do is subtract fifteen. Similarly, unemployment statistics are invalid as indicators of the *number* of unemployed, for they omit millions of discouraged workers who need and want work but have given up looking. However, since the numbers of discouraged workers go up and down at about the same rate as the active job seekers (according to several studies), unemployment rates do reliably indicate *trends*.

An indicator is only a tool, not an end in itself. It is inherently reductionist, reducing a complex quality to a number. This is okay so long as you take its limitations into account when using it. Regretfully, it is common to present a statistical analysis of the indicator as if it were the real thing. This is called *reification*, "treating an abstraction as a concrete material object." To do so is arrogant (excessive claims to expert knowledge), lazy (avoiding inconvenience), or dumb (unaware of the discrepancy).

A good indicator meets the following criteria:

- The real objective/entity is clearly identified.
- The indicator is carefully reviewed to ensure it is accurate enough to serve the purpose.
- The user remains alert to intervening variables that weaken its reliability, where possible incorporating such variables into a revised indicator.
- It is applied only within its limits, which are openly acknowledged.

Economic Indicators: Pricing

Price is "the amount of money for which anything is bought, sold, or offered for sale." Sir Robert Walpole observed of his colleagues, "All those men have their price." The economic model goes further: *everything* has its price.

In economics, value is *market price,* whatever is actually paid for a home, a sweater, or a day's work. It is simple, neat, and by definition, avoids arguments about what a worker "really" deserves, or the "true" value of a designer dress, or the relative value of lawyers and teachers. *Vox populi*—the people have voted with their pocketbooks for the lawyer.

Conventional approaches say "a dollar is a dollar," irrespective of who gains or loses it or whether that dollar has the same value for both poor and rich. A more sophisticated approach to pricing is "the *declining marginal utility* of output to the individual" (Sillince, 1986, p. 123), based on a *demand curve.* The more you already have, the less the next increment is worth to you. A star athlete admitted to losing more than a million dollars gambling one year but shrugged it off as casual recreation. A million dollars?! Well, counting endorsements, that was only 3 percent of his income, approximately the same percent I spent on my somewhat more modest recreation that year. Based on declining marginal utility, his million meant as much to him as my thousand or two to me. *This economic concept is central to issues about distribution of tax load among different income groups.*

Whereas a reading test score may be closely related to reading, pricing intangibles in dollars tends to be more distant and indirect and therefore less reliable. On the other hand, dollars are convenient, widely accepted, and can be compared almost across the board with everything else under the sun. A key dilemma: in each case, how much accuracy are we prepared to trade off for convenience?

WELFARE ECONOMICS

Developed by such economic thinkers as Pigou (1932), Little (1957), and deGraaf (1957), welfare economics and its technical tool, cost-benefit analysis, has been the primary rationale for economic policy in the United States, Britain, and Canada, during the last third of the century. It is not a new idea; it dates back in writing at least to John Hanaway (1761). Historian Greg Dening reports:

> John Hanaway was a man of calculating charity. He was always compiling statistics. He had discovered . . . just how appealing the ironic realism of economics was. Complain to him that saving a foundling cost the state £85/5/- and he would counter with calculations showing that with the working expectancy of twenty-three working years, such a foundling would earn £412/7/5. Thus the nation would profit £326/5/2 on its outlay. "Political humanity," was a favorite phrase of his. (1992, p. 134)

We have seen how economists reduced happiness to having more or less money, but at least it still referred to each individual. Welfare economics carried this to its logical extreme by narrowing monetary gain/loss considerations to the aggregate (from the Latin for "to lead or add to a herd"). Such economics relates to the individual as ranching does to any particular steer: "Strict economic rationality means getting the most national income out of a given investment. The end is to increase the real GNP, no matter who receives it and the means is an investment expenditure, no matter who pays for it" (Wildavsky, 1973, p. 145).

Collectivism is a familiar systems theory approach that subordinates the parts to the whole or, in jargon, the subsystems to the suprasystem. These parts in a society include individuals, families, neighborhoods, and organizations. Public policy decisions maximize the total economy, measured imperfectly by Domestic National Product (DNP), without reference to internal distribution or what

happens to individuals along the way. That's the price of progress—
and profits. An illustration is the 1984 executive order cited in
Chapter 6 that ordered federal agencies to enforce the Occupational
Safety and Health Act only when the dollar loss to the economy of
illness, injury, and deaths exceeded the dollar cost of safety measures. The effect of the policy on particular workers was not a
consideration.

Welfare economics has been used as a rationale for reducing
employee wages, anti-inflationary monetary interventions that increased unemployment, punitive welfare reform, logging of prime-
val tracts in national forests, and downward adjustments in pension
and medical care rights of the elderly.

It has also been used to support individual human services as an
investment that pays off for the larger economy. For example, President Nixon said, "A child ill-fed is dulled in curiosity, lower in
stamina, distracted from learning. A worker ill-fed is less productive, more often absent from work. [The mounting costs] . . . place a
heavy economic burden on a society as a whole. . . . [The nation
must] accept the problem of malnourishment as a national responsibility."

Supporters have claimed that welfare economics achieves the
greatest good for the greatest number, based on Pareto's Law that the
relative distribution of income is always essentially the same. When
business and investors prosper, the benefits will *trickle down* proportionately to the middle and lower classes. Thus, everyone benefits
from every welfare economics gain. Unfortunately, it does not always turn out this way. As reported in Chapter 7, although the United
States, following welfare economics policies, has experienced substantial aggregate economic growth in the last quarter of the twentieth century, half of its individual citizens not only failed to share in
the gain but actually lost ground.

Using Welfare Economics

Although *total* reliance on welfare economics has its pitfalls and
risks, the approach is an excellent *input* to macropolicy of all kinds,
by presenting an overview of issues. It can be a check and balance
against predatory interests that regularly propose, in pursuit of their
narrow gains, policies that benefit them at the expense of the whole

society. Environmentalists, for example, have used it this way. Welfare economics also brings badly needed perspective to the loose cannon of disjointed muddling through, a common characteristic of politics and policy in North America and Great Britain.

Moreover, we *want* aggregate gain, don't we? It is clearly in the interests of all of us so long as the gains (and the costs) are fairly distributed. Many of President Roosevelt's anti-Depression measures, such as the National Recovery Act, a federal bailout of the banking industry, and subsidies to restore the agriculture industry, had an aggregate economy rationale. However, this rationale was not an end itself but rather a means to a transcendent value, universal adequacy for all Americans: "The test of our progress is not whether we add more to the abundance of those who have much; it is whether we provide enough for those who have too little" (Franklin Roosevelt, 1937).

Welfare economics perspectives are most useful in combination with other policy considerations such as:

- the value and interest premises guiding the choice,
- the winners (Who benefits most and least from the gains?),
- the losers (Who bears the costs/losses? How are they compensated?), and
- marginal utility as a guide in allocation of gains and costs.

THE PROTESTANT WORK ETHIC

Origins: Calvinistic Ethics

Definitions of sin have varied in different economic and social settings. Several of the Ten Commandments prohibit specific antisocial behaviors: Thou shalt not . . .

- kill,
- commit adultery,
- steal,
- bear false witness, or
- covet.

Plato extolled four virtues:

- Temperance
- Fortitude
- Prudence
- Justice

Medieval Catholicism had its seven cardinal sins, many of which relate to the Commandments or Plato. They are:

- pride (putting oneself up vis-á-vis other people and God),
- anger (includes killing and both physical and emotional assault),
- lust (includes adultery),
- envy (coveting thy neighbor's things),
- avarice (coveting and accumulating riches),
- sloth, and
- gluttony.

An expression of this general ethic is Cardinal Newman's statement, "I believe, O my God, that poverty is better than riches. . . . I will never have faith in riches, rank, power, or reputation. I will never set my heart on worldly success or on worldly advantages. I will never wish for what men call the prizes of life" (Seldes, 1960, p. 744). Definitely not a classical economics model!

The Puritan channel of Protestantism developed a new sin priority list, which coincided with the socioeconomic transition from the Middle Ages to the "modern" era of division of labor, trade, an emerging commercial class, and later, with the technical advances of the industrial revolution, capitalism. I call them the "four I's." With their counterpart virtues, they were particularly compatible with these new developments:

1. *Indolence* (sloth): counterpart virtue is hard work.
2. *Intemperance* (gluttony): counterpart virtue is self-discipline.
3. *Immorality* (lust, adultery): counterpart virtue is sexual propriety.
4. *Improvidence* (imprudence): counterpart virtue is thrift.

The differences are noteworthy. Sins of pride, anger, and envy drop from the "first flight." Avarice is converted, at least in part, from sin to the virtue of thrift—a moral responsibility to save, invest those savings, and thereby accumulate wealth. Plato's justice and Catholicism's emphasis (in its parallel virtues) on charity were missing.

The effect of the new ethic was *economic reductionism,* reducing virtue and sin to economic assets and liabilities. People are to be judged primarily by material productiveness. There is no place in this ethic for contemplative virtues, aesthetic creation, or vows of poverty in service to others. Reverend Thomas Malthus, in his immensely influential *An Essay on the Principles of Population* (1798), asserted, "Hard as it may appear in individual cases, dependent poverty ought to be held disgraceful" (Seldes, 1960, p. 744).

Evolution into the Protestant Work Ethic

The Calvinist social ethic was tied to a belief in the predestination of individuals to heaven or hell before they are born, as described in Chapter 6. The Protestant work ethic itself evolved from this origin into a free will reward-and-punishment system through a very human rationalizing process:

1. Poverty and the four I's were seen as this-world *indicators* that the person had probably been predestined to hell (damned), while prosperity and the counterpart virtues were probable indicators of being among the heaven bound (elect).
2. Anxious believers strived to achieve these behavioral indicators to reassure themselves by *demonstrating,* through their prosperity and virtue, that they surely must have been chosen to be elect, while the vice-ridden poor were presumably demonstrating that they had been destined to the other, damned group.
3. It was but a short step from demonstrating to a feeling of *deserving* election because of one's virtues or damnation because of one's vices.
4. One more short step moved them from deserving it to working to *earn* both worldly success and heaven through self-discipline, hard work, thrift, and moralistic behavior, while poverty was a *just punishment* earned by indolence, intemperance, immorality, and improvidence.

5. Meanwhile, the Age of Enlightenment contributed an explicit belief in pure free will and self-determination, which was implied de facto by the behaviors of stage four. This completed the blend—one part Puritan moralism, one part classical economics, a third part hard-nosed capitalism, and stir in a generous splash of secular rationalism. A potent cocktail that Max Weber (1904) called the Protestant work ethic.

This has become an integral cultural and ideological component of market economics and industrial capitalism. It (1) encourages the characteristics required to be an successful entrepreneur, (2) supports qualities most desirable for a docile, hardworking labor force, and (3) justifies minimal social responsibility toward the poor, since poverty is by definition the just consequence of the four I's.

This work ethic affects public social policies, suggesting that you should not only work hard but reap the benefits of that work. In a *USA Today* editorial favoring lower tax rates on capital gains than on wage income, Paul Beckner (1997), president of Citizens for a Sound Economy, offered a delightful if unwitting parody of its application: "Is it really too much to ask that the government allow taxpayers to keep just a little more of their *hard-earned money*" (empasis added). (The irony, of course, is that capital gains are explicitly defined as *unearned* income, as distinct from earned income, which is defined as wages, salaries, or fees received for work directly performed by a person.)

Less Eligibility

Another relevant policy area is human services for the poor. A watershed was the English 1834 Poor Law Reform Act, which explicitly shifted the rationale for poor laws from preordination and noblesse oblige to the work ethic.

It was based on an extensive study of the causes of poverty and the operation of the Poor Law, conducted by laissez-faire economist Edwin Chadwick, who called the 1834 Act, "the first great piece of legislation based on science or economical principles" (quoted in Fraser, 1973, p. 40). Historian Derek Fraser described it differently, as "in essence a piece of propaganda for a predetermined case" (1973, p. 40).

Chadwick came to this conclusion:

> Whatever inquiries have been made as to the previous condition of the able-bodied individuals who live in such numbers on the town parishes, it has been found that the pauperism of the greater number has originated in indolence, improvidence, and vice, and might have been averted by ordinary care and industry. (Chadwick, 1833, quoted in de Schweinitz, 1961, p. 126)

Based on this premise, that people are inherently lazy, irresponsible animals responsive only to economic rewards and punishments, the solution was an economic policy called *less eligibility:*

> The first and most essential of all conditions, a principle which we find universally admitted, even by those whose practice is at variance with it, is that his [the individual relieved] situation on the whole shall not be made really or apparently so eligible [desirable] as the situation of the independent laborer's of the lowest class. (Ibid., p. 127)

The harshly punitive blame-the-victim conclusions set the course of Victorian England for the next seventy-five years, despite a second Chadwick study, *Report on the Sanitary Conditions of the Laboring Population of Great Britain* (1842), which came to an entirely different conclusion. The second study blamed poverty and lowered worker productivity on health problems relating to housing, water, sewage disposal, and resulting contagious disease and promised that public health investments would pay off in better conditions for the poor, lower relief budgets, and higher profit for owners, due to higher productivity by healthier workers.

The Poor Law governors rejected the second report and fired Chadwick, but his report led to a parallel human service tradition, public health, that ignored the work ethic ideology in favor of external causes. The same dichotomy exists to this day in the United States. Indeed, the sponsors of the 1996 Welfare Reform Act might have used the same words as the conclusion of the 1933 Chadwick report:

> It will be observed that the measures which we have suggested are intended to produce rather negative than positive effects;

rather to remove the debasing influence to which a large portion of the laboring population is now subject [outdoor relief],
than to afford new means of prosperity and virtue. (quoted in
de Schweinitz, p. 126)

PART OF THE PACKAGE

Economic reductionism is one of the greatest pitfalls in social
policy: It demeans and dehumanizes; it distorts values; it shuts out
the heart and soul of life. However, this doesn't mean we should
throw out economic perspectives and tools. Quite the contrary, economics is one of the most important elements in social policy and
social well-being. Humans are not just dumb economic animals,
responding by instinct to mundane material rewards and threats.
"Man does not live by bread alone." There are many rich elements
to life. All of them must be taken into account in making social
policy decisions.

However, we are in part economic animals. We can't live without
economic activity. We can't provide for other social needs without
production and some type of money-based market system for selling what we produce and buying what we need or want. If you look
only at the economic dimension, you are nowhere, but if you *don't*
look at it you are even "more nowhere."

Cost-benefit analysis is not a panacea. It can't measure everything that matters nor dictate *any* decision. It is, however, one of the
best tools we have for understanding what inputs are needed to gain
an objective or benefit, what are the best ways of achieving it, and
what are the relative merits of our alternative choices. Cost-benefit
analysis is valuable where we can fit our noneconomic values and
dimensions into the model closely enough to be useful. It is also
useful, obviously, for the many truly economic decisions that we
make.

Welfare economics as an idol is dangerous. It can seduce us into
doing evil in the name of good. It can be manipulated, misrepre-
sented, and subverted by elite con artists who sell us their special
interests as general welfare. On the other hand, without welfare
economics, we would be in a jungle of conflicting interests, with no
means of sorting out priorities and trade-offs other than "might

makes right." Perhaps worse, we can wander around with no sense of direction and perspective and muddle ourselves into who knows what difficulties.

Similar to its tool, cost-benefit analysis, welfare economics is a cornerstone of rational social policy analysis and decision making—so long as it remains the servant, never the master. Remember the story of the sorcerer's apprentice? The magic broom under the sorcerer's control was a dandy appliance; out of control, in the hands of the sorcerer's apprentice, it was a nightmare.

Finally, the work ethic. By itself, it is at best an obsessive-compulsive neurosis. In the hands of unscrupulous leaders (or even ones who lack self-awareness), it can be a powerful tool for exploitation and an excuse for irresponsibility and destruction of community.

On the other hand, for all these caveats, the work ethic is an indelible part of our own culture. I was socialized into it as a child. I am temperate, hardworking, disciplined, prudent, reasonably thrifty, and a straight arrow in my personal life. This has served me well in my career and also in my voluntary service interests, and not just I. By internalizing motivation for hard work and/or an entrepreneurship, the work ethic has contributed greatly to the success of our nation. It has positive equity values, expecting people to pull their own weight.

As with the other "reductionism" items, if it has sole control, it can stunt our spiritual, emotional, and aesthetic growth. Nowadays, it has become a threat to family life, preempting time and energy that we believe people should use for parenting, recreation, personal development, creative hobbies, and other qualitative noneconomic human activities. But if you keep it in its place, it is, similar to the others, a tool that, properly used, improves productivity and efficiency in ways which free us up for the rest of life.

Each economic framework in this chapter is irreplaceable—in its place. Appreciate it. Use it. Keep it in proper perspective.

For everything there is a season, and a time for every matter.

Ecclesiastes 3:1

PART IV:
ECONOMIC AND SOCIAL
MARKET CHOICES

Chapter 11

The Economic Market

Imperfect products should be available because consumers have different preferences for defect avoidance.

James Miller, Federal Trade Commission

If Jesus were a football player, he'd play fair, he'd play clean, and he'd put the guy across the line on his butt.

Barry Rice, Liberty College athlete

Perhaps the most pervasive social policy area of our society is the *economic system*, including division of labor, production and consumption, distribution, employers and workers, sellers and buyers. Economic choices make a critical difference in such areas as equity, equality and inequalities, adequacy, negative and positive freedom, individualism, and social cohesion.

A MARKET ECONOMY

An isolated family or small community may be self-sufficient at a subsistence level, meeting all of its needs internally and sharing the results. A *market* emerges as soon as there is a need or desire to trade some goods or labor for other items. All markets have three characteristics:

1. *Division of labor* so that we have different things to trade
2. *A common medium of exchange* (money) so that we can compare the value of apples with oranges or an hour of work with a pair of shoes

3. *A method of setting prices* (including wages) so that we can agree on how many hours of work for those shoes

Not all markets are free. What is produced, who can produce it, who can sell it and buy it, on what terms and for what price—these can be dictated, in whole or in part, by tradition (as in medieval days) or by a central authority (such as a Communist dictatorship or a capitalist monopoly). Most democracies are semifree markets, modified by some tradition (e.g., paying women less), some government command (e.g., import quotas, minimum wage), and some private command (e.g., price-fixing).

Characteristics of a Free Market

First, we need to understand how a free market works in theory. It is regulated by the *natural law* of supply and demand, in which independent free choices of millions of individual buyers (demand) and sellers (supply) keep everything in balance. This requires the following characteristics:

- *Purely economic choice*, unaffected by social ties, union loyalties, patriotism, or where one's physician has staff privileges
- *One's own self-interest* as the sole basis for decision
- *Freedom of work, enterprise, and trade*, the right to produce and sell anything without restriction, favoritism, or discrimination
- *Open competition* among suppliers (producers/sellers), without private combinations in restraint of trade or government restrictions
- *Free and informed consumer choice* to buy what one wants from any seller in full knowledge of what one is buying, without coercion, constraint, or fraud
- *Freedom of contract*, the right to make binding commitments with each other, except where they subvert the above
- *Equal power* between buyers, who can patronize a choice of accessible sellers, and sellers, who aren't dependent on one particular buyer

The Law of Supply and Demand

Supply is what's for sale. *Demand* is the means and desire to buy. In a free market, the process is akin to haggling in a Middle Eastern bazaar—or the New York Stock Exchange. Buyers and sellers are each making counteroffers. When the bids of a buyer and a seller agree, they fix a price and the sale is made. Meanwhile, bargaining resumes for the next deal.

Price is the regulator that keeps supply and demand in *equilibrium*. If there are more buyers (demand) than available goods or services (supply), sellers hold out for higher prices. These prices discourage some potential buyers, reducing demand. At the same time, the lure of easy sales and higher profits encourages expanded production. Supply goes up, demand goes down, and balance is restored.

If it's the other way around, and the supply exceeds buyer demand, buyers get choosy. Production is cut to reduce inventory, and sellers compete for the available business by lowering prices. New shoppers, who couldn't afford the earlier prices or felt the products were not worth the cost, are attracted by the bargains. Supply goes down, and demand goes up, restoring balance.

Economic Cycles

This is how a free market works in theory. In practice, it never comes out quite right. There is a time lag between a production decision and the finished product. By the time the product hits the market, the circumstances have changed. Further, determining how much to produce is not a coordinated action but rather many independent, scattered choices. If there is undersupply, each producer optimistically hopes to win a larger share of the market from its competitors. If there is oversupply, worried producers may pessimistically cut back too far.

The overall result is that the responses tend to overshoot the mark and create a new imbalance in the opposite direction. Thus, a free market experiences a recurring *cycle,* in which inflation and expansion alternate with deflation and recession. Here is how it might apply to home computers:

1. More people want computers. Not enough are available: demand exceeds supply. This is *shortage.*
2. Prices on available computers rise. This is *inflation,* a rise in prices that reduces purchasing power.

3. Responding to the excess of customers and the prospect of high profit margins, current manufacturers increase production and new companies enter the field. Supply increases. This is *expansion*.

4. A year later, the flood of new computers reaches the market. Because some manufacturers were eager and optimistic, they made more computers than there are buyers. This is a *surplus*, caused by *overproduction*.

5. To move their high inventory of computers, companies hold sales, offer rebates and special discounts, or lower the list price. One way or another, the real price customers pay for computers drops. This is *deflation*.

6. Lower prices reduce profits. Unsold inventories cause losses. Some companies go broke; some drop their home computer line; the rest cut back production. All of them lay off workers. This is *recession*.

7. The cutbacks return us to shortage again, and we begin the next cycle.

Demand

Demand is "the desire to purchase and possess, coupled with the power of purchasing"—how much money people are ready, willing, and able to spend right now. It is the product of two factors: money times velocity.

Money

In the United States, the primary ingredient of demand is the *M1* money supply, which is cash, checking accounts, and travelers checks, all available for immediate spending. Although credit cards and other prearranged lines of credit are potentially spendable, they become M1 only when the money is actually borrowed/charged.

There are three additional measures of money supply that add other, less immediate, funds.

M2 is M1 plus "short time" investments, chiefly regular savings deposits and money market demand accounts. Because these additions can be quickly converted into spendable cash, some experts argue that M2 should replace M1 as the primary measure of demand. Defenders of M1 reply that although this is true the M2 additions are invested specifically because they are *not intended* to be spent right away.

M3 is M2 plus "large time" bank deposits and money market funds that cannot be withdrawn without penalty for a given period of time. A familiar example of this is CDs (certificates of deposit), commonly with a maturity of six months to five years.

The *L* money supply goes the next step. To M3, it adds savings bonds, short-term treasury securities (up to a year), and commercial paper (short-term loans to private corporations).

Beyond this are assets and property that must be "liquidated" (converted into cash) by selling them in the economic market. This *wealth* is not considered part of the money market because conversion takes time and the price is not assured in advance. Examples are stocks, bonds, your house, other real estate, a small business, and your equity in a pension fund. Property that is difficult to sell is called a "frozen" (as opposed to liquid) asset.

M1 money supply can be changed in two basic ways:

1. *Saving.* Spendable money is taken out of circulation through savings or investments. M1 is increased by withdrawing savings or selling assets.
2. *Borrowing.* M1 increases when you borrow future money to spend today. It goes back out of circulation when you repay it from otherwise "disposable income" on that future date.

Of course, the dynamics are more complicated. For instance, if you put savings into a credit union, which lends it to another member as an auto loan, it's a wash. He or she put back into circulation what you took out. If you make a capital investment, that money goes back into circulation to purchase machinery, build a plant, or pay development staff. This is not necessarily true for all investment. "The purchase of securities, or financial investment, merely involves an exchange of assets of differing degrees of liquidity with no addition to productive capacity" (Golob, 1954, p. 154).

Velocity

How fast money is spent (turnover) is called velocity. Each time the same money is spent, it *counts again as demand*. Let's use a simple example, following two different ten-dollar salary payments, paid on Monday afternoon by the same company to a worker and an executive.

The first $10 turns over thirteen times in five days:

1. Monday, the money is paid to the worker.
2. Worker pays barber for a haircut on the way home from work.
3. Barber buys groceries on his way home.
4. Tuesday, grocer pays neighborhood baker for homemade bread, which he sells in his grocery.
5. Baker pays his assistant.
6. Assistant spends it on beer at a local bar after work.
7. Wednesday, the bar pays its bartender.
8. Thursday, bartender buys a used table at a garage sale.
9. Seller buys gas for her car.
10. Gas station pays its part-time attendant.
11. Friday, attendant pays rent to his landlord.
12. Landlord pays teenager to mow the lawn after school.
13. Teenager goes to the movies and buys snacks.

Meanwhile, the executive deposits her $10 in a checking account and, on Friday night, writes a check to pay for groceries. That $10 is spent twice, once to her and once to the store.

$D = MV$

Demand (D) equals the money available for spending (M) times the velocity at which it is respent in a given period of time (V). In the previous example, the first $10 generated $130 of demand ($10 × 13), while the second created only $20 of demand ($10 × 2). Demand increases if money is paid to quick turnaround spenders (e.g., lower-income wages) and decreases if the same money is paid instead to a slow spender (e.g., a dam construction contract).

PROS AND CONS
OF THE "FREE" ECONOMIC MARKET

Market liberals (not to be confused with social liberals) believe that a free economic market is in everyone's best interests. Not everyone agrees. The following are some commonly expressed pros and cons.

PRO	CON
1. Stability	
Over the long run, the self-regulating system maintains approximate equilibrium and predictability.	Much undeserved hardship and suffering, in the form of unemployment and bankruptcies, is caused by the instability of recurring cycles.
2. Responsiveness to Needs	
Demand is the best determination of need as defined by consumers.	The human needs of those without adequate purchasing power are ignored.
3. Efficiency	
All production is based on demand. Competition weeds the inefficient.	Free markets are *socially* inefficient by diverting production from social priorities to affluent individuals' choices. They are *economically* inefficient because recessions waste both capital and human resources.
4. Flexibility	
The market reacts automatically to change.	The market reacts slowly to change, has problems coping with rapid changes in environment and technology, and usually does so at major cost to individuals.
5. Fairness	
It is equitable, rewarding diligence and initiative.	It is inherently unequal, and it takes no responsibility for undeserved disservices it causes.
6. Morality and Social Responsibility	
Dispersion and competition contain and limit the effects of unethical behavior and unwise decisions.	The system converts a "deadly sin" (avarice) into a cardinal virtue. Competition and conflict are rewarded at the expense of cooperation, mutual support, and commitment to public interest.
7. Liberty	
A free market offers negative freedom.	It subverts positive freedom, especially for the working classes.
8. Motivation	
Competitive self-interest is the strongest motivator.	It is a disincentive for noncommercial social contribution, and discourages the majority who are not winners.

TRADITIONAL ECONOMIES

Robert Heilbroner identified two alternatives to a market economy:

> Societies can trust to the guiding hand of tradition for the maintenance of a fixed configuration of activities; this is the "system" of tradition by which primitive societies secure their continuance. Tradition will not, however, arrange things when the environment changes, or when new technologies enter or when growth is sought (the latter two cases unlikely in a tradition-bound milieu). The coordinating mechanism then becomes "command"—the conscious direction of social energies by some individual or institution empowered to allocate effort, determine levels of consumption, etc. (1982, p. 176)

A traditional economy maintains things the way they always have been. It may be egalitarian or hierarchical.

Traditional *egalitarian* economies tend to be small, self-contained societies with a common identity, as symbolized by legends about tribal origins. They have relatively simple, consensual divisions of labor and share a modest production with little surplus for luxuries or accumulation of wealth.

Traditional *hierarchical* economies, such as feudalism, typically accept some kind of preordination that defines economic roles and interactions. A *just price* is established by long usage and usually imbued with natural law or divine sanction, as in Aristotelian philosophy and Thomistic theology.

The traditional economy can thrive only where there is economic, social, and technological stability and high consensus about production and distribution. As a society advances in technology, size, and complexity, tradition must give way to some kind of coordinating mechanism, either through central control or a balancing systems dynamic. We still have some traditional elements in our market society, as when we talk about "fair" prices and wages or decry "unfair" income differences between CEOs and their employees.

COMMAND ECONOMIES

Central Control

A command economy can be effective and socially responsible to the extent that it has three characteristics, without which there is a risk of chaos, screwups, or exploitation.

First, central planning requires high *technical competence:*

- A comprehensive data collection and analysis system
- Reliable forecasts of noncontrollable elements
- Ability to predict the direct and indirect effects of planning decisions
- A consistent basis for setting the price of each item in relation to all others, in the absence of either tradition or bargaining

Computerization has greatly increased our ability to manage the complexities of comprehensive rational analysis, making central planning potentially more effective than in the past. Critics counter with "GIGO" (garbage in, garbage out). The product cannot be better than its inputs, which are selective, incomplete, and programmed by fallible humans. This is not a new issue:

> The Government are very keen on amassing statistics. They collect them, add them, raise them to the nth power, take the cube root, and prepare wonderful diagrams. But you must never forget that every one of these figures comes in the first instance from the village watchman, who just puts down what he damn pleases. (attributed to Sir Josiah Stamp, Inland Revenue Department, ca. 1900)

Even if the analysis were impeccable, all the data is from the past, whereas the plan unfolds in the unknown future, about which we can, at best, make educated guesses. (For amusement sometime, look up futurist books, articles, and movies of a generation ago and compare their predictions with the actual outcome.)

Second, it must have *authority* to implement its decisions. A plan is meaningless if it can be ignored or defied. Shared ideologies and incentives go a long way, but ultimately, a command economy must use coercive powers to enforce obedience. This, of course, raises liberty issues as well as risks of rebellion, evasion, and passive-aggressive resistance.

Third, exercise of such authority requires *wisdom, altruism,* and *impartiality.* Ideally, central control more fairly distributes goods among citizens, free from exploitation, special privilege, and individual aggrandizement. This assumes that the planners and controllers are a moral and intellectual elite who transcend their own narrow self-interests and resist others who seek special privilege.

Critics reply that decisions are actually made not by wise altruists but by self-serving elites and unsensitive bureaucrats, neither of whom know nor care about the "little guy." The economic market, assuming cynically that everyone is self-serving, has a system of checks and balances among competing interests. The more optimistic central control approach lacks such defenses.

Another argument for a planned economy is that it uses capital and labor more efficiently by avoiding the costs of competition and the waste of economic cycles that periodically idle workers and equipment. One response is that, given human fallibility, planners will make mistakes. Big plans make big mistakes.

Another criticism is that central control is inefficient because it squelches initiative. A favorite worker joke in Communist countries was, "They pretend to pay us, and we pretend to work."

Leninist Marxism

The most notable experiment in central control was Soviet Communism. Karl Marx himself envisioned "dictatorship by the proletariat" (central planning and control) only as an interim stage, to establish the new social order after the overthrow of capitalism. Gradually, the utopian new era of comradeship would make government authority obsolete, replaced by an anarchist society in which the workers would get together in decentralized groups to control their own means of production and engage in honest, egalitarian trade with other groups. This would be a sort of collaborative free market featuring voluntary solidarity, in contrast with the competitive individualism of capitalism.

It didn't happen. The Marxist state fixated at the "interim" central control stage. Eventually, deficiencies in wisdom, altruism, and fairness, along with reactions to the high level of coercion required to make it work, led to a breakdown of both the economic system and the Union itself.

Private Sector Command

Market liberals see government as the enemy. However, for many people, in many places, in many eras, the greatest threat to their economic liberty and well-being has been private sector centralization of power. This was true in nineteenth-century England and in the United States from about 1850 to 1930, and it may happen again, as mergers and takeovers centralize power in fewer, larger corporations at both national and multinational levels.

To the extent that the competitive free-market system actually performs its theoretical function of decentralizing private power, private sector command is a minor worry. However, there is a natural counterforce. The primary objective of any commercial enterprise is to maximize profits. This is done, explained my father, by "dealing in livestock: buy sheep [cheap] and sell deer [dear]." The more control a company has over its pool of potential suppliers and workers, the greater its power to lower production costs by dictating the prices it pays for their inputs. The more it can control availability of its commodities to consumers, the more it can charge them. It is therefore only reasonable to strive for as much private sector command as possible.

Adam Smith, father of modern free-market economics, warned of this inevitable subversive force in *The Wealth of Nations* (1776):

> We rarely hear, it has been said, of the combination of masters; though frequently of workmen. But whoever imagines, upon this account, that masters rarely combine is as ignorant of the world as of the subject. Masters are always and everywhere in a sort of tacit, but constant and uniform, combination, not to raise the wages of labor. (quoted in Seldes, 1973, p. 943)

A secondary effect of private command is that it tends to become more like government. Historian Eugene Golob reported, "[A result of] the growth of monopoly is the transformation of the entrepreneur into a private business bureaucrat" (1954, p. 157).

Businesses can dictate production, distribution, and price, whenever they put together two conditions to create a *monopoly:*

- *Necessity:* the product is something people can't (or think they can't) do without, such as jobs, energy, or medical care.
- *Exclusivity:* they have sufficient control of supply that the need cannot be met adequately from other sources.

Monopolies come in various shapes and sizes. A loose form is a cartel, in which separate organizations collaborate to control their common market. In the 1970s, members of OPEC (Organization of Petroleum Exporting Countries) agreed to cut production, creating a shortage that enabled them to raise oil prices nearly tenfold.

In labor, the AFL-CIO, an association of independent labor unions, operates as a cartel, when all of its unions agree to honor the picket lines of each member union or to boycott the products of employers who allegedly use unfair labor practices, as in the grape boycott of the 1970s.

An *oligopoly* achieves the same thing without formal agreement. In the 1950s, the American auto industry was dominated by a few big companies and an industrywide union. The companies' costs remained similar because the union negotiated comparable wage agreements with each of them. By copying one another's price increases, they jointly passed along the costs of their high wages, high profit margins, and obsolescent technology to captive consumers.

These monopolies weakened in the 1980s, as outside competitors (new oil producers, nonunion immigrants, Japanese automakers) broke their exclusivity. In addition to the development of outside producers, OPEC had a second problem: some of its members cheated; they exceeded their production quotas and sold below the fixed price.

This can be avoided by forming a *trust,* a holding company with central coordinating authority over its subsidiary corporations. Standard Oil and AT&T were trusts until the government broke them up into smaller companies to restore competition.

The labor counterpart is a *guild,* "a union of men in the same craft or trade to uphold standards and protect the members." A plumbers' union or a bar association can become a monopoly if it gains enough power to impose a "closed shop." That is, it (1) restricts employment in its field to members and (2) controls entry into membership. (A "union shop" does only the first. It restricts employment to members but has an open policy on membership.)

Although private sector control is always motivated by self-interest, it is often argued that the results are in the public interest. Businesses say that a monopoly permits more cost-efficient production and marketing. It may. The social question is, does this lower consumer prices or just increase profits?

Fascism

Fascism is a term developed in Italy by Mussolini and applied to Nazi Germany, but it has been known in other settings by other names. It merges public and private command: there is (1) a ruling junta that exerts political and social control, usually coercive, and (2) substantial concentration of private economic power in the hands of a few corporations.

The junta and the corporations develop a mutual-benefit alliance that reinforces the priorities of each. Sometimes one side is more powerful. The Nazi government basically dictated what industry should do, resulting in low freedom but high profits for companies. In other settings, a political ruling group may be kept in power, but dominated by, transnational corporations.

MIXED ECONOMIES

There are many variants in which the economy is a blend of both free market and central command.

Selective Socialism

Socialism is government ownership and operation of the means of production and/or distribution. Selective socialism is a predominantly private economic market system, with selective governmental ownership for specific reasons. This pragmatic approach was summed up by William Beveridge in *The Pillars of Society* (1943, p. 118): "We probably need public monopoly ownership in certain fields, private enterprise subject to public control in other fields, private enterprise free of any save the general controls in yet other fields."

The 1945 platform, "Let us Face the Future," on which the British Labour Party swept into power for the first time, made social responsibility the test: "Each industry must have applied to it the test of national service. If it serves the nation, well and good. If it is inefficient and falls down on its job, the nation must see that things are put right" (Golob, 1954, p. 281).

In a mixed economy, government ownership of business is usually based on one or more of the following judgments:

- *Unsuitability for private enterprise.* This applies to businesses in which the profit motive could subvert the primary objective, such as national military security or universal health services.
- *Unprofitability.* This describes businesses in which the market revenues don't pay the full cost, such as a county hospital or a public transit system.
- *Need for a monopoly.* This exists for businesses, such as a sewer system, where free competition would be inefficient or inadequate.
- *Troubled industries.* When a number of American railroads went bankrupt, the government took over the business through public companies called Amtrak and Conrail. In other countries, "sick" coal, steel, and banking companies were nationalized. Selective socialism may resell them to the private sector after getting them back on their feet.
- *Strategic industries.* The people may choose government ownership of certain enterprises when they believe it will better serve the general welfare. Mexico took over a highly profitable oil business in order to have the revenues for social programs. The State Bank of North Dakota was established because the state's wheat farmers were losing their farms due to exploitation by "Eastern bankers" (from Minnesota).

Public businesses are usually expected to act "businesslike." Utilities and strategic industries are expected to be self-supporting through sales revenues. Operating surpluses are retained for capital improvements or returned to the treasury as profit. In troubled industries, capital investment subsidies may be provided with the long-term goal of self-sufficiency.

Mercantilism

At the end of the Middle Ages, central monarchies developed some autonomy from their feudal vassals by controlling foreign trade. This was accelerated by the discovery of the New World, which was exploited by trading monopolies owned by the king or by paying commissions to him.

Mercantilism emerged as a central control system that accumulated national (royal) wealth in the form of gold, silver, and precious stones by (1) exporting more than they imported, (2) overcharging domestic consumers through monopolistic price-fixing, and (3) plundering foreigners through conquistadors, colonialism, privateers (royally commissioned pirates), and military aggression.

Modern mercantilism is economic nationalism. The central government restricts market freedom in ways that favor domestic industry and maintain a "favorable" balance of payments (export more than you import). It uses a number of techniques:

- *Quotas:* limitations on the quantity of imports admitted.
- *Tariffs:* taxes that increase the consumer cost of imports, giving domestic industries a price advantage.
- *Export subsidies:* lowering the price to foreign buyers, thereby stimulating sales. The government may purchase the goods for resale abroad at a loss, give tax welfare or cash rebates to exporters, and/or provide free marketing services.
- *Industrial development:* direct or indirect assistance in building a new or strategic industry. These subsidies to private businesses lower the price at which they can sell their cars or airplanes in competition with those of other nations.
- *Devaluation of currency:* by making the dollar worth less in foreign exchange for yen, marks, and pounds, the dollar prices on our exports cost less in the buyer's currency, and the prices of their goods cost more to our consumers, thus encouraging exports and discouraging imports.

The pros and cons of mercantilism are somewhat muddled ideologically. On a macro level, its nationalistic approach to the "community of nations" reflects the classical capitalist ideology of competitive individualism. On the other hand, seen from the perspective of individual producers and consumers, it substitutes central control for a free market. In practice, bottom-line decisions tend to be pragmatic, not ideological. Nations tend to favor free trade when it results in a "favorable" balance of trade and mercantilistic practice when their free-trade balance would be negative.

Developing a national consensus on the balance between mercantilism and free trade is not easy. Restrictions favor industries in which foreign imports are strong, such as autos. Free trade benefits exporting industries, such as agriculture. The average person may be ambivalent, advocating for restriction when it enhances one's job security and for free trade when it lowers the cost of one's clothes. A consistent national policy on mercantilism is further complicated by the inability to control the ever-changing circumstances and practices of other nations.

Worker Ownership

Another mixed economic approach is syndicalism, "worker ownership of the means of production and distribution." It has two separate historical origins, one a radical socialist ideology and the other a capitalistic reform.

Radical syndicalism, founded in nineteenth-century France by Pierre Proudhon, believed that (1) workers were being exploited by capitalists who misappropriated the fruits of their labor and that (2) government was an instrument of that oppression. In the new order, workers would control the means of production through their unions (syndicates), which would also perform the few government functions needed in this utopian society. Marx incorporated many of their views into his writings.

In 1950, Yugoslavia's Tito broke away from Stalinist ideology and set up a form of Marxist syndicalism, which differed from original syndicalists by maintaining government ownership. Workers in each factory belonged to a Basic Organization of Associated Labor, which elected a workers' council to be the factory's board of directors. The council hired and supervised management and set wages and production targets (within limits). Until it was destroyed by ethnic civil wars, Yugoslavia was the most prosperous of all

Communist countries (but less prosperous than its capitalist European neighbors).

Bogdan Denitch praised the success of Yugoslavian syndicalism's "communitarian and consensual rather than conflictual" approach:

> It posits an economy run essentially by elected bodies of workers and other employees. These elected bodies have had ever-widening powers. They have acted—and this is crucial—not merely as institutions managing sectors of the economy, but as organs of political socialization creating a new nexus of values and links in an industrialized society. (Howe, 1982, pp. 192-193)

Time Magazine (January 6, 1986) was more cynical: "In theory the self-governing councils are 'the purest form of Marxism.' But in practice, the trade union and the management are all controlled by the local party in every big plant."

Capitalist syndicalism had its start about 1820, when Robert Owen, an English factory owner who had earlier pioneered paternalistic welfare capitalism at his New Lanark factory, proposed the establishment of *cooperative communities of producers*. Although fellow capitalists rejected his ideas, working-class groups and liberal intellectuals responded. Several short-lived utopian communities were developed in England and America as part of this ideology. More successful worker-owner enterprises (with different origins) were the Amish Amana Colony in Iowa and kibbutzim in Israel.

A parallel movement was the development of cooperatives, with roots in both inner-city settlement houses and rural populism. Among better-known cooperative enterprises today are Land O Lakes, Dairy Lea, rural electric utilities, and credit unions. Although their structure of ownership is communal, they tend to function externally as business corporations.

In recent years, workers have become overt capitalists by buying stock in their corporations. This has taken place variously, through stock options as a fringe benefit, emergency buyouts by employees to prevent a factory from being shut down, pressure on workers from financially hard-pressed management to take some of their compensation in stock instead of cash, and strategic stock purchases by union members via their pension funds. Over time, this leads to at least partial worker-owner control.

For instance, in 1994, when United Airlines was running a deficit, employee groups agreed to major cash-wage concessions in exchange for company stock. Three years later, with United earning record profits, the pilots' union, frustrated by what they felt was an unacceptable, unreasonable management position, announced that the issues went beyond wages to the company's responsiveness to the concerns of *employee-owners.*

Chapter 12

The Social State

We, the People of the United States, in Order to form a more perfect Union, establish Justice, insure domestic Tranquility, provide for the common defence, promote the general Welfare, and secure the Blessings of Liberty to ourselves and our Posterity do ordain and establish this Constitution for the United States of America.

Preamble to the U.S. Constitution

The poor have sometimes objected to being governed badly; the rich have always objected to being governed at all.

G. K. Chesterton

INTRODUCTION

According to social compact theory, free men and women "unite in commonwealth" for mutual benefit (Locke, 1690). The role of government is to protect the liberty and security of its citizens and promote the general welfare. A key question is, "How can the general welfare best be promoted?" The *social state* contributes two core democratic values—social responsibility and social justice—that are not part of the economic market as such.

The term *social state* (*Sozialstaat*) was a West German Federal Republic reaction against both its own former fascism and the communism imposed by Russia on East Germany. It was incorporated into the constitution as a companion and complement to *Rechtsstaat*, political democracy including civil rights and liberties. The German version of the social state blends the social philosophies of its two largest political blocs, *solidarity* from the socialists and *subsidiarity* from the Christian democrats. They prefer this broader concept to the more paternalistic *Wohlfahrsstaat* (welfare state), initiated by Premier Otto von Bismarck in the 1870s:

> The principal significance of the idea of the "social state" is not only that it entitles public authorities to intervene in markets but also that, within certain limits, the government is actually obliged to address social inequalities and to pursue social welfare goals which are enforceable by the courts. The state is not itself a universal provider but, rather, a *guarantor* and *overseer* of certain rights mostly fulfilled by other agencies. (Clasen and Freeman, 1994, pp. 10-11)

Pope John XXIII's 1963 encyclical, Pacem in Terris, called for such a state:

> It is therefore necessary that the administration give wholehearted and careful attention to the social as well as the economic progress of citizens, and to the development, in keeping with the development of the productive system, of such essential services as the building of roads, transportation, communications, water supply, housing, public health, education, facilitation of the practice of religion, and recreational facilities.
>
> It is necessary also that governments make efforts to see that insurance systems are made available to the citizens, so that, in case of misfortune or increased family responsibilities, no person will be without the necessary means to maintain a decent standard of living.
>
> The government should make similarly effective efforts to see that those who are able to work can find employment in keeping with their aptitudes and that each worker receives a wage in keeping with the laws of justice and equity.
>
> It should be equally the concern of civil authorities to insure that workers be allowed their proper responsibility in the work undertaken in industrial organization, and to facilitate establishment of intermediate groups which will make social life richer and more effective.

Finally, it should be possible for all the citizens to share as far as they are able in their country's cultural advantages.

This chapter examines the social state as a tool to enhance the economic market and to contain, through regulation, some of its negative social effects. Chapter 13 will discuss the other "social state" function, filling economic market gaps with a supplementary social market. Chapter 18 will relate the social state to the issue of centralization versus decentralization.

ENHANCEMENT

Enhancement seeks to improve the existing system's operation. Authoritarian countries approach that goal through central planning and control, as in the Soviet Five-Year Plans and the Chinese Great Leap Forward. It's not so simple in a free market. How do you steer those millions of separate decisions by individuals and companies in the "right" direction?

Laissez-faire policy doesn't try, preferring to endure the cyclical vicissitudes of the law of supply and demand:

- *Inflation* is a rise in prices that reduces purchasing power and undermines confidence in the system of exchange (money).
- *Boom* is an overresponse to demand by uncoordinated suppliers, creating an oversupply that triggers a production-cutting reaction.
- *Recession* is a reduction in production that causes unemployment, reduces profits, increases business failures, and lowers consumption.
- *Depression* is a deep recession in which lost buying power due to unemployment and business failures more than offsets the "normal" increase of demand caused by lowered prices, thus blocking recovery.

FISCAL INTERVENTIONS

Keynesian Economics

Into this world of cyclical market economics came John Maynard Keynes. Responding to the worldwide depression, he wrote *The*

General Theory of Employment, Interest, and Money (1936/1964) in which he developed the idea of influencing the dynamics of supply and demand. Keynes's point of intervention was demand, on the premise that *supply responds to demand:* someone will make what other people are prepared to buy. If more people are buying cars, more cars will be made. If fewer people are buying cars, automakers will cut back. By manipulating the money supply in certain ways, you can encourage individuals and businesses to make *countercyclical* decisions about buying (demand) and producing (supply):

- Increase demand to stimulate production during recession.
- Reduce demand to counter inflation and overexpansion.

An early application of this approach was the 1930s' New Deal:

> Some of Roosevelt's advisers, embracing the theory of John Maynard Keynes (and also making a virtue of necessity), had been arguing . . . that when the government, by over-spending, poured new money into the economic blood-stream, business would be stimulated and a new adjustment would be reached at a higher level, thus rendering the anguish of deflation unnecessary. The new money would "prime the pump" of business; presently all sorts of new businesses would be undertaken, there would be a boom, the unemployed would be absorbed in industry, and all would be well. (Allen, 1939, p. 180)

As it turned out, significant short-range improvements did coincide with these actions to stimulate demand, while long-range effects were less clear.

Since then, Keynesian economics has been a standard ingredient in the pragmatic capitalism of every Western industrial nation. It appears to have been most effective under relatively free supply-and-demand market conditions. It has been, predictably, less effective in dealing with such anti-free-market factors as wars, monopolies, and mercantilism.

Fiscal Policies

The word *fisc* means the government treasury. Fiscal actions involve money going into the treasury as taxes or out of it as expenditures.

Most fiscal interventions focus on the *money supply*. Taxes take money out of circulation; public spending puts it back in. If the two are equal, the money supply is not affected.

The government increases the money supply when it puts more money into circulation than it takes out through taxes in one of two ways: cut taxes or increase spending. This creates a *deficit*, covered by *borrowing*, which increases the national debt. It is similar to making a smaller payment on your credit card than what you charged this month.

The government decreases money supply by running a *surplus*, taking more out in taxes than it spends. The difference is used to reduce the national debt. This is the same as reducing your Master-Card balance.

Keynesian countercyclical economics call for deficits to stimulate demand during a recession, by increasing the money supply, and surpluses to cool inflation and/or rapid expansion, by decreasing the money supply.

Fiscal policies may also change *velocity*. Money is respent more quickly under some circumstances than others. In general, lower-income families spend faster than wealthier ones because more of their income must be respent immediately for current living expenses that can't be put off. *Wages and salaries* get respent faster than corporate revenues. Public spending appropriated for multiyear projects, such as building a new warship, trickles out slowly, while that spent on *short-term purposes*, such as food for the ship's crew, goes into circulation immediately.

In 1981, a change in government fiscal policy reduced the velocity side of demand. Tax cuts for corporations and wealthy investors, combined with Social Security tax increases for low- and middle-income workers, redistributed some of the nation's after-tax income from high-velocity workers to low-velocity upper-income groups. Meanwhile, on the public-spending side, expenditures were transferred from welfare benefits (highest velocity of all) and wage-intensive human services to long-term military hardware projects. The substantial drop in consumer demand that triggered the severe recession of 1982-1983 coincided with the implementation of these fiscal-velocity changes.

If, instead, the government had increased take-home pay for working families by raising the standard deduction—offset by closing tax shelters and eliminating loopholes—and shifted spending from long-term "Star Wars" space projects to rapid-turnaround health services, there presumably would have been a velocity-side stimulation of demand within the same fiscal-money balance.

MONETARY INTERVENTIONS

Just as public borrowing expands demand and increases the M1 money supply, so does private sector borrowing. Repaying those loans takes the money back out of circulation, as does saving, which moves money to the not-for-immediate-spending M2 and M3 categories.

Monetary policies manipulate the money supply by influencing millions of individual and business decisions concerning borrowing and saving.

The *central bank* regulates monetary policy. In the United States, this is a semiautonomous government agency called the Federal Reserve System ("the Fed"). The Fed acts as the banks' bank. Banks borrow money from the Fed and lend it to consumers at a profit.

Interest Rates

The most publicized monetary intervention is the raising and lowering of interest rates. High interest rates reduce demand in two ways:

1. They increase the "effective price" of buying on credit (the item cost plus the loan interest).
2. They make it more profitable for you to save (instead of spending).

Low rates, of course, lower real prices and make it less rewarding to save, and they can make a big difference. If your monthly take-home pay is $2,000 and you need a $60,000 mortgage to buy a house, the monthly interest on an 18 percent mortgage (a common 1981 rate) costs you $900 per month in interest alone, a precarious

45 percent of your $2,000. At 8 percent (a 1997 rate), the same mortgage costs only $400 for interest, a moderate 20 percent of your income. At 6 percent (a 1994 rate, briefly), the cost is $300, an easy 15 percent. When the rates come down, sales go up.

The same thing happens to capital investments by business. When interest rates are high, prudent businesses postpone buying new equipment until they come back down. The high interest raises their overhead more than they care to risk. Not following this prudent practice, some of my neighbors went bankrupt and lost their farms, bringing down their local savings and loan association with them. Riding a wave of optimism, they bought land, tractors, and harvesters when interest rates were high. When the price of corn settled back to "normal" a few years later, they couldn't meet the payments.

The Fed influences interest rates primarily by setting the *discount rate,* which is the interest it charges the banks. The banks, in turn, must charge you more than that to cover their administrative costs and turn a profit. In 1981, when the Fed was discouraging demand to lower inflation, the discount rate was 14 percent, and banks were charging 19 percent to their preferred customers (the "prime rate"). Two years later, needing to stimulate demand to overcome a severe recession, the Fed cut the discount rate to 9 percent, and the banks were charging customers only 11 percent for the same loans.

Several times per year the Federal Reserve Board meets to determine whether to lower interest rates to stimulate a lagging economy or raise them to "cool" inflation or the rate of expansion. Supporters credit the Fed's fine-tuning for a long period of relatively stable economic growth from the late-1980s to the late-1990s. During this period, the rate fell gradually from 7 percent to 3 percent, in the 1991-1992 recession, before climbing gradually back to the 5 percent range in 1995-1997. Critics decry such central micromanagement of the economy as an unnecessary and harmful interference in the operation of a supposedly free market. Skeptics wonder, given the many internal and external forces that affect the market, how much difference it makes either way.

Reserves

Another Fed control is the level of cash and government securities banks must maintain to back their loans. Similar to the down-payment required for a home mortgage, its original purpose was to prevent bank failure by requiring a reserve large enough to cover bad loans. After a while, the reserve ratio became primarily a tool to manipulate the amount of private-sector borrowing.

At a 10 percent level, a bank with a $1 million reserve could lend $10 million, increasing the money supply by the $9 million lent to businesses and consumers, stimulating demand by that amount.

If the Fed wanted to reduce demand, it could raise the reserve ratio to that traditional 20 percent level set centuries ago by the Bank of England and still required for conventional home mortgages. Now the bank's $1 million reserve permits it to lend only $5 million, removing the other $5 million from the money supply. At this point, the bank must drastically curtail new loans and scramble to collect on old loans to get down to the allowed level. This creates a *tight-money* situation, in which it is difficult to get a loan at any price without an inside connection; therefore, we can't buy big-ticket items, and corporations have to postpone planned capital improvements.

If the Fed wanted to stimulate demand instead, it could reduce the reserve ratio to, say, 5 percent. Now the bank's $1 million reserve lets it lend $20 million instead of $10 million. This creates a *loose-money* situation, in which banks try to increase their profit by *lending more money*. At this point, a bank that turned up its nose at borrowers when the reserve was raised is now begging the same customers, through ads, direct mail, and telemarketing to borrow its money.

In practice, the Fed, which is governed largely by people connected with the finance industry, has frequently lowered reserve requirements but rarely exercises its power to raise reserves, which would lower a bank's investment returns. The following are actual reserve levels at different periods:

- 1800s: average 20 percent
- 1929, just before the Crash: 7.5 percent (38 percent of all banks closed in next four years.)
- 1940, after Depression crises: 30 percent—once burnt, twice shy
- 1950, after looser-money World War II and postwar expansion: 13 percent
- 1980, just before the rash of bank failures that cost taxpayers more than $150 billion to cover bank losses: 3.2 percent
- 1990: 2.5 percent (Hixson, 1997, p. 55)

SUPPLY-SIDE ECONOMICS

In the 1980s, supply-side economics was widely hailed as a replacement for Keynesian demand-side economics. In fact, both are rooted in the same classical economics supply and demand theory—and both use "artificial" interventions to manipulate it. Keynes said that suppliers would respond to any increase in consumer demand. Supply-siders started on the other side, assuming that if suppliers invest in expanded production, demand will follow.

This theory was incorporated in the Economic Recovery Tax Act of 1981. Rates were cut 29 percent for capital gains and the wealthiest taxpayers. Supply-side subsidies also use such mechanisms as accelerated depreciation, investment tax credits, and deferral of taxes on income investment through IRAs and equity-based employee pension plans. Overall, the tax reduction was about $150 billion per year, most of it to affluent investors.

All this was supposed to stimulate so much economic growth that, even at the lowered rates, taxes on a much richer economy would not only offset the tax cuts but also reduce the budget deficit. Observed Leonard Silk (1984), "This simply did not happen. . . . They opened up far bigger deficit gaps than he [Reagan] had inherited from the Carter and earlier administrations."

A look at its premises may help put supply-side economics into perspective.

Say's Law

Premise

Early in the nineteenth century, Jean Baptiste Say postulated "Say's Law" that *supply creates its own demand*. The act of producing creates a demand by buying labor, supplies, machinery, and energy. This, in turn, gives the workers and suppliers money to buy what is produced. Put simply, employed autoworkers can afford to buy cars.

Limitations

The recirculation is continuous—provided the product is sold. In 1981, while supply-side fiscal policies were encouraging new investment and production, other tax, monetary, and social program policies were taking money out of circulation, from middle- and lower-class consumers through benefit cuts, unemployment caused by anti-inflation monetary policies, and a Social Security tax increase. That is, counterpolicies created gaps in the circle that lowered demand. Without a market for new production, the circle was broken, and a recession occurred. On the other hand, supply-side economics *did* work in the 1930s (aid to banks and industries) and 1960s (upper-income and corporate tax cuts), when they coincided with social programs that increased low- and middle-income buying power at the same time.

Lesson

Supply-side economics may be effective as a partner of, rather than an alternative to, demand-side economics.

Pareto's Law and the Trickle-Down Theory

Premise

In 1897, Vilfredo Pareto, a pioneer in the mathematic approach to economics, said that *the distribution of income is essentially the same everywhere.* Inequality is constant. When businesses and investors prosper, the benefits, by natural law, trickle down proportionately to the middle and lower classes.

Limitations

As discussed in Chapter 7, this didn't happen in late-twentieth-century America: the rich got richer and the poor got poorer.

Lesson

If the intent is indeed to benefit all segments of society, supply-side economics needs to be accompanied by specific distributive social policies.

The Postulate of Rationality

Premise

According to the natural-law theory of classical economics, businesses and individuals will pursue their self-interests in a manner that optimizes the economic and social orders.

Limitations

Beneficiaries of the 1981 supply-side tax revisions did pursue their self-interest rationally—maximizing their wealth and profit as they were expected to do—but in ways that did not achieve the assumed beneficial social and economic effects.

Five years later, Stern (1986) found that there was an apparent *inverse* relationship between tax breaks and supply-side productive capital investment. Forty-four companies, which showed 11 percent pretax profit increase, earned $57 billion but paid *no* taxes under the new rules, yet their capital investment and payrolls actually went *down* by 4 percent and 6 percent, respectively. Meanwhile, the forty-three highest-taxed firms increased both capital outlays and employment. Where did the money go?

The postulate assumes that socially desirable reinvestment is a natural-law consequence of greater profits, so the tax law did not, for instance, require companies to spend the savings gained from tax write-offs of old plants and equipment on modernized plants and equipment. Stern observed, prophetically, that "a firm can spend its savings as it pleases: to give its executives a raise; to increase dividends to share-holders; to buy out another company" (1986).

Lesson

Since supply-side subsidies benefit the economy only when they are used to improve and/or expand production, they should be applied selectively, within an economic development strategy. The American approach gave unrestricted tax subsidies. Japan, on the other hand, had dramatic success for half a century by providing restricted subsidies, loans, and technical assistance to industries targeted for special development.

Some experts suggest that supply-side subsidies should be "in kind" rather than in cash. Government-financed space research and alternative-energy experiments have made available knowledge and technology "free" to private enterprise. Research and technical assistance from land-grant universities do the same for farmers.

LIMITATIONS ON ALL
SUPPLY-AND-DEMAND STRATEGIES

Political Expedience

"Virtue is its own reward." It had better be, for there may be no other reward for statesmanship. Politicians must stand for reelection every two, four, or, at most, six years. They are dependent on campaign contributions from special interest groups, and they must also be careful not to offend the majority of voters. It's our system. Then-Senator John Kennedy's *Profiles in Courage* is about senators who risked their careers for the sake of moral principle, disinterested statesmanship, and broad, long-range societal interest. This is rare. Kennedy apparently found only seven such senators over a 180-year period.

Both demand- and supply-side interventions have a welcome and an unwelcome side. Keynesian economics calls for interventions to increase demand during recessions and to decrease it during periods of inflation and expansion. We like the stimulation side—lower taxes, expanded benefits, fat defense and construction contracts, and easy credit with low interest rates. The austerity appropriate to "up" times is, to say the least, somewhat less popular, with higher taxes, fewer benefits, fewer military and public works contracts, tight credit, and high interest.

Supply-side economics gives benefits to corporations and the wealthy and expects these benefits to be applied to socially beneficial investments. Corporate interests want the tax welfare but with no strings attached. Wouldn't you in their place?

Politicians are human. If they want votes, they will be tempted to do only the popular half of the Keynesian model. If they want campaign contributions, they will be tempted to do only the popular half of the supply-side model.

Cost-Push Inflation and Stagflation

The law of supply and demand recognizes *"demand-pull"* inflation. When there is a shortage, buyers will compete for the scarce item by offering higher prices. That is, demand *pulls* the price up. A dramatic example of this is what happens to the street price of cocaine when drug agents make a big bust that temporarily cuts off the supply.

Conversely, when there are fewer buyers than there are cars for sale, smart buyers bargain hard as dealers compete to clear their crowded showrooms. Inflation is not supposed to occur when there is an oversupply and weak demand—but during the 1970s, it did!

Faced with increased production costs beyond their control, suppliers *had* to raise prices. This was *cost-push* inflation. It had a predictable effect on sales: as auto prices went up, fewer people could afford new cars. Many of us had to revive that World War II advertising jingle:

> There's a Ford in your future,
> But the Ford in your past
> Is the Ford you have now,
> So you'd better make it last!

As sales dropped, companies produced fewer cars, yet pushed by costs, they raised prices again. Sales dropped more. Workers were laid off, further reducing demand, but not prices. Thus, we had *stagnation* and *inflation* at the same time. We called it *stagflation.*

Traditional countercyclical responses didn't work. Stimulating demand accelerated the inflation, while cooling demand deepened the recession. They were damned if they did, and damned if they didn't.

Monopolistic Causes of Stagflation

How did this occur? *Somebody repealed the law of supply and demand.* Stagflation can occur in a market that has been subverted by the centralized private command discussed in Chapter 11. In the 1970s' case, we can identify three contributing factors:

- *Cartels.* Energy is a major cost in nearly all production. OPEC, controlling a majority of the world's oil production, unilaterally dictated a tenfold increase in the price of energy, a cost that producers had to pass on to buyers.

- *Oligopolies.* Industries dominated by a few big corporations and industrywide unions collaborated in passing along parallel cost increases to consumers who had to pay the price or do without.
- *Cost-plus regulation.* In regulated industries, such as utilities, transportation, and hospitals, the government approved rates based on the audited cost of production—plus a "fair" profit. There was no incentive to seek more cost-effective methods.

Alternatives

Where supply and demand interventions are ineffective due to the lack of price competition among suppliers, there are three choices:

1. *Laissez-faire.* Let the chips fall where they may. By definition, this is "for the best." Best for whom?
2. *Restoration of free market competition.* Deregulate, break up monopolies, and lower international trade barriers.
3. *Stronger central control.* In the absence of competition, establish "just-price" controls on goods and wages.

REGULATION

Winston Churchill called democracy the worst possible form of government—except all others. In the same vein, both liberal and conservative pragmatists have concluded that for all its faults capitalism is still the best available system, given judicious government regulation. They differ, of course, on the specifics of when, where, why, and how.

Laissez-Faire and Monopoly

Classical economic theory assumes (1) that a free economic market is in our best interests, collectively and individually, and (2) that left to itself capitalism will perpetuate an actual free market. The correct government role is noninterference. To do otherwise would upset the delicate operation of the self-regulating natural law of supply and demand.

However, just as no existing economy is fully controlled, neither has any ever been completely free. Even in 1776, when Adam Smith wrote his free-market treatise, *The Wealth of Nations,* and the primitive state of industrial and agricultural technology kept the economy relatively decentralized, foreign trade was largely in the hands of government-sponsored monopolies, and since 1349, when the Statute of Laborers responded to the labor shortage caused by the Black Plague, English Poor Laws had restricted workers' freedom to move about and sell their labor to the highest bidder.

As the technical capacity to manage larger and more complex systems increased during the nineteenth century, *monopolistic capitalism* evolved. Through trusts and cartels, "robber baron" capitalists amassed huge fortunes by dictating lower wages and higher prices than would have been possible if they faced free-market competition. Ironically, the hands-off government policy of laissez-faire left society vulnerable to subversion of the very free market it was intended to preserve. Some modern economists fear that transnational corporations will similarly exploit the "no-man's-land" gaps between national jurisdictions.

The result, to a greater or lesser degree, is conversion of the economy from free-market to private-sector command.

Social State Regulation

Discussing abuses in his industry, a business leader expressed strong support for corrective governmental regulation, then added, with a grin, "except of course when they are regulating me." He was only half joking. Maximum gain is the stated goal of capitalism. Is it not reasonable, then, for an entrepreneur to suppress competition when it is profitable to do so? And, is it not equally reasonable for the people to use their government as the only tool powerful enough to engage big business and protect them from forces that would subvert their market freedoms. (Many would add that the reverse holds true as well. Private enterprise is one of only two forces in our society powerful enough to protect us from a comparable abuse of power by the government. The other is free and open elections.)

Richard Tawney was a realist about selective government intervention: "Fools will use it, when they can, for foolish ends, criminals for criminal ends. Sensible and decent men will use it for ends which are sensible and decent. We in England have repeatedly remade the state, and we are remaking it now, and shall remake it again" (1964, p. 169).

Among the most common interventions are:

- *preserving free-market competition* with antitrust laws;
- *setting a "just price"* for franchised utilities where free competition is not practical;
- *preventing disservices* associated with capitalistic enterprise by setting standards for safe consumer goods, occupational health, environmental protection, and the like;
- *enforcing performance standards* through licensing of physicians, safety standards for autos, pure food and drug regulation, and so on; and
- *refereeing the game* in such areas as fraud, contracts, financial transactions, and collective bargaining.

An example of the last item was the 1936 National Labor Relations Act, which legalized the right of labor to organize and bargain collectively, explicitly to protect free-market rights of employees. Its stated intent was to correct "the unequal bargaining power between employees who did not possess full freedom of association or actual liberty of contract and employers who are organized in the corporate or other forms of ownership associations."

This was not a theoretical statement but rather an empirical one. When bargaining power is unequal, the "free" market can be a cruel joke. In a Nebraska meat-packing company town a few years ago, workers were given a choice: take a 50 percent cut or be replaced by immigrants bused in from Texas. All three worker groups suffered: the ones who took the cut, the ones who had to leave their family roots to seek work elsewhere, and the ones at poverty-line wages who moved into an alien harsh-winter prairie town, without adequate housing available in their income range.

Other kinds of social state reforms have already been discussed in Chapter 3.

LEVELS OF INTERVENTION

The social state may intervene on a continuum from nonintrusive to central control (this section is indebted to Bicanic, 1967, pp. 42-46).

1. *Informative.* Provide social and economic data as input "to whom it may concern," including information on existing situations and trends.
2. *Advisory.* Make nonbinding recommendations, backed by clear rationales that include values, interests, and the situational data reported in number 1.
3. *Stimulative.* Identify desirable policies and promote them with carrot-and-stick incentives, such as tax incentives or eligibility for government contracts.
4. *Directive.* Set policies and implement them directly, as through public programs.
5. *Coercive.* Develop and enforce centrally determined policies, such as the Thirteenth Amendment (slavery) or the Eighteenth Amendment (prohibition).

Chapter 13

The Social Market

Charity is a policy as well as a virtue.

P. D. James

We cannot be content if some fraction of our people is ill-fed, ill-clothed, ill housed, and insecure.

Franklin Roosevelt

"There is no such thing as an absolute boundary line between the market and socially provided goods and services. Where a commodity that is essential to existence becomes so scarce that its distribution by the market may destroy society's norms and values and undermine law and order, the market will be replaced" (Glennester, 1995, p. 65). The question is what commodities are essential and how serious the scarcity must be to do something about it.

Reasons for a social market include a belief in basic human rights, the self-interest of "have-nots" in adequacy, and the self-interest of "haves" in a secure, stable society. Otto von Bismarck pioneered social market programs in 1870s' Germany for the last reason—as a successful strategy to defuse a serious radical socialist threat of revolution. Franklin Roosevelt initiated them in 1930s' United States for the first reason—emergency relief to meet dire needs, then long-term social insurances to prevent future deprivation.

ECONOMIC AND SOCIAL MARKETS

Economic and Social Market Values

The *economic market* (EM) is the sum total of self-interested individual choices. It expects you to buy medical care or day care,

221

instead of something else, if you want it enough. If you do, providers will emerge in response to the profit opportunity. If you don't, why should anyone give it to you? As a social welfare policy, this assumes three things:

1. You *know* what you need and have the good sense to get it.
2. You can *afford* to buy it.
3. You can *evaluate* and choose among competing providers.

Unfortunately, this is not always the case. Young children, Alzheimer's disease patients, and unconscious accident victims may not be competent to decide. Tens of millions of Americans do not have enough money to live on, let alone the discretionary income to choose between psychotherapy and a Porsche. Few of us can evaluate doctors, marriage counselors, or hospitals in advance.

The *social market* (SM) is a response to these inherent economic market deficiencies. Whereas the economic market assumes self-interested individualism, the social market assumes that we care for each other's others' well-being. This may be the most fundamental social policy value choice today:

> In American society, where the egoistic equity values are dominant, economic debate most frequently evolves about the role that is to be assigned to the social value systems. . . . The intensity of opposition is out of all proportion to the demands they make on social resources and must be understood as the result of a conflict between two acknowledged ethical standards that find coexistence difficult. (Kuenne, 1993, p. 19)

"Moderates" walk a tight line which affirms the legitimacy of self-centeredness in the economic market, provided there coexists a social market which adequately supplements it.

A Summary of the Two Markets

Conceptually, the distinction between economic and social markets is simple:

> In the economic market the criterion is one of utility, or price; in the social market the criterion is one of need. Within the

economic market there is discrimination between like cases of need in terms of price. Those with an equal ability to pay can enjoy equality of provision. Within the social market the allocation of welfare provision is governed by the principle that like cases of need should be treated in a like manner. (Pinker, 1979, p. 224)

In analyzing the two markets, we need to look at both the consumer (demand) and the provider (supply) sides, as they affect human services.

Economic and Social Markets

	Consumers	Providers
Economic	Ability to pay and want it enough	Competitive sale to able buyer
Social	Need unrelated to ability to pay	Subsidized by government or charity

The Consumer Side

In the EM, two factors determine whether a consumer gets a needed or wanted service. One is ability to pay for it. If not, forget it. If ability exists, this second factor opportunity cost (see Chapter 10). Do you need/want family counseling or straight teeth enough to scrimp on food and clothing for six months or, at a higher income level, to make do another year with the old car?

By contrast, the SM basis for receiving is need and/or ability to benefit unrelated to ability to pay. My late wife, a PhD professor, grew up poor in New York City. By qualifying on a tough entrance exam, she received an outstanding secondary education at the Bronx High School of Science, then rode the subway to a tuition-free city university.

The Provider Side

An EM provider sells its services, in competition with other providers, to able buyers, as in music lessons, most orthodontics, and some day care.

An SM provider is subsidized to provide free (or below-cost) service to persons with qualifying need. A family service agency can serve you regardless of your ability to pay because it is subsidized by the United Way. The tuition at a community college is low because two-thirds of the cost is paid by public funds. A private college offers need-based scholarships financed by government grants and alumni gifts.

Hybrid Markets

There are four possible demand-supply combinations in the human service field. Two are simple and obvious. When both are economic market, we have a normal business situation of consumer-buyers and commercial sellers. Both are social market when subsidized public and voluntary agencies accept clients on the basis of need.

This leaves two hybrids. One is SM payer/EM provider. This is called "purchase of service," a method used by Title IV (child welfare), Title XVIII (Medicare), Title XIX (Medicaid), and Title XX (social services) of the Social Security Act. The patient or client receives the service on the basis of need, and the government pays for it. However, instead of providing it directly through its own subsidized agency, such as a Veteran's Hospital, the SM payer buys it from competing sellers in the economic market, which may include private entrepreneurs, large corporations, and "businesslike" nonprofit organizations. When it is purchased from commercial providers, it is called "privatization." Many "welfare state" opponents support this on the grounds that if you can't stop government spending at least you can route it through the EM, where business can profit from it.

The other hybrid is EM payer/SM provider. An affluent couple who can afford to buy marriage counseling in the EM chooses the SM United Way family service agency anyway because of its good reputation but pays an EM rate that covers the full cost of service, preserving the subsidy for other clients.

DISWELFARES AND THE ECONOMIC MARKET

In the normal circumstances of life, we may suffer harm that is completely or partially beyond our control to avoid. In economics, this is called a loss, in social policy, a *diswelfare*. If it is caused by someone else or society as a whole, it is a *disservice*. There is no specific mechanism within the economic market to address these issues.

Individual Disservices

Traditionally, economic market rules let you seek compensation for disservices, provided you can:

- prove specific damage and establish a dollar value,
- prove specific parties to be responsible,
- prove they were negligent,
- engage in adversary litigation, and
- not be outmaneuvered by an opposing lawyer.

Even if the source of the disservice is clearly identified and found responsible, you may not collect. You may be denied compensation if both parties are to blame, "however small that blame may be on one side." The proven disservice may be excused on the grounds that it is normal and acceptable behavior in our society, as was the case in several early lawsuits against sellers of cigarettes. Awarded damages may not be paid because the responsible party has filed for bankruptcy protection, is in jail, or has hidden his or her assets in an offshore bank.

No-Fault Diswelfares

What about diswelfares that can't be pinned on one identifiable culprit? Some seem to be nobody's fault, such as when a hailstorm destroys your wheat crop, a flood ravages your home, or arthritis destroys your ability to work as a watch repairer. Our normal life cycle creates "no-fault" needs: child rearing puts an extra financial burden on young families; in old age, earning power diminishes and medical needs increase.

In other cases, "we have met the enemy, and he is us" (Pogo). We know what causes the acid rain that reduces your bushels of corn per acre, deteriorates your house, and aggravates your sinusitis, but there are literally millions of contributing industrial and auto-driving culprits, including you and me. You can't take us all to court.

The culprit may be the system itself. The economic market system inherently creates hardship for millions of people in the course of its ups and downs. Further, it defines employees as impersonal economic units. A business is expected to terminate employees, lower wages, or move jobs overseas, whenever it is more profitable to do so. Even good personnel practices must be justified by a bottom line which shows that they pay off in more productive workers.

Own-Fault Needs

I have a friend who is paraplegic, as a result of a street fight he initiated. Another friend had to quit work and receive expensive treatment because of emphysema caused by her two-pack-a-day cigarette habit. Their conditions were no less grim because they had been imprudent.

"Let the Loss Lie Where It Falls"

In all of these situations, regardless of cause or fault, the diswelfares are real and need relief. Lord Blackburn, in an 1884 British trial, pronounced what became a famous precedent, "The loss lies where it falls." The economic market agrees: that's the way the cookie crumbles!

Needed: Something to Fill the Gaps

The social market exists because most of us are not this callous; it matters to us what happens to others. For many of us, it is also enlightened self-interest. One day the cookie that crumbles may be yours or mine. A lot of us have already been there. Anti-SM government leaders during the past quarter century, in the United States, Britain, Canada, and elsewhere, have cut services to low-income subgroups but could make little inroad on broad-based social insurances. Why? Recent trends in our society have led millions of citizens to rediscover their vulnerability. They know that even if they are on the high road now, the odds are that they will need social market programs sometime, someplace, probably more than once. Among those developments are the following:

- Downsizing of long-term employees, many at senior levels, lowers confidence in career security.
- Longer life expectancy means people who retire at sixty-five now average seventeen years of postsalary life.
- Millions of late-middle-age Americans, trying to secure their own retirement years, are burdened with care and costs of parents who, in past generations, would have already died.
- A 1997 prediction by the Center for Disease Control and Prevention states "that if current smoking patterns continue, about 25 million people now living will die prematurely"—nearly one-tenth of us. Most will endure expensive medical needs in the process and leave behind relatives burdened with increased economic and social problems.
- Both new and older workers are discovering that their high school education may no longer ensure an adequate job. Millions are seeking further education at SM community colleges and universities.

PRIVATE SOCIAL MARKET SUPPLEMENT: CHARITY

The private social market is strong in the United States. It includes:

- charities that offer care, personal services, and material aid, many of them church-related and/or supported by the United Way;
- organized volunteers, often under the auspices of a charitable agency;
- philanthropic support for arts and education from foundations, corporate donations, and individual large donors;
- cooperatives and other mutual assistance organizations;
- person-to-person aid and caregiving, mostly to relatives, friends, and neighbors (the more traditional the culture or subculture, the greater this appears to be); and
- public interest advocates for persons with special needs, such as the Children's Defense Fund.

German and Japanese medical care presents an interesting gray area. On the one hand, it is purchased by private employers and employees from private insurers who pay private providers. On the other hand, the buyers are required to do so, and the insurers and providers must meet rigorous government standards.

When all is said and done, the private social market is a large, indispensable sector of American society—which has never been able by itself to close the gap between the needs of citizens and what the economic market alone provides. This leads us to the next sector.

PUBLIC SOCIAL MARKET SUPPLEMENT: THE WELFARE STATE

Sometimes it seems as if the welfare state is nobody's friend. It is constantly damned for being too much or too little. Conservatives have called it socialist because it increases public intervention. Socialists have called it "an attempt by the Establishment at soaking up unrest while leaving basic structures of power unchanged" (Clasen and Freeman, 1994, p. 162), "a kind of ambulance service for capitalism" (Townsend, 1975, p. 28).

These charges are not new. The first social insurances were enacted by the British Liberal Party during 1908-1911. Socialist Kier Hardie, founder of the Labour Party, campaigned for fundamental economic reforms. "No say the Liberals, but we will give you the Insurance Bill. We shall not uproot the cause of poverty but we will give you a porous plaster to cover the disease that poverty causes" (speech to miners at Merthyr Tydfil, 1908, in Fraser, 1973, p. 151).

In defending the programs, Prime Minister Lloyd George in a 1911 campaign speech, proudly acknowledged that it was indeed an ambulance service:

> I am in the ambulance corps. There are men who tell me I have overloaded the wagon. I have taken three years to pack it carefully. I cannot spare a single parcel, for the suffering is very great. There are those who say the ambulance is half empty. It is as much as I can carry. Now there are those who say I'm in a hurry. I am in a hurry, for I can hear the moanings of the wounded. (speech at Birmingham, reported in the *London Times*, June 11, 1911, quoted in Fraser, 1973, p. 257)

According to the dictionary, the welfare state is everybody's friend, "a state in which the welfare of its citizens, with regard to employment, medical care, social security, etc., is considered to be the responsibility of government."

In 1942, Ernest Bevin, Minister of Labor, in *Social Insurance and Allied Services,* a report which greatly influenced Britain's postwar welfare state development, summarized the goal as "total abolition of that part of poverty which is due to interruption or loss of earnings" (quoted in Fraser, 1973, p. 199).

The Council of Europe (COE, 1993, p. 6) defines "nine branches" of the welfare state:

- medical care,
- sickness benefits [sick leave],
- unemployment insurance,
- old age benefits,
- employee injury benefits,
- family benefits,
- maternity benefits,
- invalidity [disability],
- survivor benefits.

Individual Benefit Objectives

Welfare state objectives fall into two categories: well-being for individual citizens and collective societal interests. Depending on whom you talk to, these are complementary or conflicting.

One objective is *adequacy.* The welfare state may seek to ensure a minimum standard of nutrition, housing, health care, education, etc. Our society, if it chose, could entirely eliminate poverty as we currently define it.

Another objective is *equity.* If equity means getting what you deserve, a logical extension of the concept is *not getting stuck with what you don't deserve.* Said Richard Titmuss (1958, p. 117):

> Services in kind and in cash . . . may represent not a benefit at all but a compensation for disservices caused by society and especially those disservices (or social costs) where the causal agent, or agents, cannot be identified, legally held responsible,

and charged with the costs. . . . Unless the social costs of these disservices are to lie where they fall (as they did in nineteenth century Britain and as they do to a large extent in the United States today) then we have to find ways and means of compensating people without stigma.

A third objective is *temporal equality.* Retirement pensions and family allowances are intended to equalize a person's standard of living over her/his lifetime, while unemployment insurance tries to even out cyclical ups and downs.

Fourth, because unemployed, retired, disabled, orphaned, and chronically ill beneficiaries usually have lower private income than the average taxpayer, a by-product of welfare state benefits is to *reduce overall inequality.* In the United States from 1933 into the 1970s (but not thereafter), social market redistributions were just sufficient to offset increases of pretax inequality that were occurring in the private sector.

Perhaps the most important objective is *security,* not only on the material level, but also the psychological security of knowing that these benefits are available if and when they are needed. A worker, for instance, may look forward to retirement with pleasant anticipation instead of fear.

There is no single consensus guideline for welfare state programs. Denmark's five principles come as close as any to expressing the intent:

1. *Proximity,* decentralization of delivery, as near and accessible to the citizen-consumer as possible.
2. *Single service,* multiservice health and welfare "one string centers."
3. *Universal.* "Chronic disorders are regarded as a major risk for which the entire community assumes responsibility."
4. *Least disturbing,* services organized and provided to keep a person, in order of preference, in (1) one's own home, (2) local sheltered housing, or (3) local nursing home, with hospitalization, institutionalization, or relocation only as last resorts.
5. *Help people to help themselves,* through services that enable as much independence and self-care as possible, avoiding practices

which foster external or psychological dependency. (COE, 1993, p. 126)

Collective Interests and Social Control

Benjamin Disraeli, later to become prime minister of England, described current social conditions in his 1845 political novel, *Sybil*:

> Said Egremont, slightly smiling, "but say what you like, our Queen reigns over the greatest nation that ever existed."
> "Which nation?" asked the younger stranger, "for she reigns over two."
> The stranger paused; Egremont was silent, but looked inquiringly.
> "Yes," resumed the younger stranger. "Two nations; between whom there is no intercourse and no sympathy; who are as ignorant of each other's habits, thoughts, and feelings, as if they were dwellers in different zones, or inhabitants of different planets; who are formed by a different breeding, are fed by a different food, are ordered by different manners, and are not governed by the same laws."
> "You speak of . . . " said Egremont hesitantly.
> *"The rich and the poor."* (quoted in de Schweinitz, 1961, p. 128)

To Joseph Townsend (1786), this was good social policy: "When hunger is either felt or feared, the desire of obtaining bread will quietly dispose the mind to undergo the greatest hardships, and will sweeten the severest labours."

Some critics accuse welfare state programs of subverting capitalism by weakening this "work or starve" social control. Others casually dismiss humanitarian considerations in the name of "general welfare":

> It is in the interests of all that, under a free system [of national health care], those with full earning capacity should often be rapidly cured of a temporary and not dangerous disablement at the expense of the aged . . . who will never again contribute to the [economic] needs of the rest. (Hayek, 1960, pp. 299-300)

A more sophisticated Establishment viewpoint sees Disraeli's dual society as a breeding ground for rebellion and revolution. In 1895, Conservative Prime Minister Lord Alfred Balfour blended responsibility and pragmatism in an early, classic rationale for welfare state programs:

> Social legislation, as I conceive it, is not merely to be distinguished from socialist legislation, but it is its most direct opposite and its most effective antidote. Socialism will never get possession of the great body of public opinion . . . if those who wield the collective forces of the community show themselves desirous to ameliorate every legitimate grievance and to buy Society upon a proper and more solid basis. (1895 campaign speech, quoted in Fraser, 1973, p. 129)

More recently, Robert Morris's intercountry review of welfare state policies concluded:

> The idea of a welfare state has popularly been treated as if it were an end in itself, but in actuality governments seem much more concerned with the production of welfare for their citizens by any means in order to preserve national stability. The welfare state is more reactive than proactive. (1988, p. 7)

Mary Switzer, longtime head of Vocational Rehabilitation, was a master at blending individual benefit with collective interests. She got increases, even in retrenchment periods, by stressing the dollar payoff from restoring disabled workers to economic productiveness.

Some social justice advocates oppose parts of the welfare state for this very reason. Piven and Cloward's classic critique of public welfare, *Regulating the Poor,* said it was a deliberate instrument of oppression:

> This book is about relief-giving and its uses in regulating the political and economic behavior of the poor. . . . Historical evidence suggests that relief arrangements are initiated or expanded during the occasional outbreaks of civil disorder produced by mass unemployment, and are then abolished or contracted when political stability is restored. . . . Expansive relief

policies are designed to mute civil disorder and restrictive ones to reinforce work norms. In other words, relief policies are cyclical—liberal or restrictive depending on the problems of regulation in the larger society with which the government must contend. (1971, p. xiii)

HOW MUCH SOCIAL MARKET CAN WE AFFORD?

Even if we agree (which some do not) that (1) we share social responsibility for each other and (2) that government is an appropriate instrument to handle the shortfalls caused or permitted by our economic market system, there is still a matter of how much caring we can afford.

The Pessimistic View

A traditional belief is that welfare state programs depress the economy. In 1983, Neil Gilbert, a respected economist who is also a leading expert on social welfare, warned:

> How much social welfare can society afford? . . . . The welfare state is nonproductive. Social welfare provisions [may be] investments in human resources which are conducive to economic growth. But these welfare provisions are created and sustained by surplus produced in the market economy. This dependence on economic surplus places a practical limit on the size of the welfare state. Since the 1960s the American welfare state has been approaching this limit; some might say it has been crossed. (p. 139)

There is a practical limit to social welfare programs. In Bangladesh, where the per capita income is below our definitions of adequacy, no amount of redistribution will meet the need. In marginal economies, basic food and shelter needs may take priority over other human services. Where does the "practical limit" of the United States lie?

We are not now talking about value and interest choices on how we use the economic surplus, how much of it we wish to accumulate privately, and how much of it we wish to share through social programs. We will discuss that later. The question here is what we could *afford*—if we chose—to spend for education, health, housing, old-age pensions, and help for those on whom the diswelfares of our system fall unevenly.

Intercountry Comparisons

Is our economic surplus really too small to support even what we are already doing? In 1983, Gilbert thought so—but this pessimistic conclusion was at odds with intercountry comparisons. Total federal, state, and local public social welfare spending at that time, including education and housing, added up to 19 percent of the gross domestic product (GDP). The comparable social expenditures were 33 percent in Germany and higher in Belgium, Netherlands, Denmark, France, and Sweden (Morris, 1988)—yet during that period, they had higher economic growth rates and had surpassed us in nearly every vital statistic from the cradle (infant mortality) to the grave (longevity).

Perhaps, far from damaging an economy, welfare state investments well above those of the United States may enhance the economy. We don't know positively in either direction because of intervening variables, such as the following:

- An era of general prosperity in Europe and America accompanied expansion of social welfare programs in the 1960s.
- Although social expenditures remained fairly constant in the 1970s, Europe and America experienced inflation and economic slowdowns. This was also the period when the OPEC cartel raised oil prices to ten times what they had been.
- The 1980s was a period of lowered inflation and gradual economic recovery, along with a political turn to the right in several countries, but relatively little change in total social expenditures. It was also the time when oil prices were cut by more than half.
- West Germany was a preeminent model of both social insurance and economic market growth, but it struggled to balance both, after merging in 1991 with an inefficient excommunist economy and extending all entitlements to the impoverished East Germans.

- While Japan was rapidly expanding its welfare state programs and its competitors were capping theirs, it became the world leader in economic growth. It was also reinvesting more of its corporate profits into capital expansion, subsidizing selected economic development, and imposing mercantile policies that gave them great advantages over their trading partners. (A 1990s' slowdown, during a stable welfare state situation, coincided with countermercantile responses.)

In 1991, the social welfare spending of all twenty-six members of the Council of Europe, including both high and low social program nations, averaged 25 percent of their GDPs (COE, 1993, p. 6).

Economic Surplus*

Due to technological advances, most U.S. "production" is in "surplus" categories. In 1995, only 25 percent of employed persons worked in agriculture, mining, manufacturing, and construction combined, down from 32 percent in 1980 and 38 percent in 1970.

From 1980, on which Gilbert based his analysis, to 1994, the nation's per capita income increased by 25 percent. The gain did not fall evenly. Median income was up only 1 percent. The top one-fifth families' share of all national income rose 13 percent, while the shares of the other four-fifths dropped, the bottom fifth by 18 percent. Thus, the net economic surplus that can finance social programs has increased by one-quarter, going primarily to those on the upper end of the income scale.

Based on Gilbert's criterion of economic surplus, how much social expenditure can we now afford? We don't really know, but certainly more than ever before. The key question is how much do those who received the gain choose to share?

The Special Case of Longevity

The Council of Europe studied the effect of increasing life spans on present and future funding of Social Security. By the year 2050,

---

*Unless otherwise indicated, data in this chapter is from the Census Bureau and the Bureau of Labor Statistics, printed in a useful one-stop government reference, *The American Almanac*, 1996-1997. It is updated annually.

the cost of pensions in constant dollars is expected to double world-wide. For the United States, they estimate a 115 percent increase.

The "dependency rate" includes persons over sixty-five and under eighteen. The percentage increase projected for those over sixty-five will be partially offset by a lower percentage in the under-eighteen dependency group, yielding lower child care, family, and education costs. COE estimates that, in 2050, overall U.S. social expenditures to maintain its existing programs will increase 65 percent.

To cover this increase, our per capita economic growth rate must average a little less than 1 percent (0.84 percent) per year in constant dollars. The comparable growth rate needed in Canada is 1.05 percent, United Kingdom, 0.16 percent, and Germany, *minus* 0.05 percent. The average U.S. per capita growth rate for 1980-1995 was 2.5 percent. The Organization for Economic Cooperation and Development (OECD) and the International Monetary Fund (IMF) both estimate that economic growth will readily cover the increases (COE, 1993, pp. 40-41).

There are, of course, factors not included in these estimates. The projections assume that programs will remain unchanged except for population and inflation changes. This may not occur. For example, we may expand per capita spending for higher education due to increasing numbers of adults, ages eighteen to sixty-five, pursuing further education. Experts expect this will be offset by their higher productivity. They're probably right, but we don't know for certain.

Another well-documented trend not taken into account is earlier retirement. The percentage of men age fifty-five to sixty-four not in the labor force increased from 28 percent, in 1980, to 34 percent, in 1995, higher in Europe. On the other hand, the decision to raise Social Security eligibility from age sixty-five to sixty-seven wasn't factored in either.

Another countertrend is employment of wives, which was up from 41 percent in 1970 to 61 percent in 1995. Under Social Security, a wife gets half of what her husband receives if she is not employed, substantially more if/when she is widowed. Wives pay the same payroll tax as single persons, but they gain in benefits only the amount, if any, by which their personal entitlement exceeds their spousal entitlement. Trend result: extra revenue without an equivalent benefit payout.

Where does this leave us? We are:

1. sobered by the increasing cost of maintaining existing programs due to demography;
2. less fearful of the catastrophe predicted by gloom-and-doomers;
3. optimistic that we can not only maintain but improve average lifetime well-being for our people, through affordable social programs—*if* we choose to use our resources to do so; and
4. humbly aware that, with the system so complex and the future so uncertain, things may turn out better or worse than projected.

COE warns us about simplistic solutions: "So called privatization of public pension systems does not automatically reduce the financial burden on society measured in terms of the share of national income devoted to it, but rather tends to yield another distribution of pensions coverage" (1993, p. 23).

"Privatization" takes many forms, including: (1) direct public expenditures to buy services from private vendors, (2) mandatory private pensions with public tax welfare subsidies, (3) mandatory private pensions without public subsidy, or (4) elimination of public programs on the (empirically unfounded) assumption that the private sector will voluntarily pick up the slack. Whatever their merits, none of these changes can eliminate the problem of demographically based societal costs. The first three do not affect the cost; they merely shift it from one sector to another. The fourth is almost certain to lower the standard of living for millions of people. The only foolproof cost solution is a policy of genocide at age sixty-five and involuntary termination of the chronically ill!

These are no grounds for complacency. The outlook is not sufficiently rosy to shrug at inefficiencies, profiteering, and user-abusers in our social programs. We cannot afford not to be more cost-effective. This doesn't mean cutting benefits: tt means getting more benefits/ services per dollar. COE Secretary General Catherine Lalumiere said:

> I am often struck by the fact that patients—or their families— adopt solutions that are extremely costly for the social security system, not out of choice, but simply because they are the only solutions available to them, or at least those which involve the least red tape. (COE, 1993, p. 7)

Among the culprits were overuse of hospitals, nursing homes, and sheltered care, for which she identified two contributing reasons: (1) lack of less costly home service alternatives and (2) separation of health and welfare services, "an institutional barrier to rational guidance on the most cost-effective solution" (Ibid., p. 7).

SOCIAL MARKET ECONOMIC EFFECTS

The Effect of Redistribution

Gilbert accurately called transfers from one person to another via taxation and social welfare benefits "*non*productive." This is correct but should not be misread as meaning *counterproductive*. It is an essentially *neutral internal transfer,* within the aggregate economy, similar to an inheritance, an allowance from one's parents, or a contribution to charity. It changes who spends the money and probably what it will be spent on, but it does not change the amount of money available to be spent (see Chapter 11).

Economists say that redistribution may have marginal effects by moving some money, directly or through in-kind benefits, from upper- to lower-income persons. One school says that this depresses the economy by reducing the pool of money potentially available for capital investment in favor of consumption by lower-income groups.

Another school says that the redistributed money stimulates demand because more of it is spent quickly for basic consumer needs (higher velocity). This in turn means higher sales and profits for business, thereby making further capital investment attractive and profitable. Most capital investment comes, they say, from retained corporate earnings and through borrowing money that is repaid by increased future sales.

Who's right? Perhaps both. If so, the overall effects could offset each other.

Using Surplus Productive Capacity

The traditional definition of economic surplus is that which is produced over and above basic necessities. That surplus may be used for:

1. *discretionary consumption goods,* such as VCRs, sport utility vehicles, wine, designer jeans, and vacation homes;
2. *services that* contribute to quality of life, such as education, entertainment, a lawn service, therapy, and surfing the Internet; and
3. *nonconsumption goods,* such as nuclear missiles. (At least we hope they will never be "consumed"!)

Benefits to meet basic human needs and human services are choices in competition with conveniences, entertainment, military hardware, luxuries, and all other possible uses of surplus productive capacity. Although the choices are *socially* significant, it matters little to the overall *economy* whether meals and maid service are provided in a luxury resort or in a nursing home or whether one buys the "product" of a psychologist or a pop singer.

The key elements in making the choice, then, are ethical and social rather than macroeconomic. All consumption of goods and services, whether distributed through the economic market or the social market, have economic utility ("the power to satisfy the needs and wants of humanity") because they contribute to someone's perceived needs and wants:

- What *purposes* are better than others? Is a sports car for Dad as desirable as a year of college for Sis? Is civilian health care as important as military strength?
- What uses are *effective* in achieving their purposes? Did a university education increase your income? Did cocaine make you happy?
- *Who* should get what and why? To what extent should amenities be unequal due to merit? Or aggressiveness? Or luck? Or inheritance? Who says so?

On the other hand, it appears that *nonconsumption* goods absorb resources without providing utility. This may explain why the average standard of living during the Cold War went up faster among our allies than in the United States—and among the USSR's allies than its own people. Many observers attribute the USSR's economic collapse to excess military expenditures at the expense of consumer goods and services. It certainly wasn't due to their meager human services!

Stability

As discussed in Chapter 11, a recurring problem in the economic market has been cyclical swings in supply and demand. During recessions, income, and therefore demand, goes down due to unemployment, reduced wages, and lower profits. In the other direction, too fast an increase in demand can trigger a boom which sets us up for another fall.

Two kinds of welfare state programs stabilize the economy:

- *Cycle-proof* programs, such as pensions, health care, and public education, remain relatively constant during good times and bad. If you remove these areas from economic swings, both the ups and the downs are moderated.
- *Countercyclical* benefits, such as unemployment insurance and food stamps, expand during recessions. By restoring some of the lost demand, they lessen the recession and contribute to a turnaround. In "up" times, they go down, slowing overrapid growth in demand.

Inflation and Deficits

"There ain't no free lunch." In the good ol' days, saloons advertised free lunches of hard-boiled eggs, peanuts, and the like. However, it wasn't really free. You bought a beer or three, which more than paid for the food.

The welfare state has been accused of causing fiscal deficits and inflation. It needn't. Internal redistribution and substitution of one production-consumption choice for another are basically neutral. Still, it is not without cost. We can have universal health service, day care, and adequate welfare without inflation, but we have to balance these expenditures on the revenue side.

So it would be were it not for the human factor. Unfortunately, this simple balancing process may not entirely please upper-bracket taxpayers, who pay more than they get back. As discussed in Chapter 12 on the limits of supply and demand strategies, pragmatic politicians hesitate to bite the bullet. Each year they do their juggling act, promising to preserve and enhance social programs popular with groups with demonstrated voting power and to reduce taxes for those who finance their campaigns. The largest noncrisis deficits in our history began in 1981, after a large tax cut that was not offset by lower expenditures. (Reductions in social programs were transferred to escalating arms race spending.)

Work Incentive

The nineteenth-century principle of "less eligibility" assumed that people work only out of financial necessity. Modern believers have warned that improved social benefits will create a labor shortage because people won't work. This has not happened in any existing welfare state. Why not?

To begin with, the economic motive for work extends beyond subsistence. Work patterns in both the United States and Marxist countries suggest that *most people want more than minimum adequacy* and will work for it, as witnessed by the frequency of moonlighting, multiple-earner families, part-time work by retirees, and other efforts to supplement base incomes.

Second, "man shall not live by bread alone" (Matthew 4:4). Work motivation is not just economic. Our jobs—or having none—make a big difference in how others view us and how we feel about ourselves. A millionaire-heiress friend of mine gets her primary identity from a job as a fashion buyer, which contributes less than 10 percent of her total income. The will to work can be even stronger than that. I have worked personally with many former and potential welfare mothers who chose employment over relief, even when doing so cost them net income and health benefits.

There is another social policy angle to work incentive. Labor surplus, not shortage, has been a chronic problem most of the time since the industrial revolution. It has been exacerbated frequently by labor-saving technological advances. Since 1950, official unemployment has averaged 5 percent to 10 percent of the labor force. From 1980 to 1995, 7 million or more workers were out of work and looking for jobs at any given moment.

Our largest welfare state program, Social Security, was explicitly promoted as an *intentional work disincentive*. To make room for younger workers, it withholds up to $15,000 per year of earned benefits from sixty-five-year-olds who refuse to quit their jobs. Similarly, widows with dependent children receive Social Security only if they don't take a job.

Policies have been inconsistent over time. Originally, in 1935, the stated purpose of Aid to Dependent Children was to keep low-income mothers out of the workforce to stay home and take care of their children. In the 1960s, the program, renamed Aid to Families with Dependent Children (AFDC), decided to permit mothers to stay with their children but *encourage* them to leave the children to take jobs. Toward this end, education, training, and work-experience programs were offered to make them employable, along with interim financial incentives to ease the transition.

In 1981, in a return to the philosophy of the 1834 Poor Law Reform, incentives and assistance were replaced by punitive less eligibility strategies to *push* them into jobs. This reached its logical conclusion in a 1996 law that renamed the program Temporary Assistance to Needy Families (TANF), which simply terminates any mother who doesn't find a job after a given period of time regardless of skills, training opportunities, child care needs, or available job openings.

Irrationally, at the same time that millions of women were ordered to take jobs, the same government pursued monetary policies overtly intended to increase the unemployment rate (to hold wages down and maintain high business profits). A de facto anti-work-incentive policy also existed in the private sector. A year after TANF was established, only eight of the nation's 100 largest corporations had any program to hire people coming off welfare. Most of the others saw these people as undesirable prospects.

What is the relationship between the welfare state and work incentive? Well, it supports it, subverts it, or ignores it, depending on nonwelfare interests.

HOW MUCH SOCIAL MARKET DO WE CHOOSE TO AFFORD?

How much welfare state can this society afford? There is sufficient surplus material production to support more than we have.

The real question concerns how we choose to use that surplus. Assuming that it is not possible to optimize everyone's desires, it becomes a matter of social choices, based on moral decisions about what is fair.

Social welfare is a discretionary spending choice. Providing basic necessities for the poor reduces the net income that more fortunate taxpayers can spend on themselves. The financial design of Social Security is such that pensions of current retirees come out of the pockets of current workers, whose pensions in turn will be paid for by the next generation of workers. Money spent for medical expenses is not available for movies, Mercedes, or McDonalds.

Few Americans who are fortunate enough to have above-average incomes would accept pure equality. Few are so hard-hearted as to openly turn their backs on fellow citizens whom they personally know to be hurting. But, where do we draw the line in-between?

Beware of those who insist that the facts dictate an obvious policy. When honestly and fully presented, facts are immensely helpful in identifying alternatives. The choices within that reality are based on beliefs, values, and interests, as explored in Chapters 4 through 10.

Do people have a *right* to a minimum standard of living? If so, at what economic and quality of life level? Are such rights absolute or conditional on certain behaviors?

Does society have a *social responsibility* to ensure adequacy, security, and/or limits to inequality? If so, to what extent can they be achieved by voluntary charity and/or self-regulation? Should the government intervene in initial distribution, through regulation of wages, collective bargaining rights, and business practices? Should it redistribute via taxation and welfare state benefits after the economic market has found its "natural" level?

What are our individual *self-interests*? What social welfare benefits do you want? How much taxes are you willing to pay? And, perhaps the biggest question, do you personally expect to gain or lose?

What are our *beliefs about human nature*? Are people lazy sinners who work only to survive—or do they work better if they already have adequate nutrition, health, security, and self-esteem? To what extent are people motivated by greed? By social approval? By self-fulfillment? By altruism?

To what extent is *declining marginal utility*—the concept that the more dollars you have, the less each dollar gained or lost is worth in terms of satisfying needs and wants—a key consideration? Robert Kuenne sees it as pivotal:

> Exercise of the compassionate strand interferes with and restricts directly the [narrowly egoistic] economic welfare of individuals who are not forced in a liberal market economy to give up income. . . . What may justly be demanded of the individual for support of others in those terms inescapably depends on his or her resources. (1993, p. 21)

IDEOLOGY AND THE WELFARE STATE

There are many ideological variations regarding the welfare state. Seven somewhat simplified representative positions concerning a welfare state or its alternatives are presented in this section.

The Radical Left

In theory, because a centrally controlled economy is supposed to prevent or correct diswelfares, there is no need for a welfare state. As part of the general control, a number of services are provided either universally, such as health and general education, or selectively, on "merit," such as higher education and retirement pensions. In practice, specific individual needs go officially unrecognized and unmet. The absence of a "Western-style" welfare state structure contributed to the downfall of some Communist regimes and has been a source of problems as those countries have tried to change abruptly from command to market economies.

Laissez-Faire

Extreme laissez-faire approaches are basically nineteenth-century ideologies. Classical capitalism took the position that the collective welfare is best served in the long run by letting the "natural" system operate without "artificial" interventions. This ideology is still alive and well but is not the actual policy of any major nation today. A harsher ideology defined the poor as ipso facto unfit specimens who should suffer and die unaided to weed them out of the gene pool. The modern version stresses moral unfitness more than genetic inferiority.

A different, utopian laissez-faire ideology was radical anarchism, which believed that in a truly communal society selfishness would be replaced by a mutuality which makes governmental regulation or provision unnecessary. A recent revival was the hippie movement of the 1960s.

European Labor Parties

European labor parties had their origins in working-class experiences of economic oppression, from which government interventions partially liberated them. Their welfare state model tends to be less individualistic, more security oriented, and supportive of comprehensive national programs.

Welfare Capitalism

The Japanese, consistent with their tradition of paternalism and mutual obligation between employers and workers, prefer that welfare state types of benefits be provided as much as possible through the mechanism of occupational welfare, with government backup for those who fall between the cracks. Business leaders prefer this approach because they believe it is less costly and reinforces employee loyalty. Historically, benefits have been culturally rather than legally prescribed. More recently, certain welfare capitalism services have become mandatory for all employers, notably in health care.

American Conservatives

The conservative position mixes individualism, free enterprise, the work ethic, and negative freedom, in conflict with an ambivalent humanitarianism.

Columnist George Will (1995) summarized this position:

> American conservatism holds that government exists to secure the natural rights essential to the individual's pursuit of happi-

ness [as opposed to] a preoccupation of the paternalistic left, protecting the "little people" from the "interests" . . . [and] liberalism's emphasis on compassion.

Conservatives believe that within the economic market everyone can provide for his or her own needs through work, savings, investments, and acquisition of property. People who fail to do so lack character and have only themselves to blame. They shouldn't freeload on honest, hardworking taxpayers. This position supports policies of either "benign neglect" or measures to promote adjustment of individuals to prevailing realities, as opposed to adjusting the social and economic order to the needs of people. Conservatives may actively engage in compassionate aid to needy persons through voluntary private charity, for charity is generous giving without regard to the issue of deservingness.

A conservative compromise with the welfare state stresses tax welfare subsidies for economic development, occupational pensions and health insurance, individual retirement savings program, and personal education choices. It tends to accept, on the budget-expenditure side, earnings-related social insurances, "opportunity" programs such as public education, and minimal "safety nets," guarded by strict eligibility criteria. Where possible, this should be done through privatization rather than public administration.

American Liberals

The American liberal position reflects social justice and humanitarian liberalism in tension with the negative freedom of classical liberalism (see four kinds of liberal in Chapter 9). David Gil's summary remains accurate a generation later:

> Liberals, during this century, have gradually come to acknowledge the roots of poverty and other social and economic problems in the unequal distribution of wealth and income. However, in spite of such understanding, liberals usually do not suggest strategies to overcome the social-structure roots of these problems. They tend to promote instead reforms aimed at ameliorating the symptoms through government-adminis-

tered social services and financial assistance to those directly affected. (1976, p. 150)

The welfare state of American liberals, who are ambivalent toward centralized power, is a pragmatic, piecemeal set of social insurances, needs-based "adequacy" programs, and services to enhance individual opportunity, social adjustment, and rehabilitation. They often include an element of decentralization to states, localities, and the private sector.

"New" Capitalism

A final ideology, perhaps the most critical one for understanding late-twentieth-century social policies, is not an explicit "ism" but rather a consistent de facto frame of reference. Loren Okroi summarizes it:

> Managerial capitalism . . . involves the administrative control of huge amounts of capital . . . by gigantic economic organizations ruled by faceless technocrats. The American welfare state is so minimal because the interests of those technocrats revolved around a narrowly circumscribed agenda whose key features embody the economic preferences as well as the culture and political values typical of private bureaucracies. (1988, p. 242)

PART V:
HUMAN SERVICE DELIVERY CHOICES

Chapter 14

Benefits: Broad or Begrudged?

If, as our Constitution tells us, our Federal Government was established among other things, "to promote the general welfare," it is our plain duty to provide for that security upon which welfare depends.

Roosevelt, 1934b

Your benefits have been denied because of your death. If you believe this information is not correct, please contact Social Security.

Medicare letter, 1993

Let's assume that we want to provide "appropriate" social welfare benefits—so far, so good. Before we can carry out our good intentions, however, we must answer several questions: What service or benefit? Why? Who gets it? Who decides? On what basis? Is it fair?

A SOCIAL RESPONSIBILITY HIERARCHY

Robert Goodin (1985) defined a social responsibility hierarchy with two dimensions. The first dimension is between *justice and humanitarianism.* Justice is a negative responsibility, not harming persons or treating them unfairly; humanitarianism is a positive responsibility toward the well-being of other people, such as education, medical care, housing, and adequate income.

251

The other dimension is between *personal and general.* The personal level is how we relate as individuals to people with whom we have direct contact, including family, friends, customers, colleagues, neighbors, and residents of our own community. The general level is how we relate collectively as a community or society to all people, whether we know them personally or not.

These can be charted:

	Negative/Justice	Positive/Humanitarian
General duties	II	IV
Special obligations	I	III

The hierarchy of moral duties are ranked, from lowest to highest:

   I. *Individual justice:* don't kill, rob, cheat, or extort.

  II. *General justice:* this is fair treatment under the law, including rules of the game, due process, and laws that protect us from crime, encroachment, discrimination, exploitation, fraudulent business practices, and other unfair or predatory behavior.

 III. *Personal acts* that enhance someone's well-being: this includes family obligations, personal welfare, and voluntary charity.

 IV. *Social programs* that contribute to the well-being of all others: these are provided through systemwide mechanisms, particularly a "government of the people, by the people, and for the people," which provides, mandates, and/or subsidizes the services and benefits.

Issues of institutional versus residual approaches and of universal versus selective eligibility are affected by the extent to which we accept level IV social responsibility.

BACKWARD- OR FORWARD-LOOKING?

Goodin discussed another framework that is useful to keep in mind as we look at how we deliver human services and benefits.

A backward-looking approach focuses on *causal responsibility.* Whether and how needs are met depends on who is considered to be responsible. If you are a victim, you deserve respect and compassionate aid from the one who caused your trouble, if feasible, otherwise from a caring society. If you brought it on yourself, your needs are likely to be met minimally and grudgingly, often with punitive elements. This accounts for the difference between Social Security for widows and Temporary Assistance to Needy Families (TANF). The former's condition is seen as blameless bad luck, while the latter's is presumed to be self-inflicted by morally deficient behavior.

A forward-looking approach emphasizes *vulnerability*. The issue is not how you got there: it is what is the best way to meet current needs and to improve your future outlook. John F. Kennedy (1963) was forward-looking in his approach to world peace: "We are not here distributing blame or pointing the finger of judgment. We must deal with the world as it is and not as it might have been had the history of the last eighteen years been different."

INSTITUTIONAL OR RESIDUAL?

A popular social systems model sees society as analogous to a biological organism. In the human body, each organ—the stomach, the heart, the liver, the brain, the pituitary gland—contributes a function essential to maintain normal life and health of the total organism, which in turn must support each organ so that it can continue to perform its function.

Social institutions are "organized patterns of group behavior well-established and accepted as a fundamental part of a culture" (not to be confused with physical facilities). They are "organs" that perform the functions necessary to maintain a "normal" and "healthy" society. Examples of societal functions are:

- *material provision*, such as production, distribution, and consumption;
- *reproduction and child rearing*;
- *socialization*, creating *internalized* common identity, shared meaning and values, and mutually accepted behaviors (norms);
- *social control*, *external* enforcement of prescribed behavior, rewarding conformity and punishing violations; and

- *mutual support*, meeting special needs, which occur in the course of life in that society, such as illness, old age, and misfortunes.

Traditionalists yearn for the "good old days" before urban, industrial mass society, when a few simple institutions like the extended family and the church took care of all the necessary functions. This may be more nostalgia than fact, suggested Peter Townsend:

> There were in fact few extended families living as households in pre-industrial England, France, and America. The nuclear family was by no means cohesive, since many children went to work and lived in the households of strangers at the age of eight, nine or ten. . . . Secondly, there is evidence from contemporary pre-industrial societies which suggests, depending crucially on the size of population of such societies, that usually there are embryonic "modern" organizations not strictly tied to the kinship structure, and a more specialized role-structure than is suggested in the differentiation model. (1975, p. 15)

In any case, today, basic functions are performed, well or poorly, by a wide range of social institutions. An increasing share of child rearing is performed by day care centers. Socialization is done by public schools, 4-H clubs, Little League, *Sesame Street,* and streetcorner gangs. Control is exercised by courts, police, and regulatory agencies. Mutual support is provided through social insurance, employee assistance, clinics, and welfare departments.

Institutional and Residual Social Welfare

Harold Wilensky and Charles Lebeaux (1965) identified two distinct approaches to social welfare: institutional and residual. Donna Snell (1989) defined them succinctly:

> An institutional need is an unavoidable part of our society; i.e., the problem has been experienced by so many that it is considered a normal development. An institutional policy or program is a *normal* way to meet *normal* needs of *normal* people under *normal* circumstances. A residual need is an extraordinary

problem, not experienced by the average citizen. A residual program is a special means to meet *abnormal* needs caused by individual deficiency, deviance or unusual circumstances.

There tends to be a difference in the character of institutional and residual programs. Those presented in the following lists are generalizations:

Institutional	Residual
• Solidarity/fraternité ideology	Individualism ideology
• Leans toward full entitlement	Tends toward conditional entitlement or no rights at all
• Forward-looking	Backward-looking
• Taken for granted as a right	Receiving a benefit carries stigma
• More comprehensive and continuing	More fragmented and variable
• More stable and secure funding	Discretionary funds, more subject to changes in the economy, politics, and charitable fashions
• Higher benefit/service standards	Standards more likely to be minimal
• Middle-class oriented	Lower-class oriented

Government's Roles

Since World War II, the *institutional* approach has been central to social policy in Northern and Western Europe. In this view, government is a primary institution for performing and/or enabling such functions as mutual support (e.g., social security and health care), child rearing (e.g., day care), and socialization (e.g., public schools).

The philosophy of conservative governments in late-twentieth-century Britain and America were *residual*. Government is a third-string reserve player on the bench, behind the first team of family and market and the second team of private charity, entering the game only as a last resort.

From our colonial origins through the Hoover presidency, American social policy was overwhelmingly residual. After facing the crisis of the Great Depression, President Roosevelt (1934a) used an historical perspective on societal functions to persuade Congress that a shift to the institutional approach was necessary:

> Among our objectives, I place the security of men, women, and children first. . . . Security was attained in the earlier days through the interdependence of members of families upon each other and of the families within a small community upon each other. The complexities of great communities and of organized industry make less real these simple means of security. Therefore, we are compelled to employ the active interest of the Nation as a whole through government in order to encourage a greater security for each individual who composes it. (National Conference on Social Welfare, 1985)

Which Benefits Are Institutional and Which Are Residual?

What is considered to be institutional or residual, in any given time and place depends on a priori values and on perceptions (accurate or not) about "the facts." American culture is more residually oriented than most others.

Institutional approaches to meet human needs that we attribute to normal circumstances and risks currently include:

- retirement income from Social Security and tax welfare–subsidized private pensions;
- employee insurance benefits covering death, disability, and illness;
- workmen's compensation for occupational injury and illness; and
- education at the elementary and secondary levels.

Residual approaches are used for needs attributed to personal failings, such as:

- chemical dependency (except smoking-related health needs),
- emotional and social adjustment problems,
- family breakdown, abuse, and unwanted pregnancy,
- chronic unemployment and underemployment, and
- poverty related to any of the previous categories.

Changing Perceptions

Treatment of benefits as institutional or residual is influenced by changing beliefs, ideology, circumstances, and self-interest.

Relief was defined as institutional by President Roosevelt in the 1933 Depression crisis. Historian Walter Trattner paraphrased his rationale: "Since relief was financed on the same basis as all other public services, accepting such aid should be no different from sending children to public school or calling the fire department" (1994, p. 254).

Two years later, in the Social Security Act, relief became residual again, on the premise that, with the principal causes of poverty (old age, widowhood, and cyclical unemployment) covered by social insurance, the need for it would "wither away" to a very small safety net. Although the premise turned out to be faulty, relief has been residual ever since.

Because alcohol abuse has traditionally been seen as individual deviance, treatment has tended to be residual. As awareness has grown about genetic predisposition, psychological vulnerability, and the environmental impact of a society in which drinking is an integral part of the majority culture, employers have increasingly provided treatment as a normal employee benefit, both directly through employee assistance programs and by inclusion within their general group health insurance coverage.

Perhaps the most dramatic change has occurred in regard to day care. When most mothers of young children remained in the home full-time, day care was viewed as a residual problem of deviant mothers. Although the statistical reality of employed mothers changed during World War II and kept changing every year thereafter, day care remained clearly residual until the 1980s, when it suddenly shifted. Whereas a few years earlier, neighbors looked askance at mothers who "dumped" their children into day care, a decade later they were looking sideways at women who stayed home as full-time mothers. In tens of millions of families, preschool day care became as normal for children as elementary school. The tax code was amended to give tax credits for day care as a normal work-related expense. Thousands of corporations developed on-site day care programs to attract and keep able female employees and to increase their productive time on the job.

The Role of Self-Interest

Historian Howard Glennester, in reviewing failed efforts in the 1980s to dismantle Britain's universal health care system, concluded, "Touch those parts of the welfare state that most benefit the middle class at your peril" (1995, p. 189).

In the United States, Social Security pensions have survived repeated attacks on public human services, with less damage than most other programs. Why? There are 40 million eligible *voters* already receiving benefits, and another 50 million citizens over the age of forty-five will become eligible within less than twenty years. This resistance did not happen by chance: Roosevelt planned it that way. Criticized by liberals in his own party for using a regressive payroll tax instead of the progressive general income tax to finance Social Security, he explained that he was giving workers a sense of direct participation and ownership of *their own* retirement program to prevent his Republican opponents from gutting it after he was gone.

In general, social welfare programs for "us" (the "respectable" middle class), such as Social Security, Medicare, public schools and universities, and now day care, tend to be set up as institutional, while benefits for "them" (anybody else) are made residual.

UNIVERSAL OR SELECTIVE?

Who gets the benefit? Everyone? Anyone who asks? Whoever needs it? Only those who deserve it?

If we don't have enough to go around, how do we decide who gets preference? Those who want it most? Those who need it most? Those who offer the best economic payoff? Your brother-in-law?

Universal

Universal means "used or intended to be used by all." Universal benefits, such as public education and city parks, are equally available to every resident. Even if you choose to use a parochial school or not to play on the swings, the benefit is still *available* should you change your mind.

Some universal benefits may be limited to certain age groups, which we all (hopefully) pass through at some time in our lives, such as public education (under nineteen) and Medicare (over sixty-five). Other universalistic-type programs are not quite universal, such as U.S. Social Security, which doesn't include families who don't have a steady wage earner in a covered occupation.

Selective

The selective approach targets particular individuals or groups. Rather than serving an entire population, it sets criteria for choosing some people over others. The criteria may be based on need, justice, deservedness, payoff for society, or rejection of certain categories of people.

Pros and Cons

An institutional view of social welfare tends to support universal programs to meet normal needs such as education, health care, retirement income, cultural stimulation, and recreation, as well as needs created by flaws in the economic system, others' behaviors, and acts of nature. For example, the American College of Physicians proclaimed, "The current situation is intolerable for patients, their families, and physicians. We have concluded that nothing short of universal access to a level of basic health care will be fair in the long run" (Washington Post, April 27, 1990).

The primary argument against universalism is *seepage*. Scarce resources are "leaked" to persons who do not need them at all or who need them much less than others:

> When programs are universal, the very poor do not get their fair share. The educated and informed, or those with some resources to employ, are guilty of "creaming" what is intended as general public provision. . . . As evidence, one may cite how, historically, the very poor do not get a fair share of the best public secondary schools and colleges; how expensive tax-supported beaches can be reached only by private car owners; how the very poor mentally ill may be incarcerated in state congre-

gate-care facilities while the more advantaged receive ambulatory care and outpatient clinical service—and so on. (Kahn, 1979, p. 78)

On the other hand, selectivity may shortchange the poor even more: "Services for poor people tend to be poor services" (Ibid., p. 79). Programs targeted for relatively powerless groups, such as poor female-headed families and the chronically mentally ill, tend to be inferior in both benefits and quality of service, and they are politically vulnerable to cutbacks. Yes, reply residualists, selective programs for the poor are inferior—and should be! We may provide for the survival of failures and laggards, but we don't want to shield them from the consequences of their unsatisfactory behaviors.

Another issue area is the intrusion of universal programs on *negative freedom*. Mandatory public retirement and education programs deprive individual taxpayers of free choice in how to spend that portion of their income. On the other hand, there are few things more intrusive on freedom than a means test investigation. Universal programs promote *positive freedom* by increasing adequacy and reducing class-based unequal opportunity.

After the smoke clears, although differing widely on how much of each and in which areas, nearly everyone accepts some universal social welfare and some selective programs.

SELECTIVE CRITERIA

Eligibility to receive a benefit may be decided by one or more of a variety of criteria. For instance, college financial aid may be based on need (a Basic Educational Opportunity Grant), deservedness (a merit scholarship), residence (reduced tuition for state residents), investment payoff for the college (football scholarship), or something unrelated to any of these (a scholarship for children of Elks Lodge members). Criteria may be as objective as the computer record of Social Security taxes paid or as evaluative as a psycho-social diagnosis.

Means Test: Economic Need

Economic need is measured either by *income* alone or by *means* (income plus assets). In common usage, both methods are called a means test. This residual approach seeks to limit benefits to those who don't have enough money to pay for what they need. Whether, when, and how to apply a means test are among the most controversial issues in social policy.

Means testing may be used to determine a *variable benefit*, which fills the gap between what you need and what you have. If you qualify for SSI, your grant is the difference between the standard benefit and whatever income you have from other sources, such as employment, insurance, or a small pension. When a clinic charges you a sliding-scale fee, your charitable benefit is the difference between the actual cost of the service and what you can afford to pay. Most student aid is calculated this way.

Other means tests determine *absolute eligibility* on a yes-or-no basis to those poor enough to meet the test—no middle ground. This type of means test may create a *notch* problem, which is both unfair and a possible work disincentive. For example, in the 1980s and 1990s, many welfare recipients became even poorer when they took a low-wage job. Their net income after paying work-related expenses was lower, and they lost their Medicaid health insurance.

Under 1960s policies, this was buffered by (1) Medicaid for the medically indigent, persons up to and just above the poverty line who were presumed to be able to meet normal living expenses but could not afford to pay for medical care, and (2) AFDC work incentive provisions, which deducted work-related expenses from income that was applied to determine eligibility and also excluded a fraction of the remainder. Later, many states narrowed "medically indigent" eligibility to exclude most of the working poor, and the work incentives were repealed.

Means tests can be extremely intrusive and demeaning. As a social investigator in the New York City Department of Welfare, I was required to do a *full field investigation* for every applicant:

- Obtain and file documentary proof of income, expenses, and assets in the form of pay stubs, rent receipts, insurance policies, etc.
- Cross-check each item with employers, landlords, etc.
- Investigate and document the income of "legally responsible relatives" (at that time, parents, grandparents, and adult children) to determine how much each must contribute.

- Interview "socially responsible relatives" (siblings, aunts and uncles, etc.) to persuade, shame, or intimidate them into "voluntary" contributions.
- Require mothers to file suit for child support against absent and putative fathers and verify that they did so.
- Interrogate neighbors regarding applicants' moral character and whether their lifestyles coincided with their declared income. For an AFDC mother, we also investigated whether she had a boyfriend.

The standard application for student aid is a less extreme means test. The applicant, and anyone defined by the university as a responsible relative, fills out a comprehensive statement on income, savings, and assets, attaches a copy of his or her latest income tax return, and signs the form, subject to criminal prosecution for false statements. This is still quite intrusive but much less so than my full field investigation.

At the least intrusive level, a family service agency may ask the client only to sign a statement of family income, without requiring documentation.

We think of means tests as determining tax expenditure benefits. There are also means-tested tax welfare benefits, such as day care credits, health care deductions, and low-income tax credits. This is a relatively painless process because all the information is on your tax return anyway.

In general, the lower the social status of the clientele, the more adversary and less respectful the means testing becomes. The suspicious, punitive approach of my Harlem Welfare Center was a far cry from the friendly helpfulness of my Ivy League college financial aid officer.

Means tests deter eligible applicants. In a society in which the mere fact of economic need defines you as a failure, going through any means test is painful. A full field investigation is deeply humiliating. In my public assistance experience, most mothers would endure anything to feed their children, but many impoverished, aged persons, responsible only for themselves, preferred death before dishonor—and subsequently did die from illnesses related to malnutrition and exposure. Of 3,663,000 persons over sixty-five below the poverty line in 1994, only 1,466,000 (40 percent) received welfare benefits. To the extent that this occurs, the program has failed to accomplish its legal mandate.

Means tests are inefficient. Can you imagine what it cost the taxpayers for the investigations I described earlier? In AFDC, federal "quality control" standards did not address efficiency or effectiveness: they docked the state for any overpayment to a client—but there was no penalty for giving less than the entitlement, and there was no ceiling or review on staffing costs. This encouraged states to divert tax dollars from benefits to the salaries of investigators and bean counters.

Ironically, means tests can discourage industry and thrift:

- *Industry:* when our children were in college, my wife's entire net income after taxes and working expenses went to pay for college expenses, much of which would have been covered by student aid if she had stayed home.
- *Thrift:* the cost of a child's college education is higher for parents who prudently planned ahead and saved than for parents with identical income who spent that money on themselves.

The purpose of a means test is to identify the "truly needy." What is the point of diminishing return, beyond which administrative costs and damage to clients outweigh its positive functions of meeting real needs on a priority basis, preventing seepage, and guarding against criminal fraud? Can it be made compatible with therapeutic and developmental goals for the client?

Reverse Means Test

The economic market has a reverse means test: if you do *not* have the means, you can't get the service. Most people consider this reasonable for private providers of nonessential services.

There is less consensus about its application to health and welfare programs that perform "public utility" functions. I will never forget the day I rushed my two-year-old son to a "charitable" hospital after he drank paint remover and went limp. He nearly died when the emergency room refused to serve him until after I had completed payment arrangements with the business office! It may be the only time in my life that I threatened violence. Since then, laws have been passed that forbid hospitals to make proven ability to pay a prior condition to receiving emergency treatment. Most private hospitals still have a reverse means test for nonemergency services.

Diagnostic Evaluation: Noneconomic Need

Diagnostic intake determines your suitability for the specific benefits offered by a program. There are two basic selection criteria:

1. *Having the covered need or condition.* A Social Security orphan's pension requires a parent's death certificate. A community mental health clinic requires diagnosis of a disorder listed in the DSM.
2. *Ability to benefit.* A mental health clinic, having failed consistently in treating borderline personality disorders, stopped accepting them, even though it was a major mental health problem.

When eligible applicants exceed the number a program can handle, some basis for giving *priority* must be devised. Most human service professionals lean toward diagnostic preference, selecting either those with the greatest need or those most able to benefit from the service. It should be noted, however, that agencies often use nondiagnostic criteria instead, such as the following:

- Chronological order of application
- Ability to pay
- Cost-benefit analysis
- Most interesting for teaching and research purposes
- Squeaky wheels, to avoid hassles and lawsuits

Attributed Need: Categorical Eligibility

If most members of a group have the same condition, why check out every individual? Isn't it simpler to provide blanket coverage to the whole group?

During the War on Poverty, Project Head Start, located in ghettos, based eligibility on neighborhood residence, on the assumption that (1) nearly all residents of poor neighborhoods are poor and (2) nearly all poor children are educationally deprived. In this case, substituting attributed need for individual diagnostic and means testing had several advantages:

- *Efficiency.* What was saved by eliminating individual investigations exceeded the cost of serving the few who would not have qualified—and those few also benefited from the service.
- *Humaneness.* Means and diagnostic tests required negative judgments about parenting as a condition of eligibility. The neighborhood approach avoided such stigma and loss of self-esteem.
- *Effectiveness.* By eliminating the deterrent and negative effects, it reached more of those who needed it and served them better.

On the other hand, some years ago, a retired professor in San Francisco bragged to me about frequent trips to Berkeley for a dime on his senior citizen BART transit pass. The taxpayers subsidized him because of an historic association of old age with poverty. However, *his* income was well above average.

This raises the problem of *accuracy.* Before Social Security, more than 70 percent of persons over sixty-five were poor. As late as 1970, their poverty rate was twice the rate of the rest of the population. Today, however, they have a lower poverty rate (11.7 percent in 1994) than the population as a whole (14.5 percent). Should these senior citizens, as a group, receive a subsidy that is withheld from single-parent households with a poverty rate of 53 percent, four and a half times as high? (Note: Don't confuse such public subsidies with senior discounts in motels and restaurants, which are commercial marketing strategies to attract business from older people because they *have* money to spend!)

Even when attributed need is cost-effective and reasonably accurate, some people raise an ideological question: Is it acceptable for *any* individual who doesn't fit the intent to get needs-based benefits? In my experience, those who "seep in" also need and benefit from the service. Such was the case when a Harvard-educated national church executive sent her daughter to Head Start. She and her husband had founded the East Harlem Protestant Parish and continued to live and be active in that ghetto, so her child was blanketed into the program. It was excellent preschool education for the daughter and had a beneficial side effect: it was an enrichment experience for the other children, as she was the only Anglo child in the class.

There is also such a thing as *attributed nonneed*, categorically blanketing out persons whose needs are otherwise the same as eligible recipients. A white male youth from an AFDC family may be as disadvantaged as his minority and female counterparts but is excluded by race and gender category from many affirmative action programs. A fifty-eight-year-old unskilled worker with high blood pressure and some arthritis may be functionally unemployable despite impeccable character but is too young for old-age benefits, too healthy for disability, and has no dependent children. In Sweden, the Social Security program has the flexibility to allow for such circumstances on an individual review basis. We don't.

Investment Return

A benefit may be provided not for the sake of the recipient but for its social and economic payoff to the larger society. This is true of medical education in Nebraska. Taxpayers contribute a higher subsidy for the tuition of medical students than for other students to meet the state's need for physicians. Admission preference is given to residents because "locals" are most likely to practice in Nebraska after they graduate. Supplementary state financial aid is reserved for students who commit themselves to practice in underserved rural areas of the state after they graduate.

Since cost-benefit analysis was introduced into human services in 1965, a trend has developed toward evaluating individual benefit programs in terms of economic payoff (see Chapter 10). In a number of instances, this has led to de facto *goal displacement*, from user benefit to investment return.

Investment return as a selection policy is legitimate—if it is explicit. However, investment-based preference in a public individual benefit program may conflict with an applicant's constitutional right to equal treatment under the law. When the Supreme Court ruled that Allan Bakke had been illegally passed over for admission to medical school in favor of minority applicants who ranked lower, according to the school's official criteria, the decision was based on the university's status as an individual benefit program (U.S. Supreme Court, 1978). If California had followed Nebraska's example of explicit investment return policies, it probably could have made the commitment to serve disadvantaged populations, not race itself, a selection criterion.

Compensation Owed for Disservices

An individual may be given benefits to compensate for an undeserved diswelfare caused by society. Relocation assistance for inner-city families displaced by a new freeway for suburban commuters and disability pensions for soldiers wounded in combat are obvious examples.

A broader compensatory program was the original GI Bill of Rights after World War II, which offered several kinds of financial aid, plus bonus points added to scores on civil service exams, all of which were intended to compensate for losing years of career development, as compared with those who had stayed home.

Supreme Court Justice Thurgood Marshall applied the same principle in support of compensatory affirmative action in his Bakke case dissent. After elaborating on the history of unequal treatment and citing current statistics on the resulting inequality, Marshall concluded:

> The relationship between those figures and the history of unequal treatment afforded to the Negro cannot be denied. At every point from birth to death the impact of the past is reflected in the still disfavored position of the Negro. In light of the sorry history of discrimination and its devastating impact on the lives of Negroes, bringing the Negro into the mainstream of American life should be a state interest of the highest order. To fail to do so is to ensure that America will forever remain a divided society. I do not believe that the Fourteenth Amendment requires us to accept that fate. Neither its history nor our past cases lend any support to the conclusion that a university may not remedy the cumulative effects of society's discrimination by giving consideration to race in an effort to increase the number and percentage of Negro doctors. (Ibid.)

Earned Benefits and Deservedness

Occupational welfare provides earned benefits, which are routinely included in statistics on "total compensation" published by the Bureau of Labor Statistics and the Bureau of Economic Analysis. These officially include legally required social insurances (Social Security, unemployment insurance, and workers compensation), health insurance, retirement and savings plans, and various kinds of paid leave. This definition of earned benefits is applied the same whether the employer is private, military, or civil service.

Closely related to earned benefits is the *merit* criterion. A merit scholarship may be given as a reward for high achievement, without reference to financial need. (Sometimes this represents investment, when a university's primary intent is to enhance its quality and reputation by recruiting exceptional students.) Merit may also be combined with other selective methods. My university, for instance, awards graduate scholarships competitively on merit—but only within the pool of students who have met a means test. Another university awards scholarships based on need—but only within the pool of students who have exceeded a defined merit standard.

Another deservedness criterion may be *moral judgment*. This seems to be a rationale for the difference in treatment between the Green and the Brown families described in the beginning of this book (see Chapter 1). This moral distinction is ironic in light of another historic difference in policy toward the two groups. Before a 1968 court ruling, an AFDC mother could lose her grant for having premarital sex, while Social Security accepted a widow who lived out of wedlock with a man but took away her grant if she married him!

MIXING THE MODELS

Institutional social welfare programs bring a positive approach to human needs. They are mainly forward-looking in the sense of meeting needs regardless of how they came about. This does not preclude a backward look too, not to cast blame, but to determine a diagnostic history. The causes and processes by which one arrives at the existing situation are often essential for developing a treatment plan. This is clearly recognized in individual medical treatment, analytic psychology, remedial education, and social counseling. This is the "micro" or "host" area of intervention.

It is also important to uncover external causes, not just for treatment, as in the case of job-related stresses, but also to prevent future problems. This is the foundation of public health, epidemiology, and social reform, including the critical social problem area of *institutionalized* racism, sexism, and classism, the "macro" or "agent and environment" interventions discussed in Chapters 3 and 12.

Universal benefits and services are by their very nature institutional. This rationale was clearly expressed by Richard Titmuss, who originated the universal (versus selective) principle:

> One fundamental historical reason for the adoption of [the universal] principle was the aim of making services available and accessible to the whole population in such ways as would not involve users in any humiliating loss of status, dignity, or self-respect. . . . Hence the emphasis on the social rights of all citizens. . . . If these services were not provided for everybody by everybody, they would either not be available at all, or only for those who could afford them, and for others on such terms as would involve the infliction of a sense of inferiority and stigma. . . . The idea of prevention—the prevention and breaking of the vicious descending spiral of poverty, disease, neglect, illiteracy and destitution—spelt the critical importance of early and easy access to preventive, remedial, and rehabilitative services. National efficiency and welfare were seen as complementary. The sin unforgivable was the waste of human resources; thus, welfare was summoned to prevent waste. (1958, pp. 129-130)

Residual approaches are always backward-looking to causes because, by definition, they deal only with deviations from normal. Similarly, since they are intended to meet special needs that normal people under normal circumstances don't have, they can only be selective. It makes no sense to have a universal program for an exception.

Selective services can also apply to institutional needs that are normal risks but not affecting everyone. A percentage of us, we don't know which ones, will get cancer, and the rest will not. We pool the cost of making cancer treatment available to whomever needs it, but its actual delivery is dependent on an individual diagnostic selection. This results in programs that have both *universal* and *selective* characteristics. Rather than let "the loss lie where it falls," a universally available treatment is there for all of us but is given selectively only to those of us who actually get cancer.

Occupational welfare is an area in which programs may be *institutional* and *selective*. Pension plans are clearly institutional, meeting the normal needs of 80 percent of the population who will live past sixty-five. At the same time, both the pension itself and the size of it vary selectively according to the benefits earned, which vary according to years, rank, and/or salary.

A summary of how the two frameworks overlap is given in the following chart:

	Universal	**Selective**
Institutional	Yes	Can be
Residual	Never	Yes

Chapter 15

Rights or Alms?

When we call anything a person's right, we mean that he has a valid claim on society to protect him in the possession of it, either by force of law or by that of education and opinion.

John Stuart Mill, 1863

Imperatives of charity are morally obligatory.

Lesley Jacobs

Does every American deserve a high school education, medical care, and a retirement pension? Should a university education be within reach of every academically qualified citizen? Do we have a right to life that includes protection from starvation? Does society have a responsibility for its mentally ill members? If yes is your answer to any of these questions, to what extent are they *legal* rights? To what conditions are they subject? How can we ensure that these rights are protected?

RIGHTS

Moral Rights

Many of us believe in human rights derived from natural law, humanitarian ethics, and/or religious belief, such as those expressed in the Declaration of Independence, the United Nations International Declaration on the Rights of Children, or Pope John XXIII's Pacem in Terris. These are moral rights. They "reflect a fundamental concern either for what happens to the right-holder or for the ability of the right-holder to determine what will happen" (Jacobs, 1993, p. 11).

Utilitarianism, and its welfare economics application (see Chapter 10), has no absolute. It reduces morality to a calculation of gains and losses on a balance sheet. Any right is conditional upon the "greater good," as defined by those in power.

In contrast, moral rights tend to be universal, based on a priori values and applied absolutely to everyone. Don't confuse this with a legal right. In our country, moral rights have not made health care available to 40,000,000 uncovered citizens nor kept a quarter of our children from falling below a very minimal poverty line.

On the other hand, moral rights can make a difference. When they are aggressively pursued by advocacy groups and accepted by politicians, they may be enacted to some degree into public social policies and programs. Before Roosevelt proclaimed that a minimum standard of living was a basic human right, there was no income assistance except the notorious poorhouse and a few meager state pensions for widows and the aged.

Moral rights often carry more weight in the private sector. My father, similar to many physicians of his day, believed he had a moral duty to give medical care to whomever needed it, whether they could pay or not. (In the 1930s, a majority couldn't.) The Salvation Army, believing in the inherent worth of all God's children, cares for people whom public policy rejects or ignores.

There are legitimate needs and wants that are not actively supported as moral or legal rights, such as cosmetic surgery to enhance self-esteem or a winter vacation in Cancún to treat cabin fever. In such cases, there is still the economic market, which is willing and able to supply the service for profit.

Legal Rights

Moral rights may be sufficient, especially in such sectors as personal welfare and charitable services—but you can't "take them to the bank" (or to court). They depend on voluntary goodwill. Legal rights, on the other hand, are officially recognized under one or more of the following forms of *law* and are *judiciable*, "subject to court jurisdiction; liable for trial in court".

- *Constitutional* rights to equal treatment and due process
- *Statutes* officially passed by a legislative body

- *Regulations* and administrative rules that elaborate and apply a statute (for example, spelling out that "handle promptly" means within thirty days of application)
- *Common law,* "the unwritten law based on custom, usage, and the decisions of law courts, as contrasted with statutory law"
- *Equity,* "a system of rules and doctrines supplementing common and statute law and superseding such law when it proves inadequate for a just settlement"

FULL ENTITLEMENT

Entitlements, called citizen rights in Britain, are *claim rights:*

A claim right is a justification of a claim or entitlement held against someone else to meet some requirement. The relevant requirement might be negative in the sense that it can be fulfilled by forbearance or it might be positive in the sense that it can be fulfilled either by the performance of some action or the provision of some good. This is referred to as a duty. (Jacobs, 1993, p. 11)

Every entitlement program of governmental benefits "must be based on criteria of eligibility that are objective, clearly defined, generally understood, well administered, and considered to be fair" (Wickenden, 1984). Full entitlement programs guarantee the benefit to *every eligible person.*

Historical Origins

The first entitlement program in America was enacted in the 1600s, by the colony of Massachusetts, for disabled veterans and widows of soldiers killed in the Indian wars on the state's western frontier. It was a response to pressure from the city of Boston, to which most veterans had returned, to relieve excessive, local poor law costs.

The Revolutionary War Pension Act of 1818 entitled every poor veteran to a means-tested pension. In 1832, it became a full entitlement for all veterans and their widows, regardless of income. A similar entitlement was enacted during and after the Civil War, originally conditional upon war-related death or disability but later (1890) broadened to be a universal, veterans old-age pension. At its peak, its cost absorbed 47 percent of the federal budget, and it served more than 90 percent of surviving veterans (Skocpol, 1994).

The other major entitlement program of the nineteenth century was the 1862 Homestead Act, which guaranteed any American family a "quarter" of land (160 acres, one-quarter square mile) in the Western territories, such as Kansas-Nebraska, on condition that they worked the land for five years. Civil War veterans could count their military service toward the five-year requirement.

In the twentieth century, three large entitlement programs were enacted. One, public education, developed incrementally state by state but eventually became nationwide. Because of its gradual and nonfederal characteristics, public education is sometimes overlooked in discussions about entitlement programs.

The second was the Social Security Act of 1935, which established old-age, survivors, and unemployment insurances (later adding disability and health insurance). It also provided conditional entitlement to public assistance (later Medicaid), as well as nonentitlement child welfare and maternal and child health services.

The other important twentieth-century entitlement was the Servicemen's Readjustment Act of 1944, better known as the GI Bill. This offered, among other things, tuition and costs of a four-year college education and home mortgages without a down payment. It turned out to be the most profitable cost-benefit investment and the greatest single upward mobility policy in our history.

Universal Entitlements

Public pension programs may be universal entitlements or professional entitlements. Universal ones provide comparable benefits to all citizens. Their fairness models (see Chapter 7) are *adequacy* and *input equality*. Guaranteed minimum income for all retirees is the intent of public pension programs in, for instance, Britain, Scandinavia, Switzerland, and the Netherlands. In some cases, individual old-age incomes may be augmented by a second professional entitlement program or tax welfare-subsidized personal and company pension plans. Sweden has all of these.

Universal entitlement is also the primary approach in education and health care in most industrial nations. For example, the British National Health Service provides nearly all health care for every British subject (and even extends it on occasion to uninsured visitors), as do the Scandinavian countries.

Professional Entitlements

Professional entitlements are earned, either as part of one's "gross earnings" or through payroll deductions. Social Security, civil service, and military pensions operate on this principle. Their fairness models are *equity* and *temporal equality*.

Eligibility and benefits are cut-and-dried calculations, based upon years and level of covered earnings. There are no subjective judgments. This approach was pioneered by Winston Churchill (1911), as a sponsor of Britain's earliest social insurances: "The qualification for insurance must be actuarial. You qualify, we pay. If you don't qualify, it's no good coming to us. That is my safe and simple plan" (quoted in Fraser, 1973, p. 150).

A problem is what do you do about the pension rights of persons who are not in covered employment? Part of the solution has been to have self-employed persons pay both the employer and the employee share. This leaves us with people who are unemployed or out of the labor force. A minimalist solution is a poverty-level, means-tested safety net, such as the U.S. Supplemental Security Income program.

An emerging issue is coverage of people who make recognized social contributions outside of paid employment. Caring for children, the aged, and invalids is paid employment if it is performed in a day care center or nursing home or by a person outside the family. Giving retirement credits to a relative willing to perform the work for free is often cheaper and more socially desirable than to hire someone else to do it.

The Council of Europe recommends making credits toward old-age and invalid benefits "generally available to unpaid persons who devote themselves to household tasks of social work with non-active persons unfit for work, periods devoted to bringing up children, looking after dependents, or performing unpaid social work of common value as qualifying periods on which old age benefits are calculated" (COE, 1993, p. 25). This has been consistently rejected in American social policy but has the potential for strong support, particularly from women, in the future.

Germany additionally credits, as "productive working years," the time spent in university study because it increases the social contribution of the person for the rest of his or her working life.

PRIVATE ENTITLEMENT

Private contracts such as an employer pension fund or group health insurance are another source of entitlement. The provider (or insurer) is legally bound to deliver the benefit.

My own experience with private entitlement has been positive. My nonprofit annuity fund has always acted in my best interests and given me disinterested counsel. Most of my health insurance claims have been handled routinely well. When they weren't, my employer interceded with the provider to set things right.

Not everyone has been so fortunate. After government regulation was relaxed in the 1980s, tens of thousands of employees lost pension equities due to legal shenanigans by their employers and sometimes even by their own unions. Managed care corporations have frequently been accused of failure to deliver contracted services. Failure to honor contractual entitlements is judiciable—but it's hard for an individual to buck the legal resources and strategies of a large corporation.

Three things increase the reliability of private entitlements:

1. *The integrity of the contractor*
2. *Social state regulation:* When government regulators do their job, they prevent most problems and can help redress the few that slip through. Such regulation benefits honest contractors by curtailing unscrupulous competitors.
3. *Collective bargaining:* Large corporate contractors offer better deals and provide better delivery when purchasers are sufficiently organized to bargain equally with them, as my employer did for me in one disputed case. Other successful bargainers have been unions, professional associations, AARP, and the

insurance-buying cooperatives that are part of the German health care system.

Funding Pensions: Pay as You Go or Capitalized?

There are two methods of funding pensions, each appropriate to its sector.

Social insurance operates on a "pay as you go" plan. Today's workers support today's retirees. Tomorrow's workers will support tomorrow's retirees, who in turn will be supported by the next generation. This is feasible because the guarantee resides in *compulsory* contributions and "the full force and faith" of a stable government (on which the value of our currency is also based).

Some nations, among them the United States, maintain partial reserve funds as a cushion to preclude constant adjustments to cyclical ups and downs and to allow longer-range planning.

Occupational pensions, on the other hand, don't have this ability to guarantee future commitments. Companies may go broke or be taken over by corporate pirates who disavow the former company's commitments. The only safe solution is full capitalization, having enough money already set aside to cover your contracted pension twenty or forty years from now.

One approach is called a *fixed contribution* plan. Each month your employer deposits a contracted number of dollars into your personal account within an autonomous annuity fund. Your annuity will be based on the market value of your equity accumulations at retirement.

The other common approach is *fixed benefit*, in which the company promises a particular pension amount based on years of service and other factors. The company puts enough money each year into a restricted fund to cover all of its future obligations to all employees, based on accepted economic and actuarial projections. This restricted fund is shielded from bankruptcy and takeovers. The same principle requires insurance companies to maintain reserves sufficient to cover their commitments in a "worst-case scenario."

If the government regulates companies to protect "your" money from both peculation and speculation, full capitalization ensures an entitlement that is as reliable as the economy and the monetary system.

Inflation Adjustments

Does fairness call for maintaining pension purchasing power through some kind of adjustment to the reality of a world in which inflation has been a constant since about 1940? Nearly everyone thinks so. The alternative would be gradual but inexorable impoverishment of millions of retirees.

When social program opponents are blocked by public opposition from overt cuts in earned entitlements, their alternative strategy is to make these cuts gradually, through tactics that reduce pensions in constant dollars, such as setting adjustments lower than the actual cost of living, eliminating adjustments altogether, or devising new measures that understate the inflation experienced by pensioners.

People who support temporal equality as a fairness criterion face another issue: Should the adjustment be absolute or relative?

The present U.S. method of using the Consumer Price Index (CPI) is an *absolute* adjustment. The intent is, as accurately as it can be measured, to maintain the level of purchasing power granted at the time of retirement. The pensioner's standard of living theoretically will neither go up nor down. From 1980 to 1994, the CPI rose 80 percent.

A *relative* adjustment would be to link the increase not to prices but to *per capita income*. The rationale is that older citizens should share in the economic gains of the whole society. This would have provided a much more generous increase, 112 percent from 1980 to 1994.

Another relative adjustment would be to tie the increase to *median income* so that retired workers fare the same as the average working American. From 1980 to 1994, this was an 82 percent increase, about the same as the CPI. However, this would have lowered pensions between 1989 and 1993, as median income went *down* 6.7 percent in purchasing power. (See Chapter 7 on unequal distribution of economic gains.)

Which is fairest: maintaining one's original standard of living, sharing in the society's economic growth, or sharing a common fate with current workers? These are social policy value and interest choices.

CONDITIONAL ENTITLEMENT

Conditional entitlement is a lesser level of rights that does not guarantee routine acceptance to every legally eligible person. Elizabeth Wickenden (1984) illustrated the difference between full and conditional entitlement:

> Social insurance benefits are based on objective and hence readily recorded data: amount of wages in a covered occupation (virtually all) over a period of time. The amount of the benefit and the data that justifies it come out of a computer: a formula determines the amount of the benefit based on average earnings and, where indicated, the number of dependents.
>
> Consider, by contrast, the number of variables and the judgments involved in a means-tested benefit. Someone must determine the standard of need that will apply and the availability of appropriated funds to sustain it. Typically this involves uncertainties and competitive fiscal pressures on the legislative body at that particular time. For example, it is a well-documented fact that the pressure to reduce Federal taxes while increasing military expenditures has taken a heavy toll of means-tested programs like public assistance, Medicaid, and food stamps.

The first step away from full, routine entitlement is to make benefits conditional upon proof of a specific need. An example of this is Social Security disability insurance. Any person covered by Social Security is eligible, subject to official diagnosis of a disability that interferes with earning a living. Physical disabilities are clearly defined, and physicians are quite consistent so disagreements tend to be settled amicably by getting a second opinion. Mental disabilities have been more problematic because definitions are less precise and evaluations more subjective.

A step further away from full entitlement are public assistance, Medicaid, and food stamp programs, as described previously by Elizabeth Wickenden. Although the review standards and procedures were often punitive, hostile, and politicized, service for those who passed was mandated and supported by an open-ended federal-matching grant. (Since 1996, Medicaid and public assistance to families are no longer entitlements. Funding is capped, and states are released from the obligation to serve qualified applicants.)

Another level of conditional entitlement is to add *behavior* to documented need as a condition. Unemployment insurance requires both evidence of need *and* acceptable behavior (actively seeking a new job).

As we descend the entitlement ladder, the bottom rung is the Fourteenth Amendment, which requires *equal treatment under the law*. It does not ensure either the availability or the quality of the service. It does guarantee equal consideration for whatever is available from public programs and private ones that receive direct or indirect public subsidies. This includes "privatized" health care programs which receive third-party payments from Medicaid or Medicare, colleges which give federal Pell grants to students, and charitable organizations which receive contributions subsidized by tax welfare. It is not yet clear whether equal treatment is also required if the tax welfare device is tax credits that reimburse the individual purchaser after the fact.

Another conditional entitlement limitation may be *quality*. Nebraska's otherwise strict licensing of psychologists exempts public agencies. Thus, state law guarantees certain psychological services to school children and mental patients but not the competence of those services. A similar quality condition occurs de facto when child protection services are mandated by law but are staffed largely by persons who lack professional qualifications for the task and who carry unrealistic caseloads. These failures may, of course, be challenged in court. Precedents so far have tended to support entitlement to competence only for services involuntarily received, such as treatment of a patient committed by the court to a mental hospital.

Accessibility

Accessibility factors can subvert an entitlement. In the Harlem welfare center where I worked, clients who were aged, disabled, or had small children with them had to walk through a crime-ridden warehouse area, climb to the third floor, and wait for hours in a dingy lobby to see workers who openly despised them.

By contrast, when I was widowed, a Social Security worker, routinely informed by the funeral director, called me within a week, expressed sympathy, and reviewed all possible benefits to which I might be entitled. Based on my answers, she filled out the application form for me and mailed it out with a return envelope for my signature, in case I was not literate enough to do it myself.

One of these financial aid programs reaches nearly 100 percent of eligible persons; the other, less than 50 percent. Guess which is which!

The following are factors that affect the accessibility of services and benefits:

- *Quantity.* Is there enough to go around or will some come away empty—or sit for months and years on a waiting list?
- *Quality.* Are the standards such that the program delivers what it promises?
- *Location.* Can clients get there via available transportation? Are there ramps and elevators for disabled users?
- *Schedule.* Can ordinary people use the program without risking their jobs?
- *Information.* Do people understand what is available and how to apply?
- *Affordability.* Can all "eligible" people afford the fees and such indirect costs as transportation, baby-sitting, and lost wages?
- *Acceptability.* Is it provided in a respectful, supportive manner compatible with the client's culture? For example, is kosher food available in the hospital?

ADMINISTRATIVE APPEALS

In universal full entitlements with simple, objective criteria and professional entitlements with cut-and-dried calculations, eligibility decisions are largely routine and impartial. People know what they are entitled to and receive it in an atmosphere of mutual respect and courtesy. If a client questions the decision, it is resolved amicably in one of three ways:

1. The agency satisfactorily explains its decision.
2. The agency discovers and corrects its error with a courteous apology.
3. The client supplies missing information.

Unfortunately, in conditional entitlements, as subjective elements come into play, the impartiality of administration and the effectiveness of "friendly" appeals diminish. The rules are less precise. There are gray areas in diagnostic and/or evaluative judgments that permit honest differences between the agency and the client. Differences arise on how the law is interpreted and applied. This is exacerbated under antiwelfare administrations that disagree with the law or when agency staff have ethnic, class, or gender biases against their clients, as they did in my welfare center.

Conflict of Interest

Administrators are reluctant to undercut staff morale by reversing questionable but defensible adverse decisions. Both workers and their supervisors have a career self-interest in denying or covering up errors caused by negligence, indifference, or incompetence.

The agency wears three hats in reviewing a conditional entitlement appeal: defendant, judge, and jury. This inherent conflict-of-interest situation is exacerbated by unequal power. For example, an appealing welfare mother usually:

- needs the agency more than it needs her,
- has a dilemma regarding how to make a strong case without offending her judges,
- worries about potential future reprisals,
- has less education and verbal skill than opponents,
- has lower status,
- has less technical knowledge about policy and her rights, and
- lacks legal counsel, while the agency routinely uses it.

Given the stacked deck, few low-status clients exercise their right to appeal regardless of the merit of their case, and even fewer succeed.

Reducing Conflict of Interest

The conflict of interest can be lessened if the agency procedures call for a neutral third party to preside over the hearing, and/or the decision is made by a diverse appeals committee. For instance, a university grievance committee may include students, faculty, staff, and administrators. Recently, one of my students won a well-founded grievance against an unscrupulous university administrator because of this quasi-independent review procedure.

To ensure a fair hearing, the power imbalance must be reduced by such means as a good lawyer and/or the backing of an effective advocacy group that can expose and challenge any deviation from impartiality. My student would not have won without the pro bono services of an outstanding lawyer, who effectively countered the legal maneuvers of the administrator and the initial bias of the committee in favor of a longtime colleague against a "brash young troublemaker."

In a Bronx welfare center, grievances had been a futile exercise for clients. After the New York City welfare director permitted the National Welfare Rights Organization to place a trained volunteer advocate at a table in the lobby, nearly all grievances were settled quickly and fairly. A beneficial side effect of the successful appeals was that supervisors began to lean on their workers to get it right the first time.

In the 1980s, the government terminated legal aid to the poor, on the grounds that it was "improper" to finance complaints against itself. A counterview is that legal aid to poor clients, by improving the performance of public employees, enhanced the government's ability to carry out its legislative mandates. After all, a public agency in a democracy has only one legitimate purpose, to make the best possible services available to every person for whom they were intended. Any other behavior is a subversion of the law.

Privatization adds two more pitfalls. One is that it removes the client another step from the accountable government entity. This tends to dilute commitment, weaken enforcement, and make adjudication a longer route with more potholes. The other is that for-profit insurers and providers have an inherent pecuniary interest in denying every appeal they possibly can.

COURT ADJUDICATION

Public agency policies and practices affecting rights and entitlement stand unless challenged in court. Challenges may be made in three areas: (1) interpretations and applications of the law, (2) procedures for determining eligibility and benefits, and (3) findings of fact in a given case.

Federal courts handle issues involving federal laws, the Constitution, interstate matters, and international affairs. Under the Tenth Amendment, everything else belongs to the state courts.

Determining Facts

Trial courts decide disputed facts. A kitchen worker left her job and applied for unemployment benefits. These were denied because her employer said that she quit without provocation. She said that she had been forced out because the chef sexually harassed her and threatened her with violence when she refused his advances. The State Employment Service rejected her appeal so she went to court to obtain her entitlement. It was an issue of fact. Whose version was true? The court decided hers was. Is that what really happened? Probably, but it no longer matters. Legally, the facts are whatever the court decides they are. Accurate or not, the factual issue is settled once and for all.

Due Process

Under the Constitution, your house and bank account cannot be taken from you without due process protections because they are *property rights*. Similarly, a social welfare entitlement is a dollars-and-cents property right; it can't be taken away from you without due process. You can challenge (1) whether agency procedures conform to the right of due process, (2) whether they are carried out properly by the staff, or (3) whether all applicants and clients receive equal treatment under the law.

Under the law, a diagnostic examination determines eligibility for a Social Security disability benefit. This eligibility continues indefinitely unless a reexamination determines that the disability no longer exists. In the early 1980s, under a presidential directive, Social Security arbitrarily terminated coverage of tens of thousands of disabled persons without any reexamination. The courts found that these persons had been denied due process, ordered reinstatement of benefits, and reprimanded the agency for willfully violating citizen rights.

Points of Law: Interpretation and Application

If you and the agency disagree on the interpretation of the law, you may ask the court to decide who is right. Title IX of the Higher Education Act barred sex discrimination in colleges that receive federal funds. A recipient college discriminated against a female student in an unaided program area. There was no issue of fact. The college agreed that it was treating her differently because she was female but said it was none of the government's business because the law applied only to the specific programs that were aided by the tax dollars. She claimed their action was illegal because the law barred *all* sex discrimination by a college that accepted *any* federal aid. The court had to decide which was the correct interpretation.

The *intent of the legislators* is a key factor in the court's decision. What did the sponsors say they intended when they wrote it? What did the committee report say? What was assumed about the bill in arguments for and against it in the debate? In the Title IX case, despite testimony to the contrary by the original sponsors of the law, the court ruled that the college was right about the original intent. As with facts, whether or not it is historically accurate, the intent is whatever the court says it is. (Congress responded by amending the law to *explicitly* prohibit all discrimination by recipient colleges.)

Another possible point of law is its *constitutionality.* For decades, most states required a year or more of residence to qualify for AFDC. This was *legal until a client challenged it.* In 1968, the Supreme Court ruled it was unconstitutional (1) because the Constitution gives us citizenship in a state the moment we make it our legal home and (2) because the Fourteenth Amendment requires a state to treat all of its citizens equally.

Judicial Appeals

All disputed cases go to a trial court. A *trial* is "the formal examination of the facts of a case by a court of law to decide the validity of a charge or claim." The decision is binding on all involved parties. Litigants can't appeal the finding of facts. However, they may appeal alleged errors in due process or points of law. There are three categories of appeals court response:

1. *Refuse to review:* the appellant failed to establish reasonable doubt about the interpretation of law or due process. The trial decision stands.
2. *Review points of law:* the courts either affirm the earlier interpretation or *reverse* the decision based on a different interpretation.

3. *Review due process:* the courts either affirm the trial court action or *vacate* the decision due to procedural errors. The case may be retried under the corrected procedures dictated by the appeals court.

In the federal system and most states, there are two levels of appeal. The lower level settles most cases. The state and U.S. Supreme Courts focus on (1) conflicting decisions among lower appeals courts and (2) cases that present broad issues which need to be clarified. Each appeals court interpretation of the law guides future court trials within each court's own jurisdiction (a region, a state, or the nation), unless and until superseded by a subsequent ruling.

Precedents

When interpretations and applications of points of law or due process are challenged, the court tends to be guided by precedents from past judicial decisions in similar or analogous cases. Such guidance follows some general rules:

- *Higher-court* precedents carry more weight than lower courts'.
- If the precedents are *strong in one direction*, the court usually follows them unless there is a persuasive argument for change.
- If there is a *trend* over time, the court usually leans toward the emerging directions and rationales.
- If the precedents are *mixed*, the court may be more open to equity and social arguments.

Although the judge is expected to do his or her own homework, the lawyers for each side search out the precedents that are most favorable to their side and cite them to "help" the judge decide in their direction.

Note: legislators, administrators, professionals, and the general public are also inclined to be influenced by precedents. In nonjudicial arenas, social policy advocates would do well to emulate their legal colleagues by researching precedents.

Chapter 16

Public, Voluntary, or Commercial?

The state's necessary and appropriate role is to support good and curb evil. To this end, it establishes and maintains structures to achieve justice and order and to promote the general welfare.

National Lutheran Council, 1961

The greatest of these is charity.

I Corinthians 13:13 (KJV)

Should delivery of human services be part of the commercial sphere to the fullest extent feasible, or are they different from "normal" business? Should the government "of the people, by the people, and for the people" deliver these services? Should private altruists provide them through voluntary nonprofit charities? There is no clear consensus in the United States today.

In a market economy, there is a presumption in favor of competitive, for-profit free enterprise. Historically, human services fell to the public and charitable sectors by default; that is, the commercial sector didn't want them:

Men who find their duties to the public interfere somewhat inconveniently with their selfish purposes club together and ask the government to relieve them of obligations they would fain get rid of. All they want is to be left at liberty to acquire wealth or employ it without being burdened with the heavy responsibilities which its possession involves. (unsigned article, *The Nonconformist*, September 3, 1846, quoted in Fraser, 1973, pp. 110-111)

Commercial social welfare enterprises emerge, however, whenever a potential profit center develops, such as in the areas of retirement and health.

LEGAL DISTINCTIONS

Service providers fall into three categories: *public* (government), *voluntary* (private nonprofit) and *commercial* (private for-profit). The legal distinctions between these sectors are clear and mutually exclusive.

Commercial human service agencies operate for profit, including corporate hospital and managed care chains, proprietary nursing homes, and private practice partnerships.

Public agencies are owned and operated by government. There are several types:

1. *Line agencies,* such as a county health department or a state employment service, have authority delegated from, and are accountable to, the elected chief executive (mayor, governor, president).
2. *Autonomous public agencies,* such as local school districts and state universities governed by independent boards, are authorized where a buffer from normal partisan politics is desired.
3. *Public service corporations,* such as the five-county Eastern Nebraska Human Service Agency, may be established for specific functions.
4. *Public businesses,* such as Amtrak, the State Bank of North Dakota, and the Omaha Public Power District, are set up to benefit citizens but are rarely involved in the area of traditional human services.

Voluntary charities are defined by Section 501(c)(3) of the Internal Revenue Code, as nonprofit organizations that use all of their income for educational, cultural, social, and health services. They are accountable to the general public through an annual outside audit of their finances, and must be nondiscriminatory according to constitutional standards.

Charities cannot engage in partisan political activity. The Internal Revenue Service has added nonpartisan lobbying in the public interest on such topics as services to children, welfare reform, safety and health regulations, civil rights, and environmental protection. Strictness of enforcement is politically influenced, varying with the agency's level of popular support and the extent to which the current administration agrees with the cause. (A commercial provider is not subject to these restrictions. Lobbying is subtracted from taxable income as a normal business expense.)

Voluntary organizations engaged in social policy advocacy are placed in a separate category, Section 501(c)(4), which exempts them from paying taxes on contributions but denies to donors the personal tax deductions that Section 501(c)(3) gives. The difference between nonprofits engaged in host interventions and those engaged in agent or environment interventions reflects a traditional conservative-American preference for adjusting people to the existing situation rather than reforming it.

If an organization wants to engage in more than one sector, it typically sets up a separate corporation for that purpose. A social advocacy group may have a separate 501(c)(3) corporation to perform purely educational or service functions for which tax deductible contributions are allowed. Because contributions to public agencies are not deductible, state universities sponsor private charitable foundations to receive alumni gifts. A tax-exempt religious order establishes a taxable business subsidiary for its winery.

TRADITIONAL VIEWS OF EACH

This section presents the traditional pros and cons of public, voluntary, and commercial agencies. They represent a mix of empirical evidence, ideological projection, and myth.

Public Agencies

PROS:

- Equal treatment under the law, enforceable rights
- Coverage and accessibility
- Relatively stable and secure funding, as opposed to depending on altruistic impulses

- Economies of scale, avoiding waste due to duplication and competition
- Savings, by eliminating such commercial cost areas as profit to owners, advertising, and highly paid corporate officers

CONS:

- Rigidities, weak on adapting to individual differences
- Bureaucratic, inefficient, mediocre
- Impersonal, uncaring, disrespectful toward poor people
- Agencies often underfunded and overextended
- Avoidance of needed but controversial services
- Less innovative, slow to respond to emerging needs and changes
- Low priority to less-common special needs

Traditionally, the government has been perceived to be in the best position to finance and guarantee universalistic entitlements, such as Social Security, but to be less effective for personalized social services.

Voluntary Agencies

PROS:

- Higher professional standards, lower caseloads
- More personal warmth and caring
- Diverse agencies geared to different cultural, religious, ethnic, and linguistic subgroups
- Can fill gaps ignored by other sectors as unprofitable, unimportant, or controversial
- Can pioneer services and methods that other sectors later adopt
- Cost-effective due to hardworking dedicated staff, less red tape, no profits taken out, lower administrative charges than commercial
- Preserve and enhance the voluntary spirit

CONS:

- Creaming, leaving the tougher cases for public welfare
- Traditional, tending to do things the way they always have done them

- Impose the cultural biases of their givers and sponsors
- Timidly avoid controversies that might affect their fund-raising
- Inefficient small agencies headed by persons with limited administrative skill
- May substitute zeal for competence
- Fund-raising expenses

Traditionally, voluntary agencies have been perceived to be best for personal social services, cultural and religious subgroups, and serving people who are ignored or unwanted by the other two sectors.

Commercial Agencies

PROS:

- Business efficiency
- More emphasis on state-of-the-art technology and ambience because they must compete for clients who may freely go to another seller
- Pay top dollar, get top people

CONS:

- Reduction of human need to a market commodity
- Client's best interest is secondary to profit motive
- Commercially motivated management policies that restrict professional judgments and service options
- Creaming those who can pay and have less serious problems, dumping the poor, chronically ill, and multiple-problem clients onto the other sectors
- Phony cost-effectiveness claims relative to the other two sectors due to its creaming and dumping

Traditional commercial rationales were based on free-economic-market ideologies and beliefs. Pros and cons are changing, as large corporations increasingly dominate this sector. These tend to be more bureaucratic, anticompetitive, dependent on government purchase of service, and more powerful than earlier commercial human service ventures. Some groups seek antitrust protection to preserve or restore competition and consumer market choice. Others accept the private centralization as a fait accompli and call for a regulated public utility model, with public purchase limited to services for which objective standards and outcomes can be defined and measured.

IDEOLOGIES

There are a number of conflicting ideologies about the role of each sector in social welfare. These coexisting currents sometimes create a *riptide* ("a tide opposing another tide or other tides, thus producing a violently disturbed area of water").

Classical Liberalism and Free-Market Economics

Classical liberalism opposes any concentration of government power. President Hoover (1931) said, "You cannot extend the mastery of government over the daily lives of the people without at the same time making it the master of their souls and thoughts" (quoted in Trattner, 1994, p. 278). Society operates best through a free market regulated by supply and demand, with open, profit-oriented competition among suppliers/sellers and freedom of choice for consumers/ buyers. Why should social welfare be an exception? If someone wants a benefit enough to buy it, someone else will find it worth supplying. Some guidelines are:

- open and equal competition among private commercial providers;
- maximum financing of services from (1) personal income, (2) private insurance systems, and (3) charitable contributions, in that order; and
- public welfare provision, if unavoidable, through mechanisms such as tax welfare, cash benefits, and vouchers, which maximize consumer choice and provider competition.

Pluralism

Pluralism affirms Thoreau's "different drummer." It recognizes with John Stuart Mill the fallibility of the majority. Multiple cultures and lifestyles are a desirable characteristic of American life. African-American comedian Dick Gregory asserted that he was "as American as *cherry* pie." Zingo! As a traditional American treat, apples are a nineteenth-century "Johnny (as in Appleseed)-come-lately," compared to the legendary cherry tree young George Washington is supposed to have chopped down about 1740. Today, pizza and french fries are more universally "American" than either.

Social welfare must relate to diverse groups on their own grounds and avoid imposition on others of any one subgroup's "right way." This calls for a diversified system of providers that serves cultural and lifestyle minorities as well as the mainstream. Public, voluntary, and business providers are all welcome as parts of this mix. The best avenues for public social welfare are financing private sector benefits through tax welfare, purchase of service, and flexible subsidies.

Limitations of Capitalism

The core of capitalism, by its own definition, is the profit motive. Many who support it as our basic system question whether it is compatible with human services. Neil Gilbert made such a distinction:

> The structure of governance in nonprofit organizations tradition-ally involves boards of directors and advisory groups composed of people expected to promote the social welfare interests of the community. . . . In contrast to nonprofit organizations, the direc-torship of profit making agencies is concerned with protecting the financial interests of the ownership group to which they usually belong. This is as it should be. Investors, staff, and the general public *expect* the governing bodies of profit making agencies to act in their self-interest. This is not to say that these bodies are oblivious to community welfare or devoid of public spirit. At the bottom line, however, abstract considerations of these sorts rarely take precedence over the hard and clear requirements of profit-and-loss statements. (1983, p. 14)

Institutional Primacy of Government

In this view, government, as the primary institution in society for the mutual support function, has bottom-line responsibility "to promote the general welfare." Other rationales for this role include its fiscal power and an ethical belief in universal human rights. About the same time that President Hoover (quoted earlier) rationalized nonintervention in the Great Depression, New York Governor Roosevelt expressed an institutional view to his legislature: "Modern society acting through its government owes the definite obligation to prevent the starvation or dire waste of any of its fellow men and women who try to maintain themselves but cannot" (quoted in Trattner, 1994, p. 279).

Some would add a religious imperative: A government official is a secular minister of God to carry out His will.

Applications of these beliefs may include:

- bottom-line public responsibility for planning, guaranteeing, funding, and ensuring standards for basic human services and benefits;
- a central public role in funding and/or direct provision of benefits;
- an independent voluntary sector that serves as a gadfly and critic, provides controversial services, fills gaps, and pioneers services for later public adoption;
- a supplementary role for the commercial sector, to provide a second tier of nonessential services on a private-pay basis; and
- pragmatic partnerships of government with the voluntary and business sectors in specific areas.

Sphere Sovereignty

Nineteenth-century Dutch neo-Calvinists asserted that God had established separate spheres, notably the family, the church, and the state. Within its own sphere, each is sovereign, with God-given functions, responsibilities, and authority. It is improper for one sphere to interfere with another. In the Netherlands, sectarian programs provide most personal social services, paid for by the government. A modified version of this has been traditional in several northeastern states that have preferred to purchase adoption and foster care services from sectarian agencies wherever possible in lieu of direct provision.

Problems arise when citizens disagree on spheres. Nebraska law made education of children a government sphere and set standards for curricula and teachers. A rural sectarian school refused to follow the state curriculum or to hire certified teachers, arguing that education was inseparable from religion and therefore exclusively in the family and church spheres. (After the state's sovereignty was affirmed, it pragmatically revised its rules to accommodate more pluralism.)

Social welfare application of sphere sovereignty can take as many forms as there are viewpoints. The following are three traditional views:

- All economically viable provisions belong to the business sphere; unprofitable services are in the public and voluntary spheres.
- "Objective" financial benefits (such as Social Security) are in the public sphere, while "personal" services belong to the voluntary.
- Delivery of child, family, and aging services is a sectarian sphere, while financing them is in the public sphere.

Subsidiarity

Although the term is seldom used in the United States, subsidiarity may be our most popular ideology. It views society as organized in successive levels from the smallest and most primary groupings to the broadest formal structures. Each "higher" (broader) level is *subsidiary* ("acting as a supplement, especially in a secondary capacity") to the smaller and more personalized ones. Applied to social welfare, the order of preference would resemble this:

1. Informal assistance from relatives, friends, and neighbors
2. Mutual assistance and support groups
3. Voluntary agencies, preferably nonbureaucratic and decentralized
4. Independent local business enterprises
5. Public financing of other sectors
6. Direct public services, as decentralized as circumstances permit
7. Central government interventions in the overall social environment

When Pope Pius XI enunciated the principle of subsidiarity in 1931, he stressed the negative freedom values of classical liberalism:

> It is a fundamental principle of social philosophy, fixed and unchangeable, that one should not withdraw from individuals and commit to the community what they can accomplish by their own enterprise and industry. So too, it is an injustice, a grave evil, and a disturbance of right order for a larger and higher organization to arrogate to itself functions which can be performed by smaller and lower bodies.

Thirty years later, Pope John XXIII further developed subsidiarity by elaborating the responsibility of higher levels to perform positive freedom and social justice functions that lower levels cannot adequately carry out:

> The state should leave to these smaller groups the settlement of business of minor importance. It will thus carry out with greater freedom, power, and success the tasks belonging to it, because it alone can effectively accomplish these, directing, watching, stimulating, and restraining, as circumstances suggest or necessity demands. (1963)

BLURRING OF DISTINCTIONS

Traditionally, the three sectors have been legally and ideologically distinct. However, trends over the past few decades have gradually blurred some of the differences in practice.

Commercialized Charity

In the past, because they cost more than their users could pay, most human services were provided by subsidized public and voluntary agencies. Obviously, you can't run a business at a loss—at least, not for long!

Beginning in the 1930s and accelerating after 1950, unions spearheaded a movement that made health insurance standard for all large employers and many smaller ones. In 1965, public insurance was added for the aged (Medicare) and poor (Medicaid).

As public and private insurance began to pay in full for their clients, health care was transformed from a money loser to a potential profit center. It did not take long for alert businesses to begin serving insured patients. Because insurers used cost reimbursement as the basis for payment, costs and revenues increased and decreased together. Cutting corners didn't increase profits, and providing more expensive services didn't reduce them. Under these circumstances, businesses behaved similar to traditional voluntary agencies. In fact, it paid to do so. (A later change that reversed the incentive—and the behavior—will be discussed in the next chapter.)

Meanwhile, nonprofit and public hospitals became *quasi-commercial.* They were also being paid in full. Contributors and legislators, expecting hospitals to pay their own way, reduced or ended operating subsidies. When I headed the national health and welfare board of my denomination, contributions covered only one-tenth of 1 percent of the operating costs of our affiliated hospitals, mostly for chaplaincy services, which were not reimbursable. Naturally, as they became dependent on sales revenue, they became "business-like" in their charges and collection practices. They began to deny services to persons who could not guarantee payment and to discharge or transfer patients who could no longer pay their bills.

Similarly, homes for the aged became commercialized. Traditionally, they were religious charities for indigent widows, but Social Security and private pension plans created a new market of retirees who could pay their own way. Re-created as "retirement communities," businesses moved into the field. Meanwhile, traditional religious sponsors themselves shifted to more luxurious, self-supporting retirement homes limited to paying customers.

The bottom line: in areas where consumers pay the bill directly or through insurance, you may have trouble telling from its behavior whether an agency is public, voluntary, or commercial.

Quasi-Public Voluntary Agencies

Broad-based voluntary organizations such as the United Way or a community hospital have always had public characteristics, such as:

- commitment to serve the entire community,
- expectation of general community support,
- indirect public funding through tax exemption and tax deductible gifts, and
- pragmatic accommodation to the priorities and biases of the majority (or of the local power structure).

The boundary has been further blurred by another trend over recent decades. Many of those agencies began to receive a substantial percentage of their operating income both from purchase of service and from project grants. In the process, these voluntary agencies have taken on both positive and limiting characteristics of the public sector.

Comprehensive Community Mental Health Centers are a classic case of quasi-public agencies. They were authorized by public legislation to achieve public objectives through a government-planned national network of "catchment areas." The centers were set up and maintained with public subsidies, subject to public regulation, and were required to have local public officials serve on their boards. They tended to receive little or no charitable subsidy. Yet each center was legally incorporated as a voluntary charity!

The logical extreme of quasi-public agencies may be the nonprofit organizations that perform, within Germany's universal health insurance program, the same functions of receiving mandatory premiums, negotiating with providers, and purchasing care, as provincial governments do within Canada's otherwise comparable system.

Although their unique voluntary qualities have diminished, these hybrids seem to perform successfully in broad, mainstream service areas.

Professionalism Crosses the Lines

Richard Tawney (1921) distinguished between the business person and the professional: "Both professionals and businessmen provide service and get a reward for doing so, but the professional puts the emphasis on the service, while the businessman puts his on the reward."

Definitions of "profession" usually include (1) an identifiable body of knowledge, (2) a specified level of competence in practice skills, (3) a high code of ethics, and (4) a commitment to serving other people.

Traditionally, voluntary agencies are expected to operate with high standards of staff altruism, individualized caring, self-direction, and professional competence. Public agencies are expected to be standardized, bureaucratized, and less professional. Businesses are expected to give profit precedence over service. There is a significant thread of truth in these sector distinctions.

The distinction is not that clear-cut in programs traditionally dominated by professional cultures. Are public university professors less dedicated, less competent, less free academically, less collegial in governance—or less idiosyncratic and persnickety—than private university professors? I can't tell any difference. In good ways and bad, they have more in common with their peers in another sector than with other staff within their own organization.

Although there is growing evidence of management differences among sectors in setting policies and priorities, I have personally encountered little difference in the competence, dedication, and caring demonstrated by the direct service nurses, physicians, and social workers at the direct patient-care level among public, voluntary, and commercial hospitals. Have you?

The same crossing of the lines can be seen in private practitioners of medicine, counseling, and therapy. They are by choice commercial entrepreneurs, yet I have known more than a few cases in which middle-class patients received more dedicated service, with a gentler approach to fee collection, from a private practitioner than from a nonprofit clinic. Also, many practitioners quietly give at their own expense a higher percentage of charitable ("pro bono") service than the average nonprofit hospital, where these decisions are made by nonprofessional business administrators.

CHURCH AND STATE

Since so many voluntary health, education, and welfare agencies have some sectarian identification, church-state questions are inevitably tied to the subject of public-voluntary relationships.

Kinds of Sectarian Organizations

There are three basic patterns of religious organization:

- *Sects*, such as the Amish, Pilgrims, Hasidic Jews, and some evangelical churches, are "called apart" through strict membership qualifications and practices.
- *Churches* are more inclusive, often blanketing people into membership by birth or even nationality. For example, Catholic, as in Roman, Greek, or Anglo, means "all inclusive." Churches are integrated into the larger society as basic institutions.
- *Associational* organizations, such as Jewish Federations and many historically church-related liberal arts colleges, are autonomous but are "in fellowship" with religious bodies or with their members.

Strictly defined by the dictionary, "sectarian" refers only to the first category. However, in this discussion, we will follow common usage and apply it loosely to all three.

Domination

Religious bodies tend to relate to the state through domination, partnership, or separation.

Church and state may be merged in a *theocracy*, "government by priests claiming to rule with divine authority." Typically, a sect, convinced that its particular beliefs, interpretations, and applications are the infallible word of God, becomes strong enough that instead of withdrawing from a sinful world it sets out to transform its part of that world into its own image. This was the pattern of Puritans when they moved from Anglican England to a colony in the new world, Mormons when they emigrated to Utah, and Shiites when they overthrew the shah of Iran.

A *secular creed* may operate the same way. Since it has no "theo" (God), perhaps we should call it *credocracy*. In the Soviet Union, from 1920 to 1990, Communist party "priests" ruled with the transcendent authority of Marxist ideology. Traditional religions were suppressed and persecuted as competitors inherently subversive to the True Faith. Eugene Golob, in his study of *Isms*, recognized that

"Marxism has become a religion and as such is completely accepted as a whole while any part may be objectively invalid. Few Marxists examine Marx" (1954, p. 223).

A more subtle domination is *nonsectarian sectarianism*, in which de facto religio-cultural content is consistently followed and even imposed, sometimes unwittingly, through secular programs that have no formal religious connection at all. While nineteenth-century American Catholic and Jewish minorities were developing extensive sectarian social welfare systems, "mainline" middle-class Anglo-Protestant churches did not. Why should they? Basic social institutions such as public schools, child welfare, and charity organization societies already embodied *their* beliefs and values. Nonsectarian sectarianism is at the heart of issues over public school prayers, crèches on the city hall lawn, and the Alabama judge who threatened lawyers or plaintiffs with contempt of court if they objected to opening their trials with prayers by ministers of his sect.

Partnership

Religions which believe that both the church and the state are instituted by God to carry out divine purpose in society lean toward one of the following forms of partnership and collaboration:

- *One established church*, as in Britain, Saudi Arabia, and many "Catholic" and "Lutheran" countries, has special privileges and responsibilities. It often receives public subsidies for its education and social welfare programs. Other religions may be either tolerated or repressed.
- *Multiple establishment* evolved as a compromise approach in Germany and the Netherlands. Divided on whether to establish a Catholic or a Protestant church, they established both.
- *Nonestablishment* permits a friendly, cooperative attitude between church and state, with neither privileges nor restrictions. Religious bodies have the same right as secular organizations to advocate economic justice, right to life, or any other social policy and to engage in partisan politics. Sectarian agencies have no more nor less access to public subsidy than nonsectarian ones.

Separation

Separation calls for church and state to have as little to do with each other as possible. It may be advocated from opposite directions: On one side, sects want separation of church and state to protect their sovereign sphere from government intrusion. On the other side, secular citizens want separation to protect them from sectarian intrusions on their freedom.

Another reason for separation is purely pragmatic. A religious group, unable to prevail, may opt for separation to prevent any other church from dominating. Should they gain sufficient power, pragmatic separatists tend to shift their policy preference to partnership or domination. John Robinson, pastor to the Pilgrims, candidly observed:

> Protestants living in the countries of the papists [Roman Catholics] commonly plead for toleration of religions: so do papists that live where Protestants bear sway: though few of either, especially of the clergy, would have the other tolerated where the world goes on their side. (quoted in Massachusetts Council of Churches, 1961)

PUBLIC FUNDING OF SECTARIAN SERVICES IN THE UNITED STATES

The First Amendment

At one time or another, several colonies had established churches: Congregational in several New England states, Reformed in New York and New Jersey, Anglican in Virginia, Roman Catholic in Maryland. Others, founded by and for victims of persecution (Quakers in Pennsylvania, Baptists in Rhode Island), distrusted any established church. Unable to agree on one religion for the United States as a whole, they compromised on neutrality: "Congress shall make no law respecting an establishment of religion, or prohibiting the free exercise thereof."

What did they intend in 1789: "Nonestablishment" or "wall of separation"? What should it mean now? The Supreme Court itself cannot seem to decide. Its decisions have gone both ways, leaving an unsettled and ambiguous gray area of policy.

Content, Impact, or Auspice?

A central issue concerning public funding for sectarian health, education, and welfare services is whether religion, for First Amendment purposes, is determined by:

1. specific religious content,
2. general religious impact, or
3. structural church-relatedness.

In each case, there are gray areas that make the exact boundary of "fundability" uncertain.

The *content* approach is least restrictive. The government will not subsidize chaplaincy services in a Catholic hospital but sees no problem with paying for an appendectomy. Sometimes the boundary is elusive. In a parochial school, bible study is religious and math is not, but what about a literature course which religiously censors the reading list or a biology course which excludes empirical information for religious reasons?

A stricter test is religious *impact*. Is there a difference between a nun teaching arithmetic to first-graders in a room that has a crucifix and a professor teaching statistics in a Baptist college? Court decisions have tended to take impressionability of the student into account, applying more restrictive standards to elementary schools than to universities, whose students are presumably sophisticated adults.

The most restrictive approach may be *auspice*, on the premise that the simple fact of being related to a religious body makes every activity inherently religious, regardless of content, objectives, or impact. (Opponents counter that discriminating among otherwise identical nonreligious services solely on the basis of auspice violates equal protection under the law.) Even here, there are gray areas. Is there a difference between a parish-owned parochial school and a Jewish community center that is an autonomous secular corporation?

A related issue has been how the First Amendment applies to public employment of ordained clergy and members of religious orders. Since separation of church and state prohibits the government from legally recognizing internal church status, those individuals have a constitutional right to equal treatment under the law, without discrimination related to their free exercise of personal religion outside the job. Thus, a minister can be president, a nun can teach in a public school, and a priest-psychologist can be reimbursed for psychotherapy services. A gray area is whether they can wear ecclesiastical uniforms during publicly paid working hours.

No one, lay or ordained, can act as an agent of a church or perform religious rites in his or her capacity as a government official, and the priest-psychologist cannot be reimbursed for spiritual counseling. What they do off the job is their private business, protected by the First Amendment. (An exception is military and prison chaplains, paid by the government to provide religious services to "captive" citizens to protect their First Amendment right to religious observance.)

Kind of Funding

By and large, government funding and the conditions attached to it lean toward a nonestablishment interpretation. The rigor with which separation is applied varies with the funding method.

Direct *subsidy* of an agency budget is scrutinized the most. Any or all of the three criteria may be applied. Once a boundary is established, whatever it may be, direct subsidy seldom crosses it.

For *purchase of service*, on the other hand, auspice alone is seldom a legal issue. Generally, the government uses a content test for health services, with the consumer choosing the provider, and an impact test for education services.

Church and state issues are often ignored entirely in areas of *tax welfare*. This applies both to *indirect public purchase* (e.g, tax credits for payments made to sectarian day care centers) and to *indirect subsidy* (tax deductions for contributions to religious groups). Supporters argue that even though the sectarian provider benefits the subsidy is technically to the individual.

Direct or indirect government aid to church-related services does not come without strings. To be eligible, a sectarian health and welfare agency must agree to meet the same professional standards and Section 501(c)(3) requirements as nonsectarian charities and to obey the Constitution. A South Carolina religious college lost its tax deductibility because it insisted on racial segregation.

There is another, seldom-recognized consideration in this partnership: if the government subsidy or payment for service is less than the agency's cost, then the sectarian agency is actually *subsidizing the state*, which would otherwise have had to bear the full cost itself.

WHAT SECTOR WHEN?

How do you decide who should do what? On the average, each sector has certain assets and liabilities. Yet as we have seen, in any given case, "it ain't necessarily so." It may be useful to look at it from three different angles before deciding which way to go:

1. *Ideology.* Do you, or someone else who matters, have ideological objections to some auspices and relationships or preferences for others? How important are they?
2. *Pragmatism.* How well does each get the job done, with what costs and drawbacks? The answer may differ among program areas, regions, and specific agencies.
3. *Legality.* What you consider to be ideologically and/or pragmatically desirable may be legal in one nation and illegal in another.

Or, you can follow the traditional American approach to these questions:

Just muddle through.

Chapter 17

Paying for It

He who pays the piper can call the tune.

Old Adage

Said the pieman to Simple Simon,
"Show me first your penny."

Nursery Rhyme

A social welfare benefit isn't created out of thin air. Someone pays for it. This is done in many ways, but it boils down to two basic approaches: subsidize the provider or sell the product.

RESTRICTED AND UNRESTRICTED SUBSIDIES

A subsidy is given to an organization to cover the cost (fully or partially) of providing a service or material aid. It may be public money, directly through budget expenditure or through tax expenditure. It may be charitable donations, bequests, or endowments. It may be in the form of in-kind goods and volunteer services. Some subsidies are unrestricted; others are narrowly designated for a specific purpose.

Unrestricted

Unrestricted subsidies give an agency the flexibility to use the money wherever it will do the most good, within the legal boundaries of its charter. Donors who agree with the agency mission and trust its leadership usually allow this flexibility. These subsidies are not normally given to commercial providers, who could legally pocket unrestricted funds as extra profit.

Legally Restricted

Donor-restricted subsidies are earmarked by the giver for specific purposes. They apply what Saul Alinsky used to call his golden rule: "He who has the gold, makes the rule." Through restricted funding, private donors persuade the agency to give priority to their special interest, be it research on a rare disease, abortion counseling, or a weight room for the football team. The federal government pursues national priorities with decentralized administration by offering grants to state, local, and nonprofit bodies willing to provide designated services.

In-kind gifts may be donated goods, such as food for a "pantry" service or used dental equipment for a neighborhood clinic. They may be free use of equipment, such as a loaned van for transporting clients or access to a mainframe computer. Volunteers donate work as scout leaders, hot line counselors, or by giving free legal counsel to the agency. An in-kind contribution is inherently restrictive. We rarely feed our volunteers to hungry clients or assign donated computers to lead a therapy group.

In-kind contributions may be partial. If a shopping mall offers reduced rent space for a family service agency branch, the difference between the commercial rental value and the charged rent is an in-kind gift, as is 50 percent of the service performed by a teaching sister who *voluntarily* works for half the pay of lay teachers.

Most agencies would prefer *cash* to in-kind subsidies. The volunteer or equipment may not be as satisfactory as what the agency could have bought. However, similar to other restricted giving, it is usually a "take it or leave it" choice. Volunteers may have time but not money to offer, and a business's donation of equipment may offer tax advantages over an equivalent cash gift.

From an agency perspective, the ideal in-kind subsidy either replaces an otherwise essential cash expenditure or adds needed equipment or services that the agency budget couldn't support. If the agency has to transport clients, the loaned van directly saves the cost of buying one. Teaching sisters enabled many parishes to have parochial schools that they otherwise couldn't afford, as demonstrated by school closings when this source dried up.

For the donor, control is an obvious advantage of restricted giving. From the agency perspective, the biggest disadvantage is loss of flexibility. The agency doesn't necessarily get what it needs most. The alumni gift for the football team's weight room, however welcome, can't be used for a more urgent need to upgrade an inadequate library.

"Following the money" changes agency priorities, sometimes at the expense of its primary mission. From 1964 to 1974, community action programs were gradually drawn by restrictive grant opportunities from their original empowerment and social development legislative intent to become multipurpose direct service agencies. Similarly, pursuit of research grants has displaced education as the top priority of more than a few academic programs.

Restricted subsidies usually cost more to administer. There are extra costs to train and supervise volunteers or, in the case of cash, to prepare proposals, maintain separate accounting systems, and write project reports. Nevertheless, they can be a great benefit to agencies to the extent that they (1) coincide with agency objectives, (2) add to rather than displace agency priorities, and/or (3) force greater accountability upon a sloppy agency.

"Morally" Restricted

For an auditor, there is no middle ground. Either the funds are legally restricted or they aren't. However, within the legally unrestricted category, there is a middle ground, *board designated funds.* This is unrestricted income that has been set aside by the agency board for an earmarked purpose. However, the agency can "unrestrict" it again if it chooses.

There are often nonbinding understandings between agency and donor. At its simplest level, an agency normally leans toward honoring funders' preferences, especially if it plans to ask for money again next year.

More shrewdly, verbal agreements have been used to circumvent IRS regulations that deny tax deductions for contributions to support social advocacy. A wealthy liberal wanted to support a social justice movement, but direct contributions were not deductible. A wealthy ultraconservative encountered the same problem in promoting his economic policies. The first made an unrestricted contribution to her church mission board, whose executive informally assured her that an equal or greater amount from another part of the board's budget would be allocated to her cause. The other endowed a university professorship of economics, with an unwritten agreement that it would be filled by someone who shared the donor's ideology.

Complicating the issue of moral restrictions is the dilemma of *multiple accountability*. Which should take precedence:

- The preferences of direct donors?
- The values of indirect donors, the general public who pay the tax welfare share of that deductible gift?
- The well-being of those served?
- The perceived collective best interests of society?

Is there one universal "right" answer, or does it vary with the particular situation? If the latter, you need general principles to guide your choices.

FEDERAL SUBSIDIES: GRANTS

The federal government participates in social welfare through direct administration, purchase, indirect subsidies, and grants.

Grants vary in their degree of control. The most controlled is the *project grant* to state, local, and nonprofit agencies for time-limited periods in specific areas such as research, training, demonstration, and start-up of new programs. The grantor typically writes a statement of its objectives and invites proposals that detail (1) the applicant's concrete project and how it furthers the grantor's objectives, (2) how the results will be measured and evaluated, (3) the plan of operation, and (4) an itemized budget.

Categorical grants are usually given to states for ongoing programs. Their objectives are broader than project grants but still targeted to a defined need and population. There have been hundreds of categorical grant programs in such areas as public assistance, child welfare, rehabilitation, employment services, agricultural extension, education, and public health.

The federal government publishes guidelines on program objectives, priorities, and standards. It requires from the grantee (1) a state plan compatible with the guidelines, (2) financial and program accountability, and usually, (3) commitment of matching state funds. Entitlement program grants require plans to meet minimum federal standards and provide equal access to all residents.

Most categorical grants distribute funds among the states through a formula based on population and/or relative need. A few programs designed to meet critical needs that are variable and unpredictable have been open-ended.

A *block grant* is simply a broader category with looser conditions. It offers more flexibility and self-determination, with weaker federal control over priorities, standards, and consistency. Its premise is that state and local government leaders have high ethics and competence, are in close touch with the human needs of their people, and are committed to their well-being as a first priority. Because of its loose nature, a block grant cannot guarantee entitlements.

In 1967, the pioneer block grant combined nine existing categorical public health "disease" grants—and *all* their funding—permitting each state to allocate purposes among the nine, according to its own particular regional needs.

In the 1970s and 1980s, the consolidation of categorical programs into block grants accelerated and took on a different ideology, federal withdrawal from their accumulated social welfare role. They largely eliminated federal priorities and were funded at a substantially lower level than the sum of categorical grants they replaced.

In 1974, categories that had been targeted for slum clearance and low-income housing were blended into an urban development block grant. My city used the funds to beautify the business district, including building an artificial lake. The mayor explained that his choice benefited Omaha as a whole more than slum clearance. This was consistent with the intent of permissive decentralization to the local power structure.

The ultimate block grant is *revenue sharing*. Taxes are collected centrally and disbursed on a formula basis as an unrestricted subsidy to state or local governments. Carried to its logical extreme, it could shift social welfare from a quasi-universalistic nationwide system to a hit-or-miss patchwork quilt of local choices. In the early 1970s, a modest revenue-sharing scheme was implemented briefly to cushion the loss of revenue that occurred when many War on Poverty categorical and project grants were phased out.

FEDERAL SUBSIDIES: TAX EXPENDITURES

Tax Exemption

Nonprofit social welfare organizations are tax exempt. The government does not collect income taxes on the agency's program-related revenue. Many states and cities waive property and sales taxes as well. This is tax welfare: any taxes forgiven have the same effect on net usable income as a government cash contribution in that amount.

Tax Deductibility

The charitable deduction is a tax expenditure subsidy to voluntary service agencies of more than $30 billion per year. Here is how it works. A and B have each decided to give $100 from their gross income to a charity. For lower-middle-income A, income taxes take $18 of this ($15 federal plus about one-fifth of that amount, $3 for state): A contributes the net amount of $82. Income taxes in an upper bracket take $47 from upper-income B ($39 federal, $8 state): B gives the net amount of $53.

We pass a law that makes these gifts deductible. A still pays $82 out of her pocket, and the governments contribute their $18 of taxes along with it. B puts in the $53 she would have had, with the governments contributing their $47.

There's more. B has appreciated stocks or real estate. If B sells a stock bought at $50 for $100, she pays $12 ($10 federal, $2 state) on the $50 of capital gain. If she donates this stock instead of cash, she gets the regular $47 deduction *plus a second deduction* of $12 on the capital gain. By giving this way, the governments' contribution rises to $59, and B's out-of-pocket contribution falls from $53 to $41. Although few working-class wage earners can take advantage of this option, upper-income donors usually do.

Everybody likes the charitable deduction. Agencies get more dollars. Contributors like it because it increases the effect of their net gifts. Humanitarians applaud its social benefits and its encouragement of the spirit of giving and caring. Libertarians associate it with greater freedom of choice. Opponents of big government like the idea of diverting some of their taxes from public welfare to private charity.

So who could criticize it? Well, it *is* regressive redistribution. In the previous illustration, for every net dollar from the modest income giver's own pocket, the government matched it with $.22 (82/18), while it matched the higher-income giver's net dollar with $1.43 (59/41). This is intentional, encouraging philanthropy by those who can afford large gifts.

Where did those gifts go? Primary recipients of the small, lower-matched gifts are churches and social services. Major recipients of the large, higher-matched gifts tend to be private universities, prep schools, and the arts. Thus, the government's charitable deduction subsidy is most generous for upscale services to upscale users. Are they desirable causes? Yes. Is it regressive redistribution? Also yes. Is the net effect good or bad? It depends on your hierarchy of values and interests.

Subsidies to Private Health, Housing, and Pensions

An even larger tax welfare subsidy goes to employer and individual purchasers of pensions, health insurance, and "fringe benefits." The 1994 federal budget reported a $66 billion tax expenditure exclusion from income tax of employer and individual dollars put into retirement plans, including employer pensions (about three-fourths of the total), Keough plans, Individual Retirement Accounts, and interest on life insurance savings. For comparison, in the same year, it made a budget expenditure of $23.5 billion to SSI, the safety net for aged and disabled persons. (Later legislation further increased tax subsidies in this area in 1998.)

The federal tax expenditure subsidy for private health care was about the same, $56 billion for exclusion of employer health insurance contributions, plus several billion more for medical deductions on individual tax returns. For comparison, the federal budget expenditure for Medicaid that year was $82 billion.

A third illustration of tax versus budget expenditure is housing. In 1994, tax expenditures for mortgage and property tax deductions on owner-occupied homes, mostly owned by middle- and upper-income citizens, were over $82 billion. The federal budget expenditure for public housing and rental assistance to the poor was $21 billion.

Other smaller amounts went for additional fringe benefits, military benefits, day care tax credits, employee parking, etc. These add up to perhaps another $10 billion. Of course, this is only for social welfare. There are also large tax expenditures for corporations unrelated to social welfare, as noted in Chapter 1, Circle 9.

Tax expenditures are the second largest social welfare funding source in the United States after Social Security. If "welfare state" means federal financing of social welfare benefits, then the middle and upper classes are by far the largest beneficiaries, when you add the quarter trillion ($264 billion in 1997) tax welfare expenditures they received to the half trillion ($529 billion in 1997) paid out by Social Security and Medicare, the majority of whose beneficiaries are middle class.

Other Subsidies

Although commercial human services do not have tax exemption or deductibility, they have access to a different set of government subsidies. Unable to find funds to subsidize the operating deficit in its church-related teaching hospital, a medical school sold it to a business corporation. *Accelerated depreciation* (allowing a tax deduction greater than the actual decrease in the value of capital equipment) created "paper losses" that the corporation used to reduce taxes on earnings in its other enterprises. The tax benefit more than offset a small, real operating loss. Thus, a complicated tax welfare subsidy turned a nonprofit agency's loss into a commercial agency's gain. (In 1997, the tax expenditure for accelerated depreciation was $27 billion.)

This does not exhaust the subject of indirect government subsidy. There are many additional odds and ends. An example is the following snippet, buried in a lengthy report on the Federal budget a few years ago: "The Treasury and Postal Service appropriations bill ran over budget chiefly because an extra $820 million was provided the Postal Service to subsidize lower rates for charities" (*Omaha World-Herald*, 1985).

THIRD-PARTY PURCHASE OF SERVICE

Perhaps the most significant U.S. social welfare funding development of the second half of the twentieth century has been the growth of third-party payments. There are always at least two parties to a transaction, a consumer and a supplier. Historically in social welfare, the first party (consumer) bought the service and/or the second party (supplier) subsidized it. If someone else purchases the service for the first party from the second party, a *third party* is introduced.

Among the largest third-party purchasers of service are employers, public and private health insurance, the military, and such public social service programs as vocational rehabilitation, child welfare, and Title XX of the Social Security Act.

The businesslike purchase-of-service model in use today started in the private insurance field. The traditional insurance method had been *indemnity*, a cash payment to the insuree (or survivor) to compensate for a loss after it has occurred. This is still the practice in homeowner's, auto, and life insurance.

The indemnity approach presented problems for both the patient and the provider. Most patients did not have the cash flow to pay the hospital bill first and wait for reimbursement. Sometimes they went without. Other times the hospital provided the service anyway. Hospitals had a problem too. By the time former patients received the insurance check, they were no longer ill and often spent the money for other wants rather than pay the old bill.

In the 1930s, a group of hospitals created their own nonprofit insurance company, Blue Cross, which made the payments directly to them rather than to the patient. This guaranteed payment to the hospitals and freed patients from financial anxiety. Physicians (Blue Shield) quickly followed suit. The two became the model for third-party payments. At that time, most of the Blue Cross providers were nonprofit, and most of the Blue Shield providers were commercial (private practice).

By the 1990s, this health services model, which treated for-profit and nonprofit providers the same and which used business-oriented cost-accounting methods, had been adopted in child welfare and other social services as well.

As both employers and government turned to *purchase of services* in lieu of direct provision, sales revenue replaced subsidy as the primary source of income for health care agencies.

This was popular for several reasons: It offered an alternative to large civil service bureaucracies. It reduced employers' administrative headaches. Unions liked that employers exerted less direct control over workers. Commercial interests discovered a new profit center in the "human service business." Users enjoyed the greater freedom of choice that, until recently, third-party payment offered.

SETTING THE PRICE

If human welfare services are to be sold, how should the price be set?

What the Traffic Will Bear

Business (including private practice) is expected to maximize profit by charging the highest price the traffic will bear. Nonprofit agencies have increasingly adopted the same view, toward the end of earning "operating surpluses" that pay for unprofitable services and capital improvements.

In a free market, competition among sellers and bargaining by buyers who have a choice of providers keep prices under control. However, social welfare seldom meets free-market conditions. The hopeful adoptive parent in a "seller's market" (shortage of available babies) is in no position to argue about fees. Sick patients may have little or no choice of hospital: They go where their physician practices, and they are in no position to haggle over price. Under these circumstances, "what the traffic will bear" can exploit vulnerable clients and patients.

Audited Cost

The law of supply and demand presumably creates a fair price, provided there is (1) direct economic competition among providers and (2) equal power between consumers and sellers. Where this is not the case, as in such public utilities as electricity, gas, and water, prices are regulated by a public utility commission, using a *cost-plus* method, that is, the audited cost of producing the product plus an extra percentage to provide a "fair" profit. Public and private health insurances followed this precedent in paying for hospital care.

Except to the extent that it may be subverted by political pressure, indirect bribery through campaign contributions, or other favoritism, this method protects the consumer from the perils of "traffic-will-bear" pricing. What it lacks is a substitute for the competitive marketing pressure to achieve cost-effectiveness. Indeed, under cost-plus, higher costs due to inefficiency actually increase one's profit.

The basic building block is an *itemized* bill. A service is broken into its component parts (a drug dose, an hour of therapy). The direct cost of each item is calculated, and a pro rata share of "overhead" (administration, depreciation, utilities) is added in.

This method assumes that the itemization is meticulous, clear, and honest. Unfortunately, it has often been abused by charging exorbitant prices for such things as sanitary napkins and pills, which are bought at quantity discounts and sold to captive patients for ten or even a hundred times their normal retail price. (The explanation I have been given is that this is necessary to offset unitemized costs. Is there an inconsistency here somewhere?)

It is difficult for an individual patient to review the charges. If you have ever received an itemized hospital bill, you know that the list may run to a thousand items, many identified by obscure abbreviations. How can you determine how many of them were actually used on or for you and what is a fair price for each? My wife, a hospital professional, has confirmed to me that many items charged routinely by management to all patients in her area were not regularly used or were for reused equipment that legitimately should have been divided among ten patients rather than charged fully to each.

These pitfalls are reduced when the bill is paid directly by a third-party insurer, which has a technical review staff and market power to negotiate charges. Even so, when I once actually reviewed every single item for which my insurance company paid for a family member's hospitalization, it appeared that my insurance company had been overcharged as much as 20 percent.

Clustered Costs: Per Diems and DRGs

Detailed itemization is a sensible and rational approach, but even when honestly carried out, it is cumbersome to administer, open to frequent errors, and difficult to check.

A compromise has been to *cluster* items into a standard package, with a set price based on the *average* total of all items. Per diem rates for basic room, board, and care in a hospital, nursing home, or institution are clusters. This works fairly well for large third-party payers, who annually review and bargain over both the items and the pricing on which the cluster package is based.

Later, Medicare formulated the idea of a *supercluster*. It analyzed the average cost of all hospitals within a region for an average cluster of items required in a *total treatment package* for each of several hundred diagnostically related groups (DRGs), such as appendicitis, normal childbirth, or a triple bypass. Based on this data, a set price was fixed for each DRG. The same price is paid for all normal appendectomies in that particular region. If the actual cost is lower for one patient, the provider keeps the windfall. If it is higher for another, the provider takes the loss.

The DRG is normally determined before a patient is admitted. In the case of emergencies, it is done as soon after admission as possible. The DRG average takes into account the incidence of normal variations above or below the norm. When abnormal complications occur, it is possible for the provider to apply for a revised DRG or a second DRG.

In general, clusters of all sizes work best where there is give and take between providers and payers of equal power. It is not effective for a David patient against a Goliath provider, even with a slingshot.

Ordinary and Customary Fee

Private practice charges are not calculated from audited costs. They vary from place to place according to what the market will bear. Third-party payers have usually agreed to pay up to the "ordinary and customary fee" charged in that area.

Client Ability to Pay

Social welfare programs that have both sales and subsidy income may set fees based on what the client can afford. There are three common approaches:

1. *Attributed general ability to pay.* A public university sets an average tuition rate (price) for all students at a level that middle-income families can afford.
2. *Attributed differences in ability to pay.* Above-cost YMCA "businessmen's memberships" offset below-cost "youth memberships."
3. *Sliding scale.* The fee charged to a mental health clinic patient is based on ability to pay, up to the audited cost.

Symbolic

In some programs that could offer the service free, a nominal fee may be charged for its effect on the user. Our society stigmatizes receiving charity, and we also tend to assume that what is free "can't be worth much." The symbolic payment enhances client self-esteem, respect for the service, and motivation "to get my money's worth."

A Shot in the Dark

A once-hallowed method used to be the *ignorant guess.* Before nonprofit programs were required to do program accounting, they had no idea what any specific service actually cost. Fees were simply a shot in the dark.

The old image of human service administrators as "softhearted and softheaded" is now in disrepute. In the businesslike culture of late-twentieth-century America, funders and board members want to know actual costs and require justification for any below-cost pricing. It is still okay to be softhearted (at least in the charitable sector) but not to be softheaded.

COST CONTROLS

A problem with third-party payments has been cost control. Consumers who didn't have to pay their bills directly tended to ask for the best care available, regardless of cost. Providers paid on an audited cost basis had no incentive to economize, and it cost them nothing to perform medically unnecessary testing and procedures to cover themselves in case of malpractice suits.

Since other cost factors, such as longer life expectancy, expensive new drugs and technology, and lifestyle choices exist in all countries, pricing/payment differences appear to be the reason that the United States has by far the highest health costs, despite its lower coverage, among the Organization for Economic Cooperation and Development's twenty-six member nations. In 1994, U.S. health expenditures were 14.2 percent of our total gross domestic product. Rates for countries with *universal health insurance systems* included Canada, 9.8 percent (second highest in the world after the United States), Germany, 8.6 percent, and Japan, 7.3 percent. Among those with *nationwide public health care delivery systems*, Sweden was highest at 7.7 percent, Britain, 6.9 percent, Denmark, 6.6 percent, and Norway, 5.5 percent. The United States also had the highest rate of increase (35 percent) between 1980 and 1994 (U.S. Census Bureau, 1996-1997).

One response to rising costs has been *withdrawal* from responsibility. Both public and private U.S. insurers have made incremental cutbacks in eligibility and covered services. Asked about unmet needs, they cluck sympathetically. In recent years, some of these actions, such as "drive-through birthing," have triggered public outrage and the beginnings of health care regulation.

A companion strategy is to require extensive review and preapproval for surgery, hospital stays, and many diagnostic procedures, except in emergencies, such as a heart attack or an auto accident. This screens out unneeded procedures, as well as gray areas in which the need is clear but they judge it not serious enough to warrant the cost of treatment. These "hoops" also save money by discouraging approvable requests as well.

Another response is for third-party payers to exert more control over services, providers, and price. Canadian provinces and German purchasing cooperatives negotiate prices through collective bargaining with the medical association and other provider groups. In the United States, Medicaid and some private insurance companies set a take-it-or-leave-it "just price" lower than the prevailing "customary" fee. Other payers are more subtle, using implicit threats that influence providers to back off from price increases.

The DRG prospective pricing system adds a profit incentive to cost control because the provider keeps any savings below the established price. The attraction is that if many providers reduce their costs this way next year's DRG price, based on this year's lower average audited cost, might be lower.

Still another popular cost reduction device is the *preferred provider* system: "I can get it for you wholesale." The payer negotiates a discount, typically 15 to 20 percent off the customary fee, from selected providers, in return for guaranteeing a large volume of business. Insurees can either have their full bill paid or their co-insurance reduced by using a designated preferred provider or exercise freedom of choice and pay the substantial difference.

Finally, several methods, such as the following, are used to *deter usage* by making it costly or unpleasant for the patient to seek services:

- *Deductibles.* The initial burden is on the consumer. (My insurer requires me to pay the first $175 of medical expenses each year.)
- *Co-insurance.* This may be a percentage of the fee or a fixed amount per unit or service. (Mine requires 25 percent of all medical charges after the deductible and a flat rate of $10 per prescription.)
- *Red tape.* Time-consuming, unpleasant, frustrating procedures, such as lengthy forms, second opinions by insurance company physicians, and written preapproval deter patients from seeking care.

PREPAID MANAGED CARE

At the Pearly Gates, Saint Peter was interviewing applications for admission to heaven. "Before I can let you in," he said, "you'll have to tell me some worthwhile thing you did for others while you were on earth." The first said, "I was a heart surgeon. I did lots of open heart surgery. I saved a lot of lives." "Fine, go straight in." The second said, "I was a nurse. I went down into the slums and worked with destitute sick persons whom no one else would help." "Excellent, go right in." Said the third, "I was the man who came up with the idea of managed health care. I saved insurance companies millions of dollars." St. Peter scratched his head. "Well, I guess it's all right. Go on in. BUT YOU CAN ONLY STAY TWO DAYS."

Prospective Payment

There are two obvious methods for buying services. The traditional method is *payment for services received.* After your car gets repaired, you receive and pay a mechanic's bill for parts and labor. After you get repaired, you (or your insurer) receive and pay a medical bill for parts and labor.

The other is *prospective payment* for future benefits. Some prospective payment contracts are for a specified benefit. Most students pay tuition in advance for a designated course. If it is canceled, they get a refund. Other prepayments buy variable benefits based on utilization. You pay a spa the same monthly rate whether you use it for four workouts or thirty. Your HMO premium buys whatever medical services you need that month.

Historic Managed Care: Insurer-Provider HMOs

A comprehensive health maintenance organization (HMO) is a smaller private version of the British Health Service. Similar to an insurance company, it collects premiums, but instead of purchasing services, it provides them directly. With administrative control over all provision, it is capable of offering security, convenience, and cost-effectiveness.

HMOs were pioneered in the 1930s and 1940s as a means of providing universal quality health care for workers. Two stand out as landmarks. One was initiated by labor unions, the other by a Fortune 500 company.

In New York City, a number of unions, led as I recall by the International Ladies' Garment Workers' Union, joined together to sponsor a comprehensive managed health care program, called HIP, and collectively bargained for employer-paid premiums as a fringe benefit.

In California during World War II, Henry Kaiser established the Kaiser-Permanente program for employees of his industry steel plants. At that time, there was a severe labor shortage, and many defense workers from distant rural settings were crowded into substandard housing in unfamiliar cities. These migrants did not know the local health providers, which were overloaded by the population increase anyway. Kaiser's guaranteed health care for workers and their families kept production up through (1) lower turnover, (2) healthier workers, and (3) higher morale.

Both HMOs were nonprofit corporations that hired physicians and other health personnel. They earned high reputations for competence, fairness, and cost-effectiveness. Most workers received better medical care than they had ever had before, delivered by medical personnel who were, for the most part, dedicated service givers. Ironically, these innovative *private* sector initiatives, paid for by *private* businesses, were attacked as "socialist."

Vertical Integration

In a market economy, combinations in restraint of trade have taken two courses. The best known is horizontal integration, gaining control of a lion's share of diamond mining, oil production, or pork bellies.

The other is vertical integration. There are several levels in the gasoline business, including exploration and production of crude oil, oil tankers, refineries, pipelines, wholesale distributors, tank trucks, and local gas stations. In an open market, each of these levels has independent businesses that compete with one another and negotiate price and service with the next higher and lower levels. A friend of mine owned his own small-town Sunoco station, which did good repair work and had a large, loyal first-name clientele. Dissatisfied with the high prices and poor delivery he received compared with city dealers, he negotiated a more favorable contract with a competitor that wanted an outlet in his town and became a Gulf dealer.

To forestall such problems, large oil companies act through acquisitions, mergers, and establishment of company-owned gas stations to control the flow of "black gold" from the well to your car. They ship their own crude oil to their own refineries in their own fleet of tankers, then send the gasoline through their own pipeline to their own regional distribution center, from which they carry it to their own gas stations in their own tank trucks.

The rationale is that this is more efficient. It usually is. They are not at the mercy of other businesses whose interests may not always coincide with theirs and who might disrupt their business because of labor problems, bankruptcy, or changes such as that made by my friend.

They are also liberated from market competition, except at the end of the line. Even there, they have forced independent competitors out of business through temporary-loss price wars and other means, ending up with local oligopolies, in which their few competitors are similar vertically integrated companies who share a common interest in avoiding price-lowering competition.

Evolution of Managed Care

Managed health care is vertical integration that is presumed to offer security, convenience, and economies of scale in exchange for market freedom.

We start with hospitals and with independent physicians who may have privileges at several local hospitals as an essential part of their practice.

Doctors with diverse specialities come together in a group practice, referring patients back and forth within the group as they need one service or another.

An ambitious hospital decides it wants all patient referrals from its affiliated medical staff. It enters into an exclusive relationship (consortium) with the group practice. In return for getting all of their patients, it gives them first call on lab and surgical facilities, which are developed in consultation with group. Anyone who comes to the hospital without a regular physician is referred to the group.

At this point, we have vertically integrated (1) primary care, (2) specialized medicine, (3) surgical facilities, (4) lab services, (5) intensive care, (6) aftercare, and other hospital services. The group also supplies the emergency room doctors (or the hospital hires them as its own employees—vertical integration either way). All participating providers have benefited.

Additional steps may be built on this basic managed care foundation. Other hospitals and group practices may join the consortium, giving it greater horizontal integration within its region. The consortium may reach out to offer a vertically integrated HMO contract to large employers in lieu of going through a middleman insurance company. The services may expand from tertiary physical medicine to include mental health services, an employee assistance program, and preventive health services. Satellite offices may be set up as the group reaches beyond the urban center to a fifty-mile radius.

As the process develops, ties become closer and perhaps more efficient. Some physicians may spend part of their time performing salaried or contracted services. An example of the latter was my son's pathologist group, which performed all of a hospital's pathology needs on site, in a lab provided and staffed by the hospital. Such contract services may call for a fixed annual payment to the group or for the hospital to collect all fees and pay a percentage to the group.

None of this is brand-new. My radiologist father entered into such a contract with a hospital in 1936. What is significant is that these things are increasingly done through structured comprehensive designs on larger and larger scales, using conventional entrepreneurial marketing strategies.

Another vertical integration may be to invite insurance companies into a joint venture. In an Omaha case, part of the package was to give the managed care group exclusive preferred provider status for third-party payments. This delivered many thousands of employer group health insurees. The captive employee groups technically retained freedom of choice, but few of us could afford the substantial economic disincentives if we should choose anyone but the company's managed care partner. Now we have arrived at the ultimate logical goal, total vertical integration.

An interesting phenomenon in the development of managed care is the mixing of sectors. Recently, my county hospital petitioned to be changed from a line agency under the county council to an autonomous public corporation, enabling them to enter into a managed care consortium with a charitable hospital and a commercial hospital.

Pros and Cons

The basic concept of managed care is better-coordinated services, at less cost, from providers that are guaranteed to meet relatively high standards of competence and accountability. The best managed care providers achieve this fairly well and are always striving to improve further. The most serious criticisms of managed care come from failure to live up to this ideal.

The accounting systems of traditional indemnity insurance, such as homeowners and auto, list premium revenue as a positive and payouts as a negative. The size of profits depends on minimizing payouts. This is appropriate and in fact desirable so long as it is done ethically. Home insurers require smoke detectors, fire extinguishers, and other preventive measures to reduce the incidence of fires. Auto insurers advocate safer roads, speed limits, seat belt laws, driver education, and tougher drunk driving enforcement, and they reward safe drivers. Their self-interest coincides with the best interest of their insurees. (There are also, of course, unethical methods, such as "lowball" damage assessments, obstructive claims procedures, and "small print" exclusions.)

For-profit health maintenance organizations have carried over the concept of *loss control* into provision of basic human services. In their annual financial reports to investors, the cost of health services delivered to members in relation to patient premiums is recorded as "medical *loss* ratios." Low benefit-to-premium ratios are highlighted as evidence of good administration. If they are higher, they promise to take steps to reduce the payout ratio.

This is a spurious transfer. *They are not indemnity insurers against occasional catastrophes. They are service agencies that give normal services to normal people under normal circumstances every day.* Service agencies are evaluated not on how little of their revenue they have to pay out but rather on *cost-effectiveness*, how much benefit they deliver per premium dollar.

There are other negatives. Transition from the old system to managed care has destroyed long-term medical ties for many patients. Advocates say that managed care replaces these with new long-term medical ties. This is true in plans that enable the member to choose, from a considerable list, an "anchor" primary care personal physician whom they see routinely and who coordinates referral for specialized services, which incidentally is the system used by the British National Health System. It does not happen in HMOs that use the clinic model where the patient takes potluck on each visit.

An independent primary care doctor told me that he recommended patients who needed orthopedic surgery to the orthopedist in the area most expert in that particular procedure, whereas a managed care colleague referred every kind of orthopedic surgery to his orthopedic partner.

A related complaint is that many programs permit patients to see specialists only for care that is beyond the competence of a primary practitioner. The principle is commendable, but many plans' medical judgments are subordinated to economic priorities. This negative is avoidable. A few plans permit ongoing primary care relationships with certain specialists, such as an OB-GYN for any woman, a rheumatologist for an arthritic, or an endocrinologist for a diabetic.

One win-win compromise has been tried with some success. Self-formed teams (group practices), which may include physicians, other health professionals, and even a hospital, are paid a team fee to care for patients with ongoing specific conditions related to that team's area of practice. The doctors work together to coordinate his or her care. The team and patient determine, *medically*, who within the team does what. When it makes medical sense, the "anchor" physician may be a specialist rather than the standard model of a generalist.

Another problem is localism. A regional managed care program is fine for people who don't travel. In an increasingly mobile society, this is becoming less common. For instance, a couple have a home in Wisconsin but spend four months each winter in Florida. A businessman based in New York spends fifty days per year traveling out of state on business and another three weeks away on vacation. What happens if they need medical attention outside their managed care area? This common problem can be mitigated by a network of reciprocity agreements among regional care organizations. That's how Sweden's network of local public health care corporations works. It's also how state "Blues" operate. Recently, I saw an Alabama doctor, who collected from Alabama Blue Shield, which in turn was reimbursed by my Nebraska Blue Shield insurer.

Finally, there is a concern about the accelerating pace of consolidation of hospitals and managed health into the hands of a few highly profitable large corporate chains. Initially, competing managed care organizations within a regional market allowed some market checks and balances. The trend toward vertical integration and consolidation creates the probability of monopolies in smaller population centers and oligopolies in metropolitan areas before long. An irony in this development is that private collectivist social programs are being developed by actors who profess a free-market ideology. This illustrates the common social policy discrepancy between stated ideology and pursuit of special interests.

When all is said and done, many health policy experts believe that on balance managed care is the way to go. In the absence of any clear national vision or leadership, the predicted default policy is that it is the way we *will* go. As noted in this discussion of pros and cons, this could be a blessing or a curse. Perhaps the difference, given human nature, will be whether managed care is recognized as a utility and regulated accordingly. This appears to be the basis for the exemplary German and Japanese systems, which will be discussed further in the next chapter.

Chapter 18

Centralized or Decentralized?

The principle business of the central authority is to give instruction, of the local authority is to apply it. Power may be localized, but knowledge, to be most useful, must be centralized.

John Stuart Mill, 1865

The states were unable to give the requisite relief. The problem had become national in area and dimensions.

U.S. Supreme Court, 1937b

One of the hottest policy issues for centuries has been centralism versus localism. What is the responsibility of the national government for social welfare? When should it provide benefits directly? When should it finance social welfare without running it? What should be left strictly to state and local government? To the private sector? To individuals? How can you allow local variations yet protect the equal rights of all citizens?

In most countries, the majority of people see their national governments as having bottom-line responsibility for the general welfare of all their citizens, including policies and programs that ensure adequacy in regard to health, social, education, food, clothing, and shelter needs. However, they may differ markedly on how they carry it out. A key variable is centralization versus decentralization, cutting across two dimensions: geographical (national/regional/local) and sector (public/charitable/commercial).

For example, nearly all industrial nations (except the United States) share the goal of ensuring universal health care as a basic human right. Great Britain uses a nationally administered health service; Sweden uses a national network of locally administered public programs. Canada has a system of provincial public insurance agencies that purchase services from local private providers. Germany mandates employer-employee funded nonprofit insurance cooperatives that collectively bargain with regional associations of private providers. Switzerland operates through canton (state) systems of compulsory commercial insurance that must meet minimum federal standards.

An overall perspective on centralization/decentralization choices for financing and delivery of human services can be summarized in a framework that identifies five general clusters:

1. Direct national administration
2. Public to public decentralization
3. Public to nonprofit sector decentralization
4. Public to commercial sector decentralization
5. Government-mandated parapublic private agencies

DIRECT NATIONAL ADMINISTRATION

Centralized administration tends to develop where one or a combination of the following commitments apply:

- *Universal*, as opposed to selective, outreach
- *Objective calculation* of eligibility and benefits, as opposed to individualized diagnostic or investment-return evaluation
- *Equality* of treatment as a transcendent value
- *Effectiveness and/or efficiency* as a higher priority than market interests and ideologies

Full Centralization: Social Security

In most countries, the national pension system is centrally administered. The United States is no exception. Old Age, Survivor, and Disability Insurance (OASDI) is operated by the Social Security Administration, with a central computerized headquarters that does the calculations, electronically deposits payment to the individual's local account, and provides a range of information via "800" telephone lines, the Internet, and mail inquiries.

The agency has internal geographic decentralization to accessible local offices in which skilled counselors, each of whom is tied into the national computer, give personalized assistance to anyone who walks in with a problem or a question about choices. Most problems get resolved and questions are answered on the spot, using the computer. If a problem is unsolved, the counselor locates the hang-up and explains how the individual can solve the problem.

Layered Decentralization: British National Health Service

The British National Health Service is run by the central government. Although its users do complain, particularly about long waiting periods for elective surgery due to underfunding of hospitals and medical specialities (one of the perils of any program supported by annual appropriations from general tax revenues), popular support squelched a 1989 move by the government to privatize the system. Even the British Medical Association, which had bitterly fought the program's establishment in 1946, lobbied to keep the NHS as it was. Reports historian Howard Glennester:

> The strong support that the National Health Service has retained throughout the period [1946-1995] derives not from any feeling of commonality or altruism but from the fact that it was a good buy. The long hard look that the Treasury gave this subject in the 1980s convinced it and a radical Tory [conservative] chancellor of the day of the fact. Ordinary people may not have done cost benefit analysis or international comparisons, but in their gut they knew that any private health care that they tried to take out to deliver the same coverages as the National Health Service would be simply beyond their reach. (1995, pp. 226-227)

The NHS operates through several layers of administrative decentralization, much as General Motors does through semiautonomous wholly owned subsidiaries. The central office holds full authority, sets program policies and standards, allocates the budget to the regional level, and has final approval for capital developments (particularly hospitals) and other major local changes.

Under its supervision, regional boards are responsible for the distribution and operation of hospitals, clinics, and other health facilities, as well as ensuring geographic accessibility of primary care physicians. Under them, local authorities manage the health care programs through governing boards composed of citizens, officials, and professionals who make decisions within the boundaries laid out by the higher levels.

At the most grassroots level, patients choose their own family physician, who makes professional primary care decisions. As with insurance companies in the United States, referrals to specialists and hospitals for major procedures may be subject to higher-level review and approval.

FEDERALISM: PUBLIC DECENTRALIZATION

U.S. Origins: A Limited Federal Role

In 1783, a loose Confederation was established for cooperation among the newly independent colonies (states), which proved unworkable due to weak central authority. Six years later, it was replaced by a federated national government, to which formerly independent member states permanently delegated certain specified functions and authority: "The Congress shall have the power to lay and collect taxes . . . to pay the debts and provide for the common defense and the general welfare of the United States" and sixteen specifically enumerated powers (U.S. Constitution, Article I, Section 8). Some of their social welfare implications are as follows:

1. *Interstate and international commerce.* This provides a rationale for national "social state" regulations discussed in Chapter 12.
2. *Military defense.* This is the rationale for federal veterans benefits, as well as for aid to Cuban and Vietnamese military allies who escaped to the United States as refugees.
3. *Foreign relations.* The Indian Health Service and Bureau of Indian Affairs social services are federal because they were

historically products of treaties with defeated "foreign" nations.

4. *Immigration and citizenship.* The national government has exclusive power to regulate immigration and grant citizenship. Under the Fourteenth Amendment, all U.S. citizens are automatically citizens of the state in which they reside and are guaranteed equal rights and entitlements to state and local as well as federal social welfare programs. The granting of legal immigrant status implies that states must also honor all rights as granted to them by Congress.

5. *The general welfare.* This will be discussed in greater detail in this section. Early applications included 1803 land grants to Ohio that were sold to finance public education, an 1819 land grant to a Connecticut school for the "deaf and dumb," the 1862 Homestead Act, and land grants to finance state universities, also in 1862.

States Rights and the Pierce Veto

In 1854, Dorothea Dix persuaded Congress to authorize land grant subsidies for state mental hospitals. In his veto of the bill, President Franklin Pierce made a strong case against federal social welfare. The United States, he claimed, was not itself a nation at all but a federation of sovereign states (nations) voluntarily banded together for limited purposes.

Pierce cited the Tenth Amendment: "The powers not delegated to the United States by the Constitution nor prohibited by it to the States are reserved to the States respectively or to the people," and then he dismissed the power given in Section 8 "to provide for . . . the general welfare of the United States," as purely rhetorical:

> Indeed, to suppose it susceptible of any other construction would be to consign all the rights of the States and of the people of the States to the mere discretion of Congress, and thus to clothe the Federal Government with authority to control the sovereign States, by which they would have been dwarfed into provinces or departments and all sovereignty vested in an absolute consolidated central power, against which the spirit of lib-

erty has so often and in so many countries struggled in vain. (Pierce, 1854, quoted in Axinn and Levin, 1982, p. 75)

He added a pragmatic fiscal argument. Federal aid to the mentally ill would set a precedent that by extension could make all illness, poverty, and need a federal responsibility. This, he warned, could overwhelm the government:

> If Congress has the power to make provision for the indigent insane . . . it has the same power to provide for the indigent who are not insane and thus transfer to the Federal Government the charge of all the poor in all the states, . . . hospitals and other local establishments for the care and cure of every species of human infirmity, and thus to assume all that duty of either public philanthropy or public necessity to the dependent, the orphan, the sick, or the needy. (Ibid.)

This (nonbinding) opinion prevailed for nearly eighty years until the crisis of the Great Depression called for a new approach.

Ebb and Flow

Since the Pierce veto, the tide of national versus decentralized responsibility has ebbed and flowed several times. Several "sovereign states," using the Pierce rationale, quit the Union. Their interpretation was overruled by superior fire power. Immediately after the war, three amendments expanded federal power to intervene internally within the states: the Thirteenth abolished slavery, the Fourteenth extended constitutional equal rights to intrastate laws and practices, and the Fifteenth mandated the voting rights of white and black males (but not women or Indians). A Freedman's Bureau was established as a direct federal education and social service program for freed slaves.

After 1870, these increases in federal power and responsibility were largely dismantled. State legislatures, powerful corporations, and judges who were identified with political and business interests ushered in an era of laissez-faire government, "robber baron" capitalism, and "Jim Crow" racism.

In the "Progressive Era," from about 1901 to 1920, the central government expanded its power and aggressiveness, primarily in the established areas of military action, foreign affairs, and interstate commerce, but also to a small degree in social policy. The U.S. Children's Bureau was established as a national social welfare advocate. Labor laws were passed to protect women and children. A federal maternal and child health program was enacted. The Nineteenth Amendment required all states to give women the vote.

The Eighteenth Amendment, Prohibition, set a radical precedent for central social control by intervening in the private behavior of individuals within the states.

In this period, perhaps the most significant social policy development went unrecognized at the time. The Sixteenth Amendment in 1912, authorizing an income tax, ultimately eliminated Pierce's second argument by giving the federal government the ability to finance a welfare state.

The "normalcy" era of the 1920s returned the nation to nineteenth-century decentralized policies and practices. Existing federal social welfare programs were repealed.

A New Deal: Providing for General Welfare

Then came the Great Depression. In one year (1929 to 1930), the Gross National Product fell 55 percent. Within the next three years:

- one-third of the labor force was out of work;
- one-fifth of the population, 27,000,000 persons, had no income at all;
- there were 1,000,000 wandering homeless men, called hobos; and
- a Pennsylvania survey found that 27 percent of school children showed physical signs of malnutrition.

Hunger was widespread. Conventional charity and local public relief were exhausted. States were near bankruptcy. President Roosevelt responded to massive suffering with considerable emergency aid. When he followed this with a long-term federal plan to meet social security needs in the industrialized mass society that America had become, he was careful to stress the continuity of this major reform with the nation's past: "Our task of reconstruction does not require the creation of new and strange values. . . . If the means and the details are in some instances new, the objectives are as permanent as human nature. . . . It is a return to values lost in the course of our economic development and expansion" (1934a).

In two precedent-setting decisions on challenges to the Social Security Act, the Supreme Court affirmed federal social welfare under the "general welfare" clause. The first decision referred to unemployment benefits:

> The fact developed quickly that the states were unable to give the requisite relief. The problem had become national in area and dimensions. There was need of help from the nation if the people were not to starve. It is too late today for the argument to be heard with tolerance that in a crisis so extreme the use of the moneys of the nation to relieve the unemployed and their dependents is a use for any purpose narrower than the promotion of the general welfare. (U.S. Supreme Court, 1937b)

In the second decision, the scope of general welfare was broadened further to include noncrisis social welfare:

> The scheme of benefits created by the provisions of Title II [old age and survivor insurance] is not a contravention of the limitations of the Tenth Amendment. Congress may spend money in aid of the "general welfare" (Constitution, Article I, Section 8). . . . The line must still be drawn between one welfare and another, between particular and general. The discretion, however, is not confided to the courts. The discretion belongs to Congress, unless the choice is clearly wrong, a display of arbitrary power, not an exercise of judgment. (U.S. Supreme Court, 1937a)

Since Yesterday

Since those 1937 interpretations, the federal government has been "here to stay" in the business of providing and/or financing social welfare benefits. The extent and nature of that participation, however, has responded to the continuing ebb and flow of ideologies about a "proper" federal, state, and private sector balance, expanding in the 1930s and 1940s, taking a breather in the 1950s, expanding again in the 1960s, and retrenching in the 1970s-1990s.

Methods of Federal-State Relations

The specific methods by which the federal government shares money and responsibility with the states have been discussed in Chapter 17. A similar pattern has been followed by other federated governments such as Canada, whose nationwide health insurance system is structured through provincial programs that meet a national standard and receive matching funds.

Rationales for Federalism

Roosevelt initially developed the federal-state partnership because it was quicker to expand existing state emergency relief programs than to develop a huge new federal bureaucracy. It also served to coopt the states into partnership instead of political opposition. Once started, it was rewarding enough to both sides that it became the new "traditional" way of operating.

Ideally, it combines advantages of both centralization and decentralization. It enables the central government to plan, implement priorities, and ensure minimum standards. Perceived federal assets are:

- stronger taxing power,
- efficient use of expertise through a small staff that provides technical assistance to all fifty states, and
- ability to ensure greater uniformity of services and benefits in a mobile society than could fifty unconnected state initiatives or thousands of local boards.

On the other hand, it is limited in its ability to adapt to the different circumstances of those states, counties, and cities. Perceived state and local government assets are:

- more flexible responses to local conditions and subcultures,
- greater administrative efficiency through smaller, less bureaucratic organizations, and
- less fear of tyranny through abuse of centralized power.

Unfortunately, these assumptions are not always accurate. The federal assets can be subverted by expedient politicians, ideological fanatics, lobbyists of powerful special interests, and bureaucrats who are indifferent, incompetent, or self-serving. State, city, and even small village governments seem to be even more susceptible to powerful vested interests, low competence, and prejudice. In my personal experience as a civil service employee in different levels of government, I found administrative efficiency and competence highest in a federal agency and lowest in a city agency.

Federalism is a conscious attempt to set up checks and balances against error, prejudice, corruption, and misuse of power by either partner. Yet it is an uneasy, imperfect, insecure compromise. There has always been a tension between centralization and decentralization, with a "moving equilibrium" that flows back and forth. Those who believe that fallibility is a universal human quality may not want this tension ever to be fully resolved.

The Swedish Pattern

Sweden, which is not a federated government, administers its "protection" programs (social, health, and relief services) through a network of semiautonomous municipal agencies that operate within national funding, policies, and standards. Every citizen has full, free entitlement to the whole range of services, integrated within the single local public agency. Each user has a permanent pilot worker to help navigate the system. This provides both coordination of multiple services and continuity of care over time. It appears to combine the best qualities attributed to both public and charitable providers.

NONPROFIT PRIVATIZATION

Howard Karger defines privatization as "the separation of governmental funding from governmental provision of human services. Specifically, while government continues to fund social services, it absolves itself of the responsibility to directly provide them" (1994, p. 111).

Sectarian Charities

In many countries, sectarian charities have performed quasi-public human services since the Middle Ages. This was part of the partnership between secular governments and established churches. For example, under the early Poor Laws, the Church of England was the public welfare agency, serving the poor in its parish area and supported by a tithe (compulsory church tax) from every resident in the parish.

For well over a century, privatization via sectarian charities, especially in health and personal social services, has also been the pattern in such multiple establishment countries as The Netherlands and Germany.

American Charities

The First Amendment has not prevented nonprofit privatization in the United States, but it has substituted purchase of care for general program subsidy. The pattern emerged first in child welfare. In the nineteenth century, child welfare services were developed, especially in the Northeast, by charitable family and child welfare services under Protestant (both official and de facto), Catholic, and Jewish sponsorship. In the 1930s, the advent of publicly funded child welfare raised two areas of conflict.

One was the vested interests of the traditional agencies. Everyone recognized a need for more services and funding. Tax-supported public welfare agencies had money, but the politically influential older programs had owned the turf for nearly a century. The compromise was for dependent children to became public wards for whom care was purchased from nonprofit agencies and institutions. The public agency was able to buy more care than it could have provided directly, and the agencies, accustomed to fully funding their services, were delighted to have part of the cost reimbursed.

The second issue was the two sides of the First Amendment. On the one hand, it guarantees religious freedom. This was interpreted to ensure that dependent children be raised in the religion of their biological parents. The problem was that public agencies weren't supposed to engage in sectarian religious activities themselves. Therefore, it was argued, they must support sectarian agencies to protect the constitutional rights of public wards. This created a dilemma because separation of church and state meant that the state couldn't subsidize church-related agencies. The compromise was a market transaction in which a product (care) was purchased. This performed the same function but was not legally a subsidy.

Later, the same rationale was used in regard to sectarian hospitals and colleges. In time, the accommodation did actually move into direct agency subsidies in those two fields, without reference to sectarian auspice, as in Hill Burton funding of hospital construction and grants to build dormitories.

Another pattern, discussed in Chapter 17 as a funding method, is tax welfare subsidies to nonprofit charities. This one method alone probably exceeds the privatization expenditures of many countries. The 1997 federal income tax expenditure for deductible charitable contributions alone amounted to $27 billion. Add to this state income tax deductions, exemption from federal and state income tax on endowment income and all other revenue except unrelated direct business activities, exemptions from school and other local property taxes, and in many cases, exemption from paying sales tax on all purchases, and the total may well be $40 to $50 billion, which is $150 or more for every man, woman, and child in America.

COMMERCIAL PRIVATIZATION

In the War of Independence, the King of England sent British redcoats to fight the American rebels in New York and New England, and Virginia. This was direct administration. He also contracted with his cousin, the Prince of Hesse, to provide (for a profit) Hessian soldiers—wearing their own uniforms, speaking their own language, with their own Hessian officers—to fight in the Pennsylvania-New Jersey war sector. (Remember Washington crossing the Delaware to attack them?) Both carried out the King's business, funded by the King's treasury.

King George wasn't the only one who resorted to commercial privatization:

> In 1775, John Adams was given the task of writing the rules and regulations for a navy. . . . George Washington cursed the notion of privateering and the contradiction it presented to military efficiency and discipline . . . [but] the American com-

munity shared [Adams'] conviction that private profit was a legitimate expectancy for public causes. (Dening, 1992, pp. 150-151)

King George didn't lessen his war effort or save money through privatization; he just substituted German soldiers for English soldiers, probably at a higher cost.

In the same way, privatization doesn't mean less welfare state. When a government pays for a human service, it is a *tax-funded public social provision,* whether the delivery mechanism is a government agency, a charity, or a business corporation. It is like building a public highway: the state can operate its own road-building department or contract it out to a private bidder.

The reasons for purchase instead of direct provision tend to fall into three categories:

- *Economic.* It is cheaper to buy small quantities of services than to provide them directly over a dispersed geographic area. CHAMPUS buys health services for military families located at small bases in lieu of running comprehensive health programs.
- *Political.* Opponents to a proposed social program may be bought off by cutting them in on the take. The AMA had successfully blocked medical care legislation for a half century. In 1965, Medicare and Medicaid were passed only after a fee-for-service system, which raised physicians' incomes, was written in.
- *Ideological.* Purchase in the economic market is preferred over direct provision or nonprofit privatization by classical economists, for whom free enterprise is the transcendent value.

Some common arguments for and against commercial privatization:

PRO:

- Market competition is a powerful cost-effectiveness incentive to satisfy customers and reduce waste.

CONS:

- Consumer satisfaction is less important. The company is motivated to satisfy the payer, not the user.

- The profit motive is an incentive to lower the quality of services.
- Consumers are poorly informed and have little or no choice of provider, which is selected by the payer. Especially vulnerable are the aged, poor, ill, and children whose payer is Medicaid.
- Contract failure is most common where the provider has incentives to shortchange users and financial data is relatively inaccessible to them.

Commercial privatization's two principle ingredients, purchase of service and managed care, were discussed in Chapter 17. As privatization has moved from an expedient to a vested interest and an ideology, the balance has shifted steadily from nonprofit toward the for-profit side, which has had more economic resources, political influence, and marketing savvy.

Interestingly, after giving serious consideration to privatizing the British National Health Service, conservative Prime Minister Thatcher abandoned the idea because she opposed *centralization*! "To divest the government of power, power has to be centralized first [from the NHS layered decentralization described earlier]. The dangers of this strategy, and the outcome, has been the state has centralized but not divested its power" (Glennester, 1995, p. 235).

PARAPUBLIC INSTITUTIONS

The social state guarantees certain rights and benefits, yet need "not itself [be] a universal provider but rather a guarantor and overseer of certain rights mostly fulfilled by other agencies." This is the approach taken by Germany and Japan. "Large areas of public life are governed independently by a heterogeneous set of parapublic institutions which merge public and private business, such as the Federal Bank, workers councils, and social service organizations" (Clasen and Freeman, 1994, p. 2).

The German approach is not exactly any of the four neat decentralization types described previously. All of them start with public funding. The "fifth" way is for the government to mandate the equivalent in private sector expenditure. In terms of your take-home pay, it doesn't make much difference whether your health insurance payroll deduction goes to a public agency or a government-regulated private organization.

Both Germany and Japan have traditions that fit this approach. Both have a far stronger culture of "solidarity" and commonality as a people than the United States. Both have historical patterns of private mutual assistance. In Germany, this pattern goes back a thousand years to the guild system developed in Hanseatic League cities.

Japan was feudal well into the last century, with the traditions of fealty, knowing and accepting one's place, and noblesse oblige. That heritage has carried over into the two-way loyalty between workers and employers within a company and a level of occupational welfare unmatched by any Western capitalist tradition.

Germany mandates *compulsory private* group health insurance. The largest sector is employee groups, with the premium split fifty-fifty between employer and employees. Although it is a "private" premium, the employee share is collected through government-ordered payroll deductions, and employer matching is equally regulated.

Instead of contributing to a single national fund, the premium goes to one of a thousand nonprofit insurance associations (down through mergers from an original 18,000 companies). Large corporations may operate their own insurance funds. Smaller companies use district cooperative insurance organizations. Another cut is occupational groups. Certain skilled trades descended from the guilds have their own, as do professional societies, police, the military, and civil servants. Retired persons normally stay with their employee group, with the government paying the employer's share of the premium. The government also pays all or part of the premium for unemployed and destitute persons, normally to a district cooperative.

Upper-income Germans have a choice between their group insurance or purchasing private commercial insurance, which may offer extra amenities. Two-thirds of them stay with the group.

All insurance companies must meet comprehensive national standards, which are high enough to rank Germany first in the quality and coverage of its medical services. Nevertheless, many large employers offer above-standard features as an incentive to retain loyal workers.

Virtually all providers are private sector, typically nonprofit hospitals and private practitioners. The insurers bargain fees with provider organizations such as the Association of Insurance Doctors. Drug prices are negotiated nationally by the federal government on a generic product basis because the insurers are not strong enough individually to bargain with multinational corporations. As you would expect, drug prices are much lower than in the United States. (A patient may opt for a proprietary brand by paying the difference in price.)

The chief flaw reported by the German system is inequity among risk pools, according to geographic and demographic makeups. For example, large employer pools obviously have fewer high-risk members, such as the poor, ill, and aged, because those groups aren't working for major corporations. Health needs tend to be higher in poor states than in affluent states. This means unequal premiums, as compared with Canada's single pool in each province.

Japan, which patterned its health insurance on the German model, has solved this problem. Its system has four types of insurance pools:

1. Large corporations
2. A government-managed cooperative for smaller employers, which includes a number of seasonal and day workers
3. Mutual associations, a mixed bag that includes self-employed persons, retirees under age seventy, and nonemployed mostly poor persons
4. A government-managed equivalent of Medicare for persons over seventy

Premiums are paid in a way similar to Germany's system, by employer, employee, self-employed person, and, on behalf of the poor and aged, the government.

Pool-risk inequities are handled in two ways. One is government subsidies, which range from 0 percent for lowest risk, type 1 above, to 38 percent for type 3, with its poor and unemployed. The other is age-related risk transfers among the plans. Type 1 naturally transfers out the most, and type 4, which has relieved the other funds of their over-seventy retirees, receives the highest transfers in (68 percent of its budget). (The equivalent intergenerational transfer in the United States occurs through Medicare's use of payroll taxes to pay for benefits to retirees.)

If the parapublic system sounds complicated, that's because it is. However, both the Germans and the Japanese have a reputation for being high-skilled in regard to complex organization and for having cultures that do not egoistically resist social sharing and seek loopholes, as American counterparts might. On the other hand, their systems may have a special attraction for Americans because they bypass both the tax expenditure and the tax welfare routes, maintaining most of the action in the nongovernment section. Although government regulation is strict, it is not oppressive, for there is high voluntary compliance.

These parapublic systems offer more professional freedom than public or privatized managed care systems. They offer relatively unrestricted consumer choice and patient-doctor relationship. Collective bargaining has cost physicians freedom to charge whatever they please, but they remain on a fee-for-service basis and have more professional freedom than in the United States since the advent of managed care, insurance company restrictions, and mandatory preapprovals—and the nonpayment rate is zero!

IN CONCLUSION

This book has been about social policy choices. There are ultimately five ingredients that go into making choices:

1. *Values.* What is right?
2. *Interests.* What will benefit you or your reference group most?
3. *Beliefs about reality,* as filtered through the lenses of traditions, cultures, personal experiences, ideologies, and selective empirical study. What are the conditions of various persons and groups, and how do the social systems function?
4. *What works.* Is one means more effective or more efficient than another for achieving a particular social goal?
5. *What the traffic will bear.* How much of a clearly desirable objective can be achieved in a given situation, and which mechanisms are acceptable, taking into account distribution of power, vested interests, tradition, current ideological fads, and the inherent amorality of the political process, optimistically defined as "the art of the possible?"

6. *Marginal utility.* Beyond what point do the costs of compromise exceed the value of what is gained?

Part I was an introduction and overview. Part II, *Foundations for Choice,* and Part III, *Fundamental Value Choices,* focused on ingredients 1 and 3 above, what's right and what's real. Part IV, *Economic and Social Market Choices,* explored ingredients 3 and 4: How do the systems really operate and what might work? Part V, *Human Service Delivery Choices,* has looked at alternative applications and patterns of implementation for goal choices based on Parts I through III, in the context of the macrosystems explored in Part IV.

Ultimately, we end with these questions. What is right? What works? What are the right values? That's for you to decide—consciously and with the ability to promote/defend your answers.

What is reality? I know what it is . . . well, I think I do . . . okay, no one is ever totally objective and disinterested. You have to work your way through to the best judgment you can reach, always open to amendment as you go along. In religion, we call this "unfolding revelation." In making policy choices, it may be almost as important to see reality through the eyes of your potential allies and opponents, since this is what they are acting on.

What works? Part V has presented a number of choices along with their rationales and beliefs. Many of them work; some are better than others. Some are better in one sociocultural/economic/political setting than in another. Some are fairly good basic ideas that could be improved upon. In twentieth-century America, this question has generated more heat than light, perhaps because our policy decisions have had more to do with a priori beliefs and vested interests than with what really works.

When we cut through the rhetoric and bluster, we discover that there is more than one way to cook an egg. You can fry it, poach it, or scramble it. It can be as plain as hard boiled or as complex as a soufflé. Each method described in this chapter has worked successfully somewhere.

Perhaps our ultimate decisions will be pragmatic, based on ingredient 5—what will the traffic bear? My *personal* bias is a deep belief in transcendent rights, human rights and the difference between rights and wrongs. In terms of human caring, there is no moral room for compromising. However, my *professional* conclusion, after a lifetime of seeking the right, is reluctantly, but firmly, to recommend Herbert Simon's answer:

> The replacement of the goal of maximizing with the goal of *satisficing,* or finding a course of action that is "good enough" . . . this substitution is an essential step in the application of the principle of bounded rationality. (1957, p. 205)

Is it better to have half a loaf than to go hungry? Is it better to compromise on a more inefficient and costly universal health program to keep vested interests from killing it, than for millions of people to suffer deprivation?

This leaves us with the never-to-be-comfortably-resolved sixth ingredient—marginal utility. We can rarely win without compromise. Indeed, many "compromises" will be imposed on us against our wishes. At what point is the gain no longer worth the negatives? As with all the other questions, there is rarely a clear-cut answer. That's why we need to do our analysis homework.

The purpose of this book is not to answer the questions but to give you the means to find some working answers for yourselves. To do that, you must (1) be clear in depth on your values, beliefs, and interests, (2) understand where others are coming from, and (3) be realistic about both technical and political dimensions of whatever policy with which you are working. All three—two out of three won't cut it.

Be as wise as serpents and as innocent as doves.

Appendix

A Framework for Analyzing
a Policy Issue

If a man will begin with certainties,
he shall end in doubts,
but if he will be content to begin with doubts,
he shall end in certainties.

Frances Bacon
(*Advancement of Learning,* BK I, IV, 8)

"Every day in every way" social policies affect you. Many of them are fine with you as they stand. For instance, you may be very pleased with the Bill of Rights and quite satisfied with the Social Security retirement program. You're resigned to a number of other less satisfactory policies. However, you feel strongly enough about a few things to want to do something. Perhaps you can!

"Doing," of course, involves many "practice" activities beyond the scope of this particular book, such as political strategies, social action, organizing, conflict management, program planning, and administration. Before strategies and tactics can do you much good, though, you must know what is, what should be, what you want to change and why, and what the terrain you'll be crossing looks like. This appendix suggests a general approach for doing so, applying insights from the book.

A simplified model for analysis proceeds in three consecutive stages:

1. *Overview of the issue:* what, who, why?
2. *Facts, factors, and actors:* analyzed within their larger contexts.
3. *Choices and direction:* long and short term.

In real life, we don't neatly follow the steps as described here. It is normal to jump back and forth, as ideas and insights hit us and as we encounter new information that makes us go back and rethink earlier analyses.

Further, the analyses themselves overlap. Perspectives given a broad stroke in the overview stage are revisited in greater depth later. Facts, factors, and actors get mixed up with one another. Historical perspective, discussed as a separate section, may in many cases be applied more effectively, within each of the key elements, and again in making judgments about the probable feasibility and effects of alternative long- and short-term choices.

OVERVIEW: WHAT'S THE ISSUE?

Defining Boundaries

In a *Peanuts* comic strip, Linus aspires to be "the world's greatest humble country doctor." Lucy tells him he can't because he doesn't love mankind. He replies, "I love mankind; it's people I can't stand." Noble as it may be, "loving mankind" goes only so far. Eventually you have to narrow it down to the specific situation/condition and the particular aspects of it that will be the focus of your energy and attention. The following are some "boundary" dimensions:

1. *What:* the subject area or condition with which you are concerned. It can be a *problem,* such as acid rain or unwanted pregnancies, or a *well-being potential,* such as holistic health or higher education. Be clear. If your concern is equal treatment on pensions, do you mean vertical equality, which would give the company president and his secretary identical pensions, or temporal equality, which would maintain the (unequal) standard of living each had during working years?
2. *Why:* your reasons for this particular concern, including your beliefs about relevant facts, values, and interests.
3. *Who:* the individuals, organizations, or groups who are, or could become, involved in one (or a combination) of the following roles:

- Hosts who are affected by the conditions
- Agents who affect the conditions
- Actors who do, or could, influence the relevant policy

4. *Where:* geographical, political, or organizational boundaries. Is your focus the United States, Arkansas, the Lower East Side, the Ottumwa school district, or St. Elsewhere Hospital? For practical reasons, boundaries are often adjusted to fit political jurisdictions, service catchment areas, or census data tracts.
5. *When:* time lines for long-term goals and immediate objectives.

The Existing Situation

At this point, a general summary of the existing condition(s) related to the subject is sufficient. This may include personal experience, anecdotal incidents, and/or statistics on hospital treatment of birthing mothers and new babies, day care, child abuse and neglect, families below the poverty line, drunk driver accidents, school dropouts, divorce, unemployment, or whatever. Full analysis will come later. (However, many of my students choose to elaborate certain "key element" areas here instead of later. This works out fine.)

The second existing situation dimension is an overview of current policies and programs related to the conditions. To narrow the focus of later policy analysis and action, it is helpful to identify what kind of policies they are (de jure, de facto, default) and the sectors in which they exist (public, organized private, implicit).

What's the Difference?

If everyone agrees with an existing state of affairs, it receives little or no policy attention. An issue is "a point, matter, or question to be disputed or decided." A policy issue may involve differences regarding:

- facts about the current situation and future projections,
- whether to change or preserve what currently exists,
- competing purposes (broad goals),
- specific applications (objectives) of a generally agreed-upon purpose, and/or
- specific means for achieving selected objectives.

Factual Differences on What Is

The roots of differences can usually be traced back to perceptions of reality (what is) and/or normative premises (what should be).

As in court decisions, the "facts" that influence social policy are not what is, but what actors think they are, influenced by inaccuracies and incompleteness of information and projections and colored by their interests, beliefs, and other selective biases.

Presidents Roosevelt and Johnson saw widespread hunger and consequently developed antipoverty and economic opportunity programs. Presidents Hoover and Reagan believed there was no hunger and rejected such policies as wasteful and un-American. Each policy fitted the president's "facts."

An AFDC caseworker told me that, where she saw vulnerable young women struggling to be adequate persons and mothers despite "the slings and arrows of outrageous fortune," her colleagues saw irresponsible, promiscuous, ne'er-do-wells. These "facts," by influencing how clients were treated, became self-fulfilling: on the average, her clients lived up to her "reality," and the others lived down to her colleagues' "reality."

Procedural "facts" also influence policy. Does commercial competition in human services improve effectiveness and efficiency, or does it lead to cutting corners at the expense of patients? Does unionization improve the operation of the free market by enabling a weak seller (worker) to bargain on a more equal basis with a powerful buyer (a large employer), or does collective bargaining subvert the free market by reducing price competition among individual sellers of labor?

Normative Differences on What Should Be

The other major source of policy difference relates to intents, based on our values and interests. Normative disagreements may be as fundamental as whether there is, or is not, an inherent right to life, liberty, and property.

Even where fundamental norms are shared, differences arise over specific *applications*. Granted a general right to life, liberty, and property, does society, acting through its government, have a clear responsibility to promote the general welfare by ensuring that all citizens will have an adequate quality of life, positive freedom, and equal opportunity in the pursuit of happiness? Or is government responsible only to protect citizens from direct predators who would steal their life, liberty, and property? May the government itself, under any circumstances, deprive citizens of life, liberty, and property? If so, for what reasons: Criminal activity? Unwillingness to work? Political dissent? National defense? The greatest good for the greatest number?

Normative differences may arise over the right *means* for achieving an agreed-upon objective. Those who support "death with dignity" for the terminally ill may still disagree intensely about whether to permit lethal injections or only "passive" actions such as withholding life support treatments. Those who favor a minimum adequate standard of living argue about whether to achieve this through universal social insurances or means-tested relief.

A more mundane basis for difference on what should be is *competing self-interests.* On the average, childless taxpayers favor lower school taxes than do parents. The 80 percent of employees who already have health insurance benefits differ from the unprotected 20 percent on the importance of universal health insurance. Electric utilities, automakers, and the oil industry, on whom the costs would fall most heavily, lobby vigorously against air quality standards that are "not cost-effective" for their profits.

How You Frame the Issue

After all this careful analysis, there is one more consideration in defining the issue. How you frame it can make a big difference in the outcome. A monk asked his superior if he could smoke while he prayed. The superior said absolutely not. Another monk asked the superior if he could pray while he smoked, and the superior said of course he could.

HISTORICAL PERSPECTIVE: SCROOGE'S THREE GHOSTS

In Charles Dickens' *A Christmas Carol,* Ebenezer Scrooge is visited on Christmas Eve by three ghosts, of Christmas Present, Past, and Future, who in combination "tell it like it is." Christmas Present shows what is happening this Christmas and Scrooge's contribution to it. Christmas Past gives him insight into how he came to be what he is today. Christmas Future shows him where he will end up if he doesn't change. Like Scrooge, we need to know (in slightly changed order) (1) *where it's at,* (2) *how it got there,* and (3) *where it's heading.*

As discussed in regard to the overview, and developed in the next section, we obviously need to know the *present* situation:

- *The condition.* What is its current status? What are the problems and needs, strengths and opportunities?
- *Existing policies and programs.* How do they affect the condition? To what extent do they meet needs and solve or prevent problems? To what extent do they create or exacerbate them? What opportunities for well-being have they responded to? With what results? What are their deficiencies?
- *Issues.* What disagreements exist relative to the condition, present policies, and/or proposed policies? Who holds each view and why? What is the level of interest, power, and energy of each actor?

"What's *past* is prologue, what is to come is yours and mine to decide" (Shakespeare, *The Tempest,* Act II, Scene I). A perspective on the past can be important in several ways for understanding the present and predicting the future:

- *Etiology of conditions.* Etiology is "the assignment of causes or origins." To choose effective social policies for problems or unmet needs, it is important to know why they exist and how they came about, so that the intervention will either address the cause or provide benefits which will not be undermined by those causes. Taking a medical history is a standard diagnostic procedure before prescribing treatment.
- *Etiology of intents.* Understanding where policies came from, what the circumstances were at that time, what values and interests they were designed to serve, and how and why they were modified over time, provides insight into their relevance today and whether to change them.

- *Precedents and trends.* Court interpretations of de jure policy lean heavily on two historical factors: (1) the original intent, such as "legislative history," and (2) precedents, past interpretations and any trend over time toward changes in them. These are prime considerations for policymakers as well.
- *Learning from experience.* By studying what has gone before, we can avoid repeating past mistakes or reinventing the wheel. "He gains wisdom in a happy way, who gains it by another's experience" (Plautus, 200 B.C.).
- *Perspective.* An objective overview is difficult to achieve from the middle of a fray in which we are emotionally involved. A more detached perspective on the dynamics of comparable situations in the past may increase our awareness of the dynamics of the present.
- *Historical determinism.* Those who believe with Roman emperor and philosopher Marcus Aurelius that, "Each thing is of like form from everlasting and comes round again in its cycle," or with Arnold Toynbee that history tends to repeat itself with variations may seek insight into the current situation by looking at its earlier prototypes. Those who hold a linear view will base their future projections on past historical trends.

Combining past experience and current information is our best shot at making *contingent predictions* about the future: (1) What will it be like if there is no change? (2) How will it be different if this or that policy change is adopted? Past experience is the foundation of nearly all planning, budgeting, and policymaking.

WHAT'S GOING ON HERE?

Key Elements

A typical social policy can, and should, be viewed from a number of different directions. Some of the more common ones are identified here. The relative importance of these several elements will vary with each situation. They may be subdivided or combined, depending on what fits the particular issue best.

1. *Description of the condition.* Sources may include:

   - collected data from the census, public health, agency records, etc.;
   - professional observation, yours and others', including case records, papers, journal articles, and books;
   - social research;
   - journalistic accounts in newspapers, magazines, and television;
   - literary depictions, such as Charles Dickens' *Oliver Twist* or John Steinbeck's *The Grapes of Wrath*; and
   - philosophical critiques, such as those of theologian Reinhold Niebuhr or organizer Saul Alinsky.

2. *Socioeconomic context.* This may include such characteristics of the hosts, agents, and actors as geographic setting, age, race, gender, socioeconomic class, ethnic identity, and how subgroups interact with one another. In the larger context, what are the effects upon the issue of technological developments, patterns of distribution within the society, and how the overall economy is functioning.

3. *Cultural context.* This addresses beliefs, values, ways of thinking, and patterns of behavior. Is there consensus, imposition by those in power, a majority view with minority deviations, or egalitarian pluralism? Are the differences among subgroups compatible or conflicting? What are the specific beliefs, values, and ways of thinking of each important actor, and how do they affect this issue?

4. *Legal context.* This includes the Constitution, statutory laws, entitlements, common law, judicial interpretations, regulations, rules, and administrative procedures.

5. *Structures of provision.* This is chiefly related to service and benefit programs and to regulation of agents. It includes such things as:

   - auspices, lines of authority, controls, accountability, sources and levels of financing;
   - intergovernmental (federal, state, local), intersectoral (public, voluntary, commercial; church and state), and interagency overlap, coordination, collaboration, and competition;

- planning and coordinating mechanisms;
- staffing types, sources, qualifications, and patterns of utilization;
- criteria and methods for selecting clients or targets; and
- methods of provision: cash, in-kind services and goods, vouchers, tax credits and deductions, incentives, sanctions, and so on.

6. *Political context.* There are two key aspects: the formal political system and the de facto operation of power and interests.
7. *What else?* In this particular policy situation, is there anything important not already covered under one of the other categories?

The Actor Factor

Who is currently involved in affecting the outcome? Who else could? How, and how much, can each influence the policy? What is your ability to relate to each?

"Actor factor" analysis, which should be applied to each important active or potential actor, starts with such obvious characteristics as status, power, energy level, intensity of interest and commitment, styles of communication and action, individual personalities, and group or organizational characteristics. Each of these elements may require quite different information and methods of obtaining it. Some data can be drawn from research and statistics. Other information may be based on direct observation or media reports. Some can only be learned from the actors themselves.

A second key area is each actor's *real* intent and the source of that intent. This enables us to evaluate the soundness of their policy positions and to develop effective strategies for dealing with opponents, allies, and other potential actors. Biasing factors include such things as:

- their actual and perceived self-interests;
- their personal history, because it has shaped where they stand now;
- sources, accuracy, completeness, and slanting of their information; and
- content, sources, and consistency of their beliefs and values.

The actor factor may be addressed as a separate analysis or integrated into the analysis of each key element.

SETTING A HEADING

In navigation, setting a heading is the choice of a compass direction. Now that you have analyzed the existing situation, including how it came about, where it seems to be going, and where the actors are coming from, you are ready to become the navigator and set your heading. You need to determine:

- the starting point (current situation),
- the destination (desired outcome),
- the relationship between the two points (the gap), and
- the course to get from starting point to destination.

What Should Be: The Desirable Situation

"What should be" is the situation or condition that you believe ideally should exist. It always entails some deduction ("reasoning from the general to the specific, or from a premise to a logical conclusion") from a priori beliefs and values about what is good or bad and what things are more or less important. It may also involve some projection from comparative study of actual situations, past and present, that are considered to be relatively "better" or "worse." Even if your ideal situation is not attainable, it is the lodestar by which you set your heading, the standard against which you compare available policy choices.

The Gap: Zero Base and Incremental Approaches

The gap is the discrepancy between what should be and what is. It is also called the problem, deficiency, disorder, unmet need, or unrealized potential. You can approach it from opposite directions:

- *Zero base* sets the destination from scratch, then compares it with the current situation.

- *Incremental* starts with what is, then considers where it should move.

Martin Luther King's civil rights crusade used a zero base *wellness* model, as expressed in his "I have a dream" speech on the Washington Mall. The approach follows this sequence:

1. *Determine what should be.*
2. *Examine what is,* empirically.
3. *Identify the gap* by comparing 2 with 1.
4. *Set outcome goals* that fill all or part of the gap.

The incremental problem-solving approach is based on the "medical model" of diagnosis and treatment. It evolves as a response to recurring problem cases that become identified as patterns of dysfunction. Administrators and true conservatives ("persons who wish to preserve traditions or institutions and resist innovation or change") normally move incrementally toward something better, through a process that Charles Lindblom (1959) called "successive limited comparisons":

1. *Examine the problem* (what is).
2. *Define health* (the desirable situation) in relation to the problem, either negatively as absence of the condition or by comparing "more" and "less" healthy existing situations.
3. *Diagnose the problem.* Infer from available data the probable causes of the deviance from 2.
4. *Set corrective outcome goals,* also known as "treatment goals," based on the diagnosis.

In real life, we often blend the two approaches. For instance, creative human service professionals are usually led to a social policy concern by diagnosis of problem cases, but once "turned on" to the issue, they may move beyond problem solving to a Robert Kennedy "why not?" wellness approach. Sometimes the dynamics of sorting out "is" and "should be" are so intertwined that it is hard to tell which came first. Hey, no problem—so long as you end up with both.

Outcome Goals

A goal is a long-term *result* (condition) toward which a social policy is directed. It may be the ideal condition or, more often, something that partially fills the gap. For example, given the gap between universal good health and current health conditions, one policy goal might be a pollution-free environment; another, more healthful eating and exercise habits; a third, universal state-of-the-art health services. Although none of these goals by itself achieves the ideal condition, each contributes toward filling the gap.

Long-term goals govern your selection of more immediate, concrete policy objectives.

WHAT CAN BE DONE?

Alternative Objectives

It would be fantastic to achieve your goal in one step, with the one available means. Unless it is a very simple, concrete goal—"you should live so long!"

Social policy is like the wilderness sport of orienteering. Having set your heading, you still have to chart a specific course over hills, across streams, around cliffs, etc. You can't just go as the crow flies. Your problem is how the crow would go if it had a broken wing and had to walk.

If you can't achieve the goal all at once, identify possible *intermediate objectives* that may be achievable within a reasonable time under realistic circumstances. An objective may achieve a piece of the final goal, provide a stepping stone toward its eventual achievement, or both.

Skilled social policy planners may develop a strategy that involves a *sequential series of stepping stones* toward the goal.

In the 1970s, a goal of the United Way of America was for its related social services to do cost-effectiveness planning and evaluation. Its first objective was to develop a program accounting system that identified agency costs in relation to each separate service program (intended effect) within an agency. The second stepping stone was to make program accounting a condition of United Way funding. This took care of measuring the cost side. A logical third stepping stone objective should have been development of reliable measures of human service success (effectiveness), followed by a fourth that required all of United Way's agencies to submit annual effectiveness reports. After a quarter-century hiatus, it appears that a Canadian team (McCready et al., 1996) may be near to making step three possible. If so, the final step would become possible, and the entire goal would be achieved!

Another astute social policy strategy is to design a *set of coordinated pieces,* each of which is independently achievable and worthy in its own right. Achievement of the whole set would accomplish the entire goal.

Let's say the goal is universal comprehensive health care. One piece might be comprehensive Medicare for all citizens over sixty-five (15 percent of the population). A second might be comprehensive Medicaid for all citizens with incomes below the poverty line (another 15 percent). A third might be to require all employers of fifty or more workers to provide private family health insurance to their employees (55 percent). A fourth might be a mandatory government health insurance program for small employers at rates comparable to those paid by large employers (10 percent). At this point, the goal is 95 percent achieved. The final piece might be achieved by extending Medicaid to cover all other nonemployed persons under sixty-five. (Percentages are illustrative, not precise.)

Alternative Means

For each objective, identify alternative means to get there. For instance, different nations achieved universal health care through such varied means as:

- direct public provision of services;
- universal public insurance, which purchases care from private providers;
- compulsory private insurance by employers, with residual public coverage for those who fall between the cracks;

- giving employers a Hobson's choice of paying taxes into the government insurance program or providing equivalent private insurance; and
- mandated provincial (state) plans that must meet national standards.

Logically, you select the objective first and then consider alternative means to get there. However, because the choice of means may greatly affect overall acceptability and effectiveness, it is often more realistic to deal with them together by identifying *objective/means combinations* for evaluation and selection. I call these "tactical plans."

A pragmatic method of keeping the number of combinations manageable is Amatai Etzioni's (1967) *mixed scanning:* do a quick scan of possibilities, from which you select the most promising few for more comprehensive analysis.

Analyzing the Opposition's Alternatives

Always review and analyze alternatives that your opponents and others have proposed—or reasonably could propose. Whether we like their alternatives or not, we need to be prepared to deal knowledgeably with them:

- *Recognize their merits.* We may want to modify our objective and/or means to incorporate their good points.
- *Identify their weaknesses.* Prepare rebuttals to use for persuasion and/or contention.
- *Look for possible compromises.* If we can't prevail, it is useful to know where we can "give a little" and where we shouldn't.

Selecting the Practical Policy

There are three criteria for selecting the specific objective/means combination: desirability, design, and feasibility. Unfortunately, there is no simple one-size-fits-all formula. How you balance desirability and feasibility, benefits and costs, effectiveness and efficiency, long-term and short-term goals, direct and indirect effects, and so forth will involve value judgments, weighing priorities, and imprecise estimates.

You can go to extremes. You can compromise with feasibility to the point that the original purpose is forgotten, as in the case of the proposed Family Assistance Plan (FAP) described in an earlier chapter. (Ironically, the FAP concessions to "feasibility" made it *in*feasible by costing it the votes of liberal senators.)

At the other extreme, the goal may be important enough to disregard conventional feasibility considerations. Two of the best-known expressions of this relate to waging war and spreading love.

In 1864 in Mobile Bay, Admiral Farragut said, "Damn the torpedoes!—full speed ahead!"

Eighteen centuries earlier, the apostle Paul said, "We have become a spectacle to the world. . . . We are fools for Christ's sake. . . . We hunger and thirst; we are ill-clad and buffeted and homeless . . . reviled . . . persecuted . . . slandered; we have become, and are now, as the refuse of the world, the offscouring of all things" (I Corinthians 4:9-13).

Most of us, most of the time, follow a middle road:

1. Eliminate objectives that turn out to be *undesirable* because they have unacceptable side effects, are too vague, or preclude further steps.
2. Eliminate means that appear to be *unworkable*. Sometimes rejection of means due to feasibility problems may lead to selecting instead a prerequisite stepping stone related to the source of the barrier. For example, a significant federal role in social welfare was not feasible until the Sixteenth Amendment authorized income taxes.
3. Eliminate means that are *unacceptable* because of cost, negative side effects, or ethical problems. However effective they might be for reducing acid rain, you probably wouldn't choose terrorist attacks against public power plants as your means.
4. Eliminate or compromise combinations that, whatever their intrinsic merit, will be *shot down* by "the powers that be" or resisted by the target hosts. (Of course, pessimistic projections are not always accurate. Farragut and Paul both won. A World War II Army Air Force slogan asserted, "The difficult we do immediately. The impossible takes a little longer.")

5. Finally, from what's left, choose the combination that best reflects, for that specific case, *your* relative weighting of desirability, design, and feasibility—seasoned with a dash of "gut feeling."

CONCLUDING OBSERVATIONS

Extent of Analysis

Think about all of the dimensions and elements outlined in this appendix. Be aware of the many factors and choices discussed throughout this book. Then *be practical.* The relative comprehensiveness of your actual analysis will depend on the importance of the issue, how much you need to know to deal with other key actors, what data are available, and how much time, energy, and resources you can afford. There is a point of diminishing returns, beyond which the gains in knowledge aren't worth the additional cost or delay.

Social Policy Is Always Evolving

Although there is a logic to the sequence of analysis outlined in this appendix, in practice, we tend to jump around. It is normal to anticipate later steps in earlier decisions and to go back to revise earlier ones in light of later considerations.

In social policy, nothing is etched in stone. It is always imperfect, evolving, and contingent upon circumstances. In the words of that baseball savant, Yogi Berra, "It ain't over till it's over."

Even if there are absolute values and principles (which I personally believe), their application in specific social policies of specific societies at specific times is always *imperfect* (due to incomplete knowledge, limited self-awareness, and rationalizations of self-interests) and *impermanent* (due to changing social, economic, geophysical, technological, and other circumstances).

What you write on a typewriter is set. Any significant change requires retyping the whole page. By contrast, when you write on a word processor, it is entered on a memory disk that you can re-edit any number of times. When you go back and change something, everything subsequent automatically adjusts. Each printout, however "final" it appears, is a draft relative to the continuing, flexible memory disk. Although social policy has specific printouts, it is *always a working draft,* always subject to review and possible revision, and never a final solution.

An old pastor once confided to me that his was the most secure profession in the world. "Our mission," he said, "is to fight sin, and there is no danger of ever working ourselves out of a job." Involvement in social policy offers the same "security"!

When thou has done, thou hast not done,
For, I have more.

John Donne, 1622

Bibliography

Aldrich, Mark and Buchele, Robert (1986). *The economics of comp worth.* Cambridge, MA: Ballinger.

Alinsky, Saul (1972). *Rules for radicals.* New York: Random House.

Allen, Frederick (1939). *Since yesterday.* New York: Bantam.

Ambert, Anne-Marie (1998). *The web of poverty: Psychosocial perspectives.* Binghamton, NY: The Haworth Press.

Axinn, June and Levin, Herman (1982). *Social welfare,* Second edition. New York: Harper & Row.

Bach, Richard (1988). *One.* New York: William Morrow.

Bartlett, John (1955). *Familiar Quotations,* Thirteenth edition. Boston, MA: Little, Brown and Company.

Bartlett, John (1992). *Familiar Quotations,* Justin Kaplan (Ed.), Boston, MA: Little, Brown and Company.

Beckner, Paul. (1997). Editorial. *USA Today,* May 7.

Beveridge, William H. (1942). *Social insurance and allied services (The Beveridge Report).* London: HMSO.

Beveridge, William H. (1943). *The pillars of society.* New York: Macmillan.

Beveridge, William H. (1945). *Why I am a liberal.* London: Jenkins.

Bicanic, Rudolph (1967). *Problems of planning, East and West.* Hague: Mouton.

Booth, Charles [1890] (1971). [A. Freed and R.M. Elman (Eds.)] *Charles Booth's London.* Hammonsworth: Penguin.

Brennan, Richard (1997). *Heisenberg probably slept here.* New York: John Wiley and Son.

Canada Government, Regional and Economic Expansion (1982). *Project management handbook.* Ottawa: Government of Canada.

Caplow, Theodore (1976). *How to run any organization.* Hinsdale, IL: Dryden.

Carnegie, Andrew (1900). *The gospel of wealth.* New York: Century.

Citro, Constance and Michael, Robert (1995). *Measuring poverty: A new approach.* Washington, DC: Academy Press.

Clasen, Jochen and Freeman, Richard (Eds.) (1994). *Social policy in Germany.* New York: Harvester Wheatsheaf.

COE (Council of Europe) (1993). *Old-age benefits and health care: Impact on present and future funding of social security.* Strasbourg, France: Steering Committee for Social Security.

Columbia Encyclopedia (1941). F. Clarke Ansley (Ed.). New York: Columbia University Press.

Columbia University (1946). *Introduction to contemporary civilization in the West,* Volumes I and II. New York: Columbia University Press.

Dening, Gregory (1992). *Mr. Bligh's bad language: Passion, power, and theater on the bounty.* Cambridge, MA: Cambridge University Press.

de Graaf, J. (1957). *Theoretical welfare economics.* Cambridge, MA: Cambridge University Press.

de Schweinitz, Karl (1961). *England's road to social security.* New York: Barnes.

Dolgoff, Ralph, Feldstein, Donald, and Skolnick, Louise (1997). *Understanding social welfare,* Fourth edition. Reading, MA: Addison-Wesley.

Dyck, Arthur (1994). *Rethinking rights and responsibilities: The moral bonds of communication.* Cleveland, OH: Pilgrim Press.

Editorial (1996). *The New York Times,* June 10.

Etzioni, Amatai (1967). "Mixed scanning: A third approach to decision making." *Public Administration Review,* 27, pp. 385-392.

Etzioni, Amatai (1996). "Why fear date rape?" *USA Today.* May 5.

France, Anatole (1909). *Penguin Island.* Reprinted in 1958. New York: Bantam Books.

Fraser, Derek (1973). *The evolution of the British welfare state: A history of social policy since the industrial revolution.* London: Macmillan.

Friedman, Milton (1962). *Capitalism and freedom.* Chicago, IL: University of Chicago.

Fulton, Jane (1993). *Canada's health system: Bordering on the possible.* Washington, DC: Faulkner and Gray's Healthcare Information Center.

Gadamer, Hans (1975). *Truth and method,* Fourth edition. New York: Seabury.

George, Vic and Wilding, Paul (1976). *Ideology and social welfare.* London: Routledge and Kegan Paul.

Gil, David (1976). *Unraveling social policy.* Cambridge, MA: Schenkman.

Gilbert, Neil (1983). *Capitalism and the welfare state.* New Haven, CT: Yale University Press.

Gilbert, Neil (1995). *Welfare justice: Restoring social equity.* New Haven, CT: Yale University Press.

Gilligan, Carol (1982). *In a different voice: Psychological theory of women's development.* Cambridge, MA: Harvard University Press.

Glennester, Howard (1995). *British policy since 1945.* Cambridge, MA: Blackwell Publishers.

Golob, Eugene (1954). *The Isms: A history and evaluation.* New York: Harper.

Goodin, Robert (1985). *Reasons for the welfare state.* Princeton, NJ: Princeton University Press.

Gould, Stephen (1991). *Bully for brontosaurus.* New York: W.W. Norton.

Gray, B. and McNerney, W. (1986). "For-profit enterprise in health care." *New England Journal of Medicine,* 314, June 15, pp. 1523-1525.

Harriman, David (1997). "Selfishness made America great." *USA Today,* April 23.

Harrington, Michael (1980). *Decade of decision.* New York: Simon and Schuster.

Hayek, Friedrich von (1960). *The constitution of liberty.* London: Routledge and Kegan Paul.

Heilbroner, Robert (1982). "What is socialism?" In Irving Howe (Ed.), *Beyond the welfare state.* New York: Schocken Books.

Hennessee, Judith (1986). "Inside a right-to-life mind." *Mademoiselle,* April.

Hewitt, Martin (1992). *Welfare, ideology, and need.* Savage, MD: Barnes and Nobles.

Hill, Michael (1990). *Social security policy in Britain.* Brookfield, VT: Elgar.

Hixson, William (1997). *It's your money.* Toronto: Comer Press.

Howard, R. (1980). "An assessment of decision analysis." *Operations Research,* 28.

Howe, Irving (Ed.) (1982). *Beyond the welfare state.* New York: Schocken Books.

Jacobs, Lesley (1993). *Rights and deprivation.* Oxford, Clarendon.

Johnson, Paul (1991). *The birth of the modern: World society 1815-1830.* New York: Harper Collins.

Kahn, Alfred (1979). *Social policy and social services,* Second edition. New York: Random House.

Karger, Howard (1994). "Is privatization a positive trend in social services?" In Howard Karger and James Midgely (Eds.), *Controversial issues in social policy.* Boston: Allyn Bacon.

Keller, Bill (1984). "What is the audited value of life?" *The New York Times,* October 26.

Kennedy, John F. (1963). "What kind of peace do we want?" Speech at American University, Washington, DC, June 10.

Keynes, John Maynard [1936] (1964). *The general theory of employment, interest, and money.* New York: Harcourt Brace Jovanovich.

Knox, Richard (1993). *Germany's health system: One nation with health care for all.* Washington, DC: Faulkner and Gray's Healthcare Information Center.

Kuenne, Robert (1993). *Economic justice in American society.* Princeton, NJ: Princeton University Press.

Lewis, R.W.B. (1991). *The Jameses.* New York: Farrar, Straus, and Giroux.

Lindblom, Charles (1959). "The science of muddling through." *Public Administration Review,* 19, pp. 79-88.

Little, I. (1957). *A critique of welfare economics.* Oxford: Oxford University Press.

Locke, John (1690). Of civil government. In *Two treatises of government.* In *Columbia Encyclopedia,* Vol. I, pp. 785-827.

Marshall, T.H. (1975). *Social policy,* Fourth edition. London: Huchison.

Marx, Karl (1848). "Manifesto of the community party." In *Columbia Encyclopedia,* Vol. II, pp. 415-435.

Maslow, Abraham (1954). *Motivation and personality.* New York: Harper & Row.

Massachusetts Council of Churches (1961). *Relations between church and state.* Boston, MA: Author.

McCready, Douglas, Pierce, Stephen, Rahn, Sheldon, and Were, Kirk (1996). "3rd gen info systems: Integrating costs and outcomes." *Administration in Social Work,* 20(1), pp. 1-15.

Merkhofer, Miley (1987). *Decision science and social risk management.* Boston, MA: D. Reidel.

Mill, John Stuart (1848). *Principles of political economy.* London: Parker and Son.

Mill, John Stuart (1859). "On liberty." In *Columbia Encyclopedia,* Vol. II, pp. 809-837.

Mill, John Stuart (1865). "Considerations on representative government." In *Columbia Encyclopedia,* Vol. II, pp. 692-710.

Mill, John Stuart (1869). "The subjection of women." In A. Rossi (Ed.), *Essays on sex equality.* Chicago, IL: University of Chicago Press, 1972.

Miller, S.M. and Collins, Charles (1996). *Growing economic fairness.* McLean, VA: Odyssey Forum.

Mills, H. (1959). *Mathematics and the managerial imagination.* Princeton, NJ: Mathematica.

Mishan, Edward (1976). *Cost–benefit analysis,* Second edition. New York: Praeger.

Morris, Robert (1988). *Testing the limits of social welfare.* Hanover, NH: University Press of New England.

Moynihan, Daniel (1969). *Maximum feasible misunderstanding.* New York: Free Press.

Murray, Charles (1984). *Losing ground: American social policy 1950-1980.* New York: Basic.

National Conference of Catholic Bishops (1986). *Economic justice for all.* Washington, DC: NCCB.

National Conference on Social Welfare (1985). *The report of the committee on economic security of 1935,* Fiftieth anniversary edition. *Washington, DC: NCSW.*

National Lutheran Council (1961). *Statement on church hospitals and the Hill-Burton Act.* New York: Author.

The New York Times (1996). News item. June 17.

Niebuhr, Reinhold (1968). *Faith and politics.* New York: G. Brazilier.

Nozick, Robert (1974). *Anarchy, state, and utopia.* New York: Basic Books.

OECD (Organization for Economic Cooperation and Development) (1981). *The welfare state in crisis.* Paris: OECD.

OECD (1988). *Aging populations.* Paris: OECD.

Okimoto, Daniel and Yoshikawa, Aki (1993). *Japan's health system: Efficiency and effectiveness in universal care.* Washington, DC: Faulkner and Gray's Healthcare Information Center.

Okroi, Loren (1988). *Economics and dissent in an age of optimism.* Princeton, NJ: Princeton University.

Overberg, Paul (1996). "Taking a worldview for keys to income inequality," *USA Today.* September 23, p. 3B.

Pearce, D. (1983). *Cost benefit analysis.* London: Macmillan.

Pigou, A. (1932). *The economics of welfare.* London: Heinemann.

Piven, Frances and Cloward, Richard (1971). *Regulating the poor.* New York: Pantheon.

Plutarch. (Translated/Annotated by Ian Scott-Kilmer) (1973). In *Age of Alexander,* pp. 104-150. New York: Penguin.

Pope John XXIII (1963). Encyclical. "Pacem in Terris."

Pope John Paul II (1991). Encyclical. "Centisimo Annus."

Pope Pius XI (1931). Encyclical. "Quadragesimo Anno."

Rawls, John (1971). *A theory of justice.* Cambridge, MA: Harvard University Press.

Reich, Robert (1997). "The unfinished agenda." *Brandeis Review,* 17(2), pp. 22-27.

Riesman, David (1993). *Market and health.* New York: St. Martin's

Roosevelt, Franklin (1934a). Message to Congress reviewing the broad objectives and accomplishments of the administration, June 8.

Roosevelt, Franklin (1934b). State of the union message, January 1934.

Rossi, A. (Ed.) (1972). *Essays on sex equality.* Chicago, IL: University of Chicago Press.

Rowley, Charles and Peacock, Alan (1975). *Welfare economics: A liberal restatement.* London: Martin Robertson.

Saul, John (1992). *Voltaire's bastards.* New York: Free Press.

Savant, Marilyn Vos (1995). "Ask Marilyn." *Parade,* April 23.

Schumacher, E. (1973). *Small is beautiful.* London: Blond.

Seldes, George (Ed.) (1960). *The Great Quotations.* New York: Pocket Books.

Sherraden, Michael (1990). A Corporation for Enterprise Development monograph. Quoted by William Raspberry in his *Washington Post* column, March 20.

Silk, Leonard (1984). "Reagan's shift on the deficits." *The New York Times,* February 1.

Sillince, John (1986). *A theory of planning.* Brookfield, VT: Gower.

Simon, Herbert (1957). *Models of man.* New York: Wiley.

Skocpol, Theda (1994). *Social policy in the United States.* Princeton, NJ: Princeton University Press.

Snell, Donna (1989). Student exam in a University of Nebraska course.

Spencer, Herbert (1884). *Man versus state.* London: Williams and Norgate.

Stern, P. (1986). "Big business is subsidized." *The New York Times,* March 19.

Swift, Jonathan (1729). "A modest proposal for preventing the children of poor people in Ireland from being a burden to their parents or country, and for making them beneficial to the public." In Wilke, Brian and Hurt, James (Eds.), *Literature of the Western World,* Second edition, Vol. II, pp. 302-308. New York: Macmillan.

Tawney, Richard (1921). *The acquisitive society.* New York: Horcourt Brace.

Tawney, Richard (1964). *The radical tradition.* London: Penguin.

Thoreau, Henry (1854). *Walden.* New York: Bantam.

Time Magazine (1986). Vol. 127, No. 1, January 6, pp. 29-38.

Titmuss, Richard (1958). *Essays on the welfare state.* London: George Allen and Unwin.

Titmuss, Richard (1967). Social welfare and the art of giving. In Eric Fromm (Ed.), *Socialist Humanism,* pp. 358-359. London: Allen Lane.

Titmuss, Richard (1976). *Commitment to welfare,* Second edition. London: George Allen and Unwin.

Townsend, Joseph (1786). A dissertation on the poor laws by a well-wisher to mankind. Reprinted 1971. Berkeley, CA: University of California Press.

Townsend, Peter (1975). *Sociology and social policy.* London: Allen Lane.

Townsend, Peter (1979). *Poverty in the United Kingdom: A survey of household resources and standards of living.* Berkeley, CA: University of California Press.

Trattner, Walter (1994). *From poor law to welfare state.* New York: Free Press.

Tropman, John (1989). *American values and social welfare.* Englewood Cliffs, NJ: Prentice-Hall.

Tropman, John, Dhuly, Milan, and Lind, Roger (Eds.) (1981). *New strategic perspectives on social policy.* New York: Pergamon.

Underhill, Francis (1996). "The Necessary Shield," column in the Hendersonville, NC, *Times-News,* May 26, p. 40.

United Nations (1996). *Human development report of 1996.*

United States Census Bureau (1997). *The American almanac,* 1996-1997.

United States Department of Health, Education, and Welfare (1966). Report to the Secretary, June 29. Washington, DC.

United States Supreme Court (1937a). *Helvering v Davis* (301-US 619). Cited in National Conference on Social Welfare. *The report of the committee on economic security of 1935,* Fiftieth anniversary edition. Washington, DC: NCSW.

United States Supreme Court (1937b). *Steward Machine Co. v Davis* (301-US 548). Cited in National Conference on Social Welfare. *The report of the committee on economic security of 1935,* Fiftieth anniversary edition. Washington, DC: NCSW.

United States Supreme Court (1978). *Regents of the University of California v Allan Bakke,* 435 US 265.

USA Today (1996). News item, July 16.

USA Today (1997). News item, March 3.

The Washington Post (1990). News item, April 27,.

Weber, MAX (1904). *The Protestant ethic and the spirit of capitalism.* (Reprinted 1958). New York: Scribners.

Wickenden, Elizabeth (1984). *Society security—Why not a means test?* New York: Study Group on Social Security, Fact Sheet 13.

Wildavsky, Aaron (1973). "If planning is everything, maybe it's nothing." *Policy Sciences,* 4, pp. 127-153.

Wilensky, Harold and Lebeaux, Charles (1965). *Industrial society and social welfare,* Second edition. New York: Free Press.

Will, George (1995). Column in the Omaha *World Herald,* October 16.

Index

Order Your Own Copy of
This Important Book for Your Personal Library!

SOCIAL WELFARE POLICY ANALYSIS AND CHOICES

_____ in hardbound at $49.95 (ISBN: 0-7890-0602-2)

_____ in softbound at $24.95 (ISBN: 0-7890-0603-0)

COST OF BOOKS _____

OUTSIDE USA/CANADA/
MEXICO: ADD 20% _____

POSTAGE & HANDLING _____
(US: $3.00 for first book & $1.25
for each additional book)
Outside US: $4.75 for first book
& $1.75 for each additional book)

SUBTOTAL _____

IN CANADA: ADD 7% GST _____

STATE TAX _____
(NY, OH & MN residents, please
add appropriate local sales tax)

FINAL TOTAL _____
(If paying in Canadian funds,
convert using the current
exchange rate. UNESCO
coupons welcome.)

☐ **BILL ME LATER:** ($5 service charge will be added)
(Bill-me option is good on US/Canada/Mexico orders only;
not good to jobbers, wholesalers, or subscription agencies.)

☐ Check here if billing address is different from
shipping address and attach purchase order and
billing address information.

Signature _____

☐ **PAYMENT ENCLOSED: $** _____

☐ **PLEASE CHARGE TO MY CREDIT CARD.**

☐ Visa   ☐ MasterCard   ☐ AmEx   ☐ Discover
☐ Diner's Club

Account # _____

Exp. Date _____

Signature _____

Prices in US dollars and subject to change without notice.

NAME _____

INSTITUTION _____

ADDRESS _____

CITY _____

STATE/ZIP _____

COUNTRY _____ COUNTY (NY residents only) _____

TEL _____ FAX _____

E-MAIL_____
May we use your e-mail address for confirmations and other types of information? ☐ Yes   ☐ No

Order From Your Local Bookstore or Directly From
The Haworth Press, Inc.
10 Alice Street, Binghamton, New York 13904-1580 • USA
TELEPHONE: 1-800-HAWORTH (1-800-429-6784) / Outside US/Canada: (607) 722-5857
FAX: 1-800-895-0582 / Outside US/Canada: (607) 772-6362
E-mail: getinfo@haworthpressinc.com
PLEASE PHOTOCOPY THIS FORM FOR YOUR PERSONAL USE.

BOF96